Nurse Practitioner
Acute Care Protocols
and
Disease Management

For Family Practice, Urgent Care, and Emergency Medicine

Nurse Practitioner
Acute Care Protocols and Disease Management

For Family Practice, Urgent Care, and Emergency Medicine

Donald C. Correll, M.D., FACEP

Acute Care Horizons

Jackson, TN

Nurse Practitioner Acute Care Protocols and Disease Management: For Family Practice, Urgent Care, and Emergency Medicine

Acute Care Horizons, LLC
Jackson, Tennessee
acutecarehorizons.com

Printed in the United States of America.

Library of Congress Control Number: 2012940144

ISBN: 978-0-9849173-9-6 (Paperback)

ISBN: 978-0-9855179-1-5 (Hardcover)

ISBN: 978-0-9855179-3-9 (E-book)

Publisher's Cataloging-in-Publication Data

Correll, Donald Charles.

Nurse practitioner acute care protocols and disease management: for family practice, urgent care, and emergency medicine / Donald C. Correll.

p. cm.

Includes index.

ISBN 978-0-9849173-9-6 (Paperback)

ISBN 978-0-9855179-1-5 (Hardcover)

1. Nurse practitioners—Handbooks, manuals, etc. 2. Medical emergencies—Handbooks, manuals, etc. 3. Emergencies—handbooks. 4. Emergency Medicine—methods—handbooks. 5. Medical protocols. I. Title.

RC86.8 .C67 2012

616.02/5—dc22 2012940144

Version
COV - 2012-05-29
TXT - 2012-10-09

DEDICATION

To the reviewers of this work.

To my brother John for his creativity and work to make this book possible.

To my mother Glenna who worked two jobs to put me through college.

To my father-in-law Joe Keller for his wisdom over the past 35 years.

To my wife Christina for her steadfast love and devotion.

To my children Joanna, Donny and Diana for bringing more meaning into my life.

PURPOSE

This *Acute Care Protocols and Disease Management* book has been created to assist practitioners who work in family practices, urgent care centers, emergency departments, and hospital practices.

This book is constructed to be concise and yet reasonably comprehensive, thereby providing a readily usable resource that practitioners can use as a management tool to further enhance patient care and safety.

FORWARD

Robert M. Blumm, MA, PA-C, DFAAPA

This is a textbook — plus much more. It's a guide that any practitioner can use when confronted with a patient who presents with a problem that has uncommon signs or symptoms. The book suggests the appropriate approach that will help to properly diagnose and treat the illness.

Having this book handy is akin to having an experienced emergency department director at your side and mentoring you as a clinician on the best approach to any particular patient.

Our profession, Physician Assistants and Nurse Practitioners, comprise a diverse range of ages, including starting clinicians, those who have practiced for ten years or longer, and those like me who will not accept retirement as a viable action. This book works for all experience categories.

I utilize this book as a refresher for Urgent Care as well as for the consulting and medical malpractice suits that I defend physician assistants for. I have 40 years' experience as a surgical physician assistant with 16 years as an ER physician assistant and five years as a clinical instructor of surgery and emergency medicine. A resource such as Dr. Correll's book will be in the pocket of my lab coat and on my bookshelf to help me become the best in my field.

I highly recommend adding it to your library and making it a part of your practice.

Bob Blumm, MA, PA-C, DFAAPA — January, 2012

CONTENTS

Dedication 5
Purpose 5
Forward 6
Contents 7
Reviewers 13
Notice 15
Guidelines of Proper Use 16
Protocol Guideline Agreement 18

General 19
General Patient Criteria Protocol 20

Cardiovascular 23
Chest Pain Protocol 24
Cardiac Dysrhythmia Protocol 35
Hypertension Protocol 51
Congestive Heart Failure Protocol 54
Syncope/Presyncope Protocol 58

Respiratory 65
Dyspnea Protocol 66
Pneumonia Protocol 75
Adult Asthma/Acute Bronchitis Protocol 79
Allergy Protocol 84

Endocrine 93
Diabetes and Hypoglycemia Protocol 94
Hypothyroidism Protocol 106
Hyperthyroidism Protocol 110

Toxic Ingestions 115
Toxicology Protocol 116

Neurology 125
Headache Protocol 126
Dizziness Protocol 135
CVA/TIA Protocol 139
Bell's Palsy Protocol 150
Adult Seizure Protocol 154

Pediatric Seizure Protocol 160
Delirium Protocol 166

Back 171
Back Pain Protocol 172
Flank Pain Protocol 176

Gastrointestinal 179
Abdominal Pain Protocol 180
CT Abdominal Scan Issues 192
Adult Gastroenteritis Protocol 195
Irritable Bowel Syndrome Protocol 201
Appendicitis Protocol 205
Antibiotic-associated Colitis Protocol 209
Inflammatory Bowel Disease Protocol 212
Gastroesophageal Reflux Disease (GERD) Protocol 216
Peptic Ulcer Disease and Gastritis Protocol 219
Gallbladder Disease Protocol 223
Hepatitis Protocol 227
Gastrointestinal Bleeding Protocol 231
Gastrointestinal Foreign Body Protocol 236
Anorectal Disorder Protocol 239
Constipation Protocol 250

Urinary and Male Genitourinary 255
Kidney Stone Protocol 256
Urinary Tract Infection Protocol 261
Chronic Renal Failure Protocol 266
Male Genitourinary Protocol 271

Electrolyte and Acid/Base Disturbances 281
Hyperkalemia Protocol 282
Hypokalemia Protocol 285
Hypernatremia Protocol 288
Hyponatremia Protocol 294
Metabolic Acidosis Protocol 299

Head Trauma and Neck Pain 303
Adult Minor Head Trauma Protocol 304
Pediatric Minor Head Trauma Protocol 309
Neck Pain Protocol 313

HEENT 317
Sore Throat Protocol 318
Otitis Externa Protocol 324
Eye Protocols 327
Nosebleed Protocol.. 344
ENT Emergency Protocol 348
Nasal and Facial Fractures Protocol 356
Dental Injury Protocols 361
Dental Pain Protocol 365

Trauma.. 367
Motor Vehicle Accident Protocol 368
Laceration and Cutaneous Wound Protocol 376
Bleeding Protocol 385
Burn Protocol 388

Extremity Disorders.. 397
Extremity Medical Disorder Protocol 398
Fracture Protocol 410
Salter Harris Fracture Protocol 423
Synovial Fluid Analysis 426
Shoulder Protocol.. 428
Shoulder and Arm Trauma Protocol 434
Elbow Protocol.. 442
Hip Protocol 446
Knee Soft Tissue Injury Protocol 451
Knee Disorders Protocol 454
Ankle Sprain Protocol 462
Hand, Wrist, and Distal Forearm Injury Protocol 465
Finger Injury Protocol 472

Pediatrics 475
Pediatric Fever Protocol 476
Benign Febrile Seizure Protocol 480
Crying Infant Protocol.. 485
URI and Sinusitis Protocol 489
Otitis Media Protocol 493
Pediatric Asthma Protocol 497
Bronchiolitis Protocol 502
Croup Protocol.. 505

Pediatric Dehydration and Gastroenteritis Protocol 509
Pediatric Diarrhea Protocol 515

Geriatrics 521
Geriatrics Protocol 522

Gynecology.. 531
Vaginal Bleeding Protocol.. 532
Pelvic Pain Protocol 536
Pregnancy Complications Protocol 544

Infectious Disease.. 553
Sexually Transmitted Disease Protocol 554
Human Immunodeficiency Virus (HIV) Protocol........... 565
HIV and Hepatitis B Postexposure Prophylaxis Recommendations 570
Endocarditis Protocol.. 576
Tetanus Protocol.. 580

Dermatology 585
Human and Animal Bite Protocol.............................. 586
Spider Bite and Insect Sting Protocol 593
Snake Bite Protocol.. 597
Cellulitis Protocol 603
Soft Tissue Abscess Protocol 607
Henoch-Schonlein Purpura Protocol........................... 611
Erythema Multiforme Protocol 614
Erythema Nodosum Protocol 618
Dyshidrotic Eczema Protocol 620
Atopic Dermatitis/Eczema Protocol........................... 622
Psoriasis Protocol.. 624
Contact Dermatitis Protocol..................................... 628
Impetigo Protocol 630
Scabies Protocol 632
Tinea Capitis Protocol... 635
Tinea Corporis Protocol... 637
Tinea Pedis (Athlete's Foot) Protocol 639
Urticaria Protocol... 641
Pityriasis Rosea Protocol 644
Herpes Simplex Gingivostomatitis Protocol................. 646
Herpetic Whitlow Protocol 648

Genital Herpes Protocol 650
Herpes Zoster (Shingles) Protocol 652
Tick Bite Protocol 655
Lyme Disease Protocol..661
Varicella (Chicken Pox) Protocol...............................665
Hand Infection Protocol 667

Hematology and Oncology 673
Venous Thromboembolic Disease Protocol 674
Sickle Cell Anemia Protocol 682
Cancer Emergency Protocol.....................................687

Psychiatric and Social 697
Adult and Adolescent Psychiatric Protocol..................698
Alcohol Intoxicated Patient Protocol..........................703
Withdrawal Protocol 707
Sexual Assault Protocol...714
Domestic Violence Protocol 717
Child Abuse Protocol...719
Elder Abuse Protocol 722

Environmental 725
Heat Illness Protocol 726
Hypothermia Protocol 732
Frostbite and Exposure Skin Injury Protocol 737
Altitude Illness Protocol 741
Near Drowning Protocol 747

Medications 751
Pain Management Protocol 752
Drug Interactions...755

Disease Management.. 759
Hypertension Management.....................................760
Coronary Artery Disease Management 768
Heart Failure Management 780
Type 1 Diabetes Mellitus Management 789
Type 2 Diabetes Mellitus Management 797
Cholesterol Management...805
Stroke Prevention Management 809
Obesity Management...814

Asthma Management 820
COPD Management 832
Ventilator Management 837
Adult Septic Shock Management 848
Depression Management 854
Headache Management 860
Seizure Management 873
Arthritis Management 881

Glossary 895

Index 903

Reviewers

Robert E. Turner III, M.D., FACEP
Emergency Physician
Jackson-Madison County General Hospital
Volunteer Clinical Instructor, University of Tennessee Family Medicine; Jackson, Tennessee

Karl E. Misulis, M.D., PhD
West Tennessee Neurosciences
Jackson-Madison County General Hospital
Jackson, Tennessee
Associate Clinical Professor of Neurology, Vanderbilt University School of Medicine; Nashville, Tennessee

Frederick (Rick) E. Barr, M.D., MSCI
Professor of Pediatrics and Anesthesiology
Division Chief, Pediatric Critical Care Medicine
Associate Director, Masters in Clinical Investigation
Monroe Carell Jr. Children's Hospital at Vanderbilt
Vanderbilt University Medical Center; Nashville, Tennessee

Timothy F. Linder, M.D., FAAFP
Family Physician
Selmer, Tennessee
Volunteer Clinical Instructor, University of Tennessee Family Medicine; Jackson, Tennessee
Past President – Tennessee Academy of Family Physicians

David Roberts, M.D., FAAFP
Medical Director Jackson-Madison County General Hospital
Family and Geriatric Medicine
Past Director of University of Tennessee Family Medicine
Jackson, Tennessee

LeAnne Wilhite, ACNP-BC
Assistant Professor of Nursing
Chair of Undergraduate Nursing
Union University; Jackson, Tennessee

E. Scott Yarbro, M.D.
Jackson Urological Associates PC
Volunteer Clinical Instructor, University of Tennessee Family Medicine; Jackson, Tennessee

Gregg Mitchell, M.D.
Program Director – University of Tennessee Family Medicine
Jackson, Tennessee
Associate Professor – University of Tennessee Department of Family Medicine

Thomas Ellis, M.D., FCCP
The Jackson Clinic
Pulmonary and Critical Care
Jackson, Tennessee

Robert Gilroy, M.D., FCCP
The Jackson Clinic
Pulmonary and Critical Care
Jackson, Tennessee

E. Lee Murray, M.D.
West Tennessee Neurosciences
Jackson-Madison County General Hospital
Jackson, Tennessee

John Baker, M.D., FACC
The Jackson Clinic
Cardiology
Jackson, Tennessee

Robert Daggett, M.D.
Rheumatology
Brentwood, Tennessee

Jacob A Aelion, M.D., FACR, CCD
Arthritis Clinic, Jackson, TN
Clinical Professor of Medicine
The University of Tennessee Health Science Center
Memphis, Tennessee

~ Read This! ~

NOTICE

The protocols and disease management guides presented in this book are *model guidelines.* Accordingly, they should be used — and, when necessary, modified — per agreement between the physician and practitioner, where applicable. Any agreement should be established *prior to use* of a protocol or management guideline by the practitioner.

The author of these protocols and management guidelines has checked with sources believed to be reliable. However, medicine is an ever changing science and art. As new research and clinical experience expand the knowledge base, changes in treatment and protocols are required.

Further, there is a possibility of human error or of changes in medical science. Neither the author nor any party involved in the preparation or publication of this work warrants that the information contained herein is in every respect accurate or complete, and they disclaim all responsibility for any errors or omissions, or for results obtained from use of the information contained in these protocols or this publication.

Users are recommended and encouraged to confirm the information contained herein with other sources and by their own experience and knowledge. This recommendation is of particular importance with new or infrequently used drugs and therapies.

GUIDELINES OF PROPER USE

The guidance and other information provided in this book are to be used *only* in accordance with the following understandings and concepts:

1. The recommendations in this book are model guidance. *Evidence-based care has been included where applicable.*

2. When deemed appropriate, each Protocol and Disease Management should be modified to reflect any authorized policies, procedures, or practices at a particular medical facility.

3. Not all patient presentations can be covered in each Protocol and Disease Management section. Those presentations not covered should be evaluated and managed according to the practitioner's training and experience, and according to the usual scope of practice of the practitioner's particular medical facility.

4. Providers should perform only those tasks that are within the practitioner's skills and competence and that are within the usual scope of practice of the particular medical facility, and that are consistent with the protection and safety of the health and well-being of the patient.

5. Any perceived potential conflict between patient safety and a Protocol or Disease Management section should be resolved in favor of patient safety.

6. Sanford Guide to Antimicrobial Therapy can be used for infections in lieu of antimicrobial treatments specified in the Protocols and Disease Management sections presented in this book.

9. Life-saving care should not be withheld because of the instructions in a Protocol or Disease Management section.

10. Suggested vital signs, lab, and age consult criteria should be viewed in the context of the practitioner's training and experience, as well as in the context of the clinical situation and the patient's condition. For example, the total WBC may or may not reflect the severity of disease.

11. Read the Notice (page 15) before applying any Protocol or Disease Management section recommendations contained herein. If you do not accept the limitations and disclaimers contained in the Notice you should refrain from using this book and the information contained herein.

PROTOCOL GUIDELINE AGREEMENT

(When applicable)

By signing this Protocol Guideline Agreement each party acknowledges that he or she has read both the Notice section and the Guidelines of Proper Use section.

Provider's signature Date

Provider's signature Date

Provider's signature Date

Provider's signature Date

Provider's signature Date

Provider's signature Date

Provider's signature Date

Provider's signature Date

Provider's signature Date

Provider's signature Date

Provider's signature Date

Provider's signature Date

Provider's signature Date

Provider's signature Date

General

Section Contents — one protocol

General Patient Criteria Protocol

When using any protocol, always follow the Guidelines of Proper Use (page 16).

GENERAL PATIENT CRITERIA PROTOCOL

When using any protocol, always follow the Guidelines of Proper Use (page 16).

Recommended conditions to notify physician during or after practitioner's initial assessment

- Acute myocardial infarction (AMI) or symptoms consistent with AMI — notify physician when AMI identified
- Acute central nervous system deficits
- Severe CHF
- Severe respiratory distress
- O2 Saturation < 90% on room air, if acute
- Hypotension
- Acute altered mental status unless intoxicated
- Adult heart rate ≥ 140
- Emergency hypertension

Recommended consult criteria with physician when:

- Age < 3 months (unless experienced with this age group)
- Moderate CHF
- SBP ≥ 240 or DBP ≥ 140 at presentation (that is asymptomatic) with preexisting hypertension history
- Adult heart rate ≥ 110 at time of disposition
- Patients sent to the ED or clinic from an outlying hospital, clinic, or from home by a medical provider
- Age ≥ 70 with systemic symptoms
- Patient receives more than one pain injection
- Patient returns ≤ 14 days for same acute complaint (Does not apply to chronic recurrent complaints unless a change in the complaint)

- Elevated BP or heart rate in pregnancy or ≤ 6 weeks postpartum
- Pregnancy complications
- Chest pain (potentially consistent with angina or anginal equivalent symptoms)
- Nonspecific chest pain age ≥ 30 with history of
    - Hypertension
    - Diabetes
    - Smoking
    - Coronary artery disease history
    - Hyperlipidemia
    - Family history of coronary artery disease by age of 60

      OR
    - Age ≥ 50 without risk factors
- Abdominal pain
    - Requiring narcotics
    - Age ≥ 70
    - Diabetic
    - Uncertain diagnosis

Lab consult criteria

- Adult WBC ≥ 15,000 or < 1,000 neutrophils
- Pediatric WBC ≥ 15,000 or < 1,000 neutrophils
- Bandemia ≥ 15%
- Acute thrombocytopenia
- Hemoglobin 8–10 gms (unless chronic and stable)
- Hemoglobin < 8 gms even if chronic
- O2 Sat ≤ 94% on room air if acute (or moderate dyspnea)
- O2 Sat 2% less than chronic levels

Vital sign and age consult criteria

Fever

- Adult ≥ 104°F or 40°C
- Pediatric ≥ 104.5°F or 40.3°C

Hypothermia

- Temperature ≤ 95°F or 35°C

Heart rate/minute

- Adult heart rate ≥ 110

- Pediatric heart rate:
  - 0–4 months ≥ 180
  - 5–7 months ≥ 175
  - 6–12 months ≥ 170
  - 1–3 years ≥ 160
  - 4–5 years ≥ 145
  - 6–8 years ≥ 130
  - 7–12 years ≥ 125
  - 12–15 years ≥ 115
  - 16 years or older ≥ 110

Hypertension

- Adult asymptomatic hypertension of SBP > 220 or DBP > 120 at time of disposition with history of hypertension
- Adult asymptomatic SBP > 195 or DBP > 115 at discharge without history of hypertension
- Pediatric hypertension — age < 14 years

NOTE: Specific protocols override this General Patient Criteria Protocol

Notes

Cardiovascular

Section Contents

Chest Pain Protocol

Cardiac Dysrhythmia Protocol

Hypertension Protocol

Congestive Heart Failure Protocol

Syncope/Presyncope Protocol

When using any protocol, always follow the Guidelines of Proper Use (page 16).

CHEST PAIN PROTOCOL

When using any protocol, always follow the Guidelines of Proper Use (page 16).

Definition

- Patient perception of discomfort in anterior chest or upper half of back

Differential Diagnosis

Pneumonia

- Cough
- Fever
- Chills
- Dyspnea
- Sweats
- Tachycardia

Pulmonary embolism

- Dyspnea
- Tachycardia
- Hypoxia
- Pleuritic chest pain
- Well's criteria moderate-to-high probability
- Troponin may be elevated in moderate to massive pulmonary embolism

Chest wall pain

- Chest tenderness
- Pleuritic chest pain
- Pain with movement

Angina/AMI

- Anterior chest pressure or tightness
- Left or right arm pain
- Jaw pain
- Right arm pain only with chest pain highly specific for cardiac ischemia

- Dyspnea (may be only presenting complaint in very elderly: age ≥ 80)
- Nausea and/or vomiting
- Diaphoresis
- Indigestion
- Angina may be exertional only

Pleurisy
- Pain occurs or worsens with breathing
- No other comorbid symptoms or signs

Pericarditis
- Pleuritic pain
- Fever
- Worse lying down
- Better sitting and leaning forward
- Diffuse ST segment elevation
- Diffuse PR segment depression
- Pericardial effusion
- Elevated C-reactive protein

Myopericarditis
- Elevated troponin
- Similar symptoms and findings as Pericarditis

Herpes zoster
- Vesicular dermatomal rash
- May have pain 4 days prior to rash

Aortic dissection
- Tearing pain
- Located or radiates to back
- Signs and symptoms above and below diaphragm frequently
- Ascending aorta most common location of thoracic dissection

Chest Pain with Respiratory (Pleuritic) or Movement Exacerbation

- May need no further testing if vital signs and O2 Sat are normal and clinical suspicion is low for cardiac or serious pulmonary disease
- Consider chest x-ray and D-dimer
- Consider EKG and troponin if diagnosis is uncertain for a non-cardiac etiology
- Consider CTA chest to evaluate for pulmonary embolism
- Apply Well's criteria

Evaluation options

- Chest x-ray
- CBC if fever or tachycardic
- BMP if diabetic or tachycardic
- D-dimer (if negative with Well's criteria 0–1 makes PE unlikely)
- CT chest (see below)
- Apply Well's pulmonary embolism and DVT criteria and chart Well's score as indicated
- Record positive or negative calf tenderness and Homan's sign

Evaluation with D-dimer

D-dimer (LIA method) — some methods currently in use not reliable

- Useful if negative at cutoff value to rule out DVT or PE
- Negative D-dimer with low to moderate probability Well's DVT or PE score largely excludes venous thromboembolic disease
- Well's DVT criteria high probability: order ultrasound scan regardless of D-dimer result
- If positive — not as useful as a negative result which usually rules out VTE (venous thromboembolic) disease
- Frequently positive with
  - Hospitalization in past month

- Chronic bedridden or low activity state
- Increasingly positive with age without significant acute disease process
- CHF
- Chronic disease processes
- Edematous states

Well's DVT criteria

- One point each:
    - Active cancer
    - Paralysis/recent cast immobilization
    - Recently bedridden > 3 days or surgery < 4 weeks
    - Deep vein tenderness
    - Entire leg edema
    - Calf swelling > 3 cm over other leg
    - Pitting edema > other calf
    - Collateral superficial veins
- Two points — alternative diagnosis less likely

High probability: ≥ 3 points

Moderate probability: 1–2 points

Low probability: 0 points

Well's PE criteria score 3 or greater consider D-dimer and CT chest PE protocol

- Suspected DVT = 3
- Alternative diagnosis less likely than PE = 3
- Heart rate > 100 = 1.5
- Immobilization/surgery past 4 wks. = 1.5
- Previous DVT/PE = 1.5
- Hemoptysis = 1
- Cancer past 6 months = 1

Well's score ≥ 6: order CTA chest PE protocol

Document positive or negative Homan's sign or calf tenderness regardless of Well's scores

Document PERC and/or Well's scores when appropriate

Pulmonary Embolism Rule-out Criteria (PERC Rule)
(Reportedly decreases significantly the likelihood of pulmonary embolism if all 8 criteria met)

- Age < 50
- Pulse oximetry > 94%
- Heart rate < 100
- No history of DVT or VTE
- No hemoptysis
- No estrogen use
- No unilateral leg swelling
- No recent surgery or trauma hospitalization past 4 weeks

Treatment

- Treat pneumonia/bronchitis per current national recommendations and Sanford Guide
- Pericarditis: NSAID's (if uncomplicated)
- NSAID or hydrocodone, or other narcotics as needed: Avoid Demerol (meperidine)
- Treat chest pain from abdominal causes or other causes as per training, experience, and protocols

Chest Pain that Could Represent Acute Coronary Syndrome (ACS) or Stable Angina

Evaluation

- EKG
- CBC
- BMP
- Chest x-ray
- Troponin

Acute Coronary Syndrome treatment (STEMI, NSTEMI and Unstable Angina) — consult physician promptly

- Aspirin 160–325 mg chew and swallow or Clopidogrel 300 mg PO once
- Nitrates prn (See nitrate contraindications and side-effects below)
- Oxygen — maintain O2 Sat > 90%
- Morphine 2-5 mg IV q5-15 minutes prn (caution if SBP < 105 mm Hg)

Short-acting nitrates

- NTG 0.3–0.6 SL prn — may repeat x 2 q5minutes prn continued ischemic cardiac pain
- May use before anginal provoking activities
    - Comes in tablets or spray
    - Tablets need refrigeration and last 3–6 months, and should tingle tongue when used
    - NTG spray lasts 2–3 years

NTG paste if needed

- 0.5-1 inch — caution if SBP < 105 mm Hg

NTG drip if needed

- Start at 10 mcg/minute IV and titrate for chest pain and limit SBP decrease to 10% if normotensive and 30% if hypertensive
- Keep SBP ≥ 90 mm Hg
- See nitrate contraindications and side-effects below

Heparin if needed

- Bolus 60 units/kg IV — NMT 4,000 units
- 12 mg/kg/hour IV drip — initially NMT 1,000 units/hour to be adjusted to PTT 50-75 seconds

OR

Enoxaprin if needed

- 1 mg/kg SQ q12hr

- May give first dose as 30 mg IV along with the SQ dose for STEMI
    - Age > 75 years give 0.75 mg/kg SQ and no IV dose for STEMI
- Dose 30 mg SQ qday for creatinine clearance < 30 ml/minute

Stable angina treatment

Short-acting nitrates

- NTG 0.3–0.6 SL prn — may repeat x 2 q5minutes prn continued ischemic cardiac pain
- May use before anginal provoking activities
    - Comes in tablets or spray
    - Tablets need refrigeration and last 3–6 months, and should tingle tongue when used
    - NTG spray lasts 2–3 years

Long-acting nitrates for stable angina

- Timing — taken at time of day that anginal symptoms or anginal equivalent symptoms (i.e., dyspnea) are most prevalent
- NTG 2.5 mg or 6.5 mg PO bid
- Isosorbide mononitrate
    - Standard dose — 20 mg PO bid given 7 hours apart
    - Smaller patients start 5 mg PO bid given 7 hours apart and increase to 10–20 mg PO bid given 7 hours apart over 2-3 days
    - Take on empty stomach 30 minutes prior to a meal or 1 hour after a meal
- Isosorbide mononitrate ER (extended release)
    - 30-120 mg PO qday
- Transdermal nitroglycerin (Nitro-Dur)
    - 0.2–0.4 mg/hr qday — remove for 10–12 hours each day
    - Max dose 0.4-0.8 mg/hr qday
    - Starts acting in 30 minutes and lasts 8–14 hours

Nitrate side–effects (some)

- Headache
- Hypotension
- Tachycardia
- Nausea

Nitrate contraindications

- Shock or hypotension
- SBP < 90 m Hg or ≥ 30 mm Hg below baseline SBP in ACS
- Bradycardia < 50 beats per minute
- Tachycardia in absence of heart failure (> 100 beats per minute)
- Acute right ventricular myocardial infarction
  - Caution in inferior myocardial infarction
- Use of erectile dysfunction medications (sildenafil, tadalafil, or vardenafil)
- Severe anemia

Beta-blockers for stable angina

- Reduce heart rate, blood pressure and cardiac contractility which decreases cardiac work and oxygen needs
- First choice usually in stable angina
- Prolongs survival and decreases second AMI incidence

Selective beta–1 blocker

- Metoprolol (Lopressor) initially 50 mg PO bid and may be increased to 200 mg PO bid
- Metoprolol (Toprol XL) 100 mg PO qday — NMT 400 mg PO qday
- Atenolol (Tenormin) 50 mg PO qday — NMT 200 mg PO qday

Beta–blocker side effects

- Bradycardia
- Hypotension
- Worsening of asthma and COPD
- Depression

- Heart failure
- Exacerbation of angina and hypertension on abrupt withdrawal (Black Box Warning)
- Worsening of peripheral arterial disease symptoms

Contraindications

- Pre-existing sinus bradycardia (< 60 beats/minutes)
- Moderate to severe left ventricle failure and pulmonary edema
- SBP < 100 mm Hg
- Signs of poor peripheral perfusion
- 2nd and 3rd degree heart block
- Asthma and COPD
- Sick sinus syndrome without pacemaker
- Untreated pheochromocytoma

ACEI or ARB added to a beta-blocker if needed in stable angina

Consult criteria

- Notify physician promptly for ACS (STEMI, NSTEMI and Unstable angina
- Consult physician for suspected stable angina

General Discharge Criteria for Chest Pain

- Benign noncardiac chest pain
- Chest wall pain
- Pleurisy or pleurodynia
- Adult heart rate < 100
- Herpes zoster
- O2 Saturation ≥ 95%
- Normal cardiac marker lab tests
- Stable and nonacute CBC, BMP and chest x-ray

Discharge instructions

- Chest pain aftercare instructions
- Follow up with primary care provider or cardiologist within 1–3 days as indicated

Consult Criteria

- Suspected angina or acute coronary syndrome
- Suspected anginal equivalent — arm, neck, jaw or epigastric pain, or dyspnea
- Acute chest x-ray abnormalities
- Pulmonary embolism or aortic dissection/aneurysm
- Pericarditis
- Severe pain in Provider's clinical judgment
- Chest pain of uncertain etiology
- Follow General Patient Criteria Protocol (page 20) for care/evaluation not covered in this protocol

Suggested age consult criteria

- Nonspecific chest pain age ≥ 30 with history of
  - Hypertension
  - Diabetes
  - Smoking
  - Coronary artery disease history
  - Hyperlipidemia
  - Family history of coronary artery disease by age of 60

    OR
  - Age ≥ 50 without risk factors

Suggested vital signs and lab consult criteria

- WBC ≥ 15,000
- Elevated troponin
- Bandemia ≥ 15%
- Increased anion gap
- Metabolic acidosis
- Significant electrolyte abnormally (see electrolyte disorders)
- Glucose ≥ 400 mg/dL in diabetic patient
- Glucose ≥ 300 mg/dL in non-diabetic patient
- Hyperglycemia with metabolic acidosis (decreased serum CO_2 or elevated anion gap)
- Chest pain with O_2 Saturation on room air < 95% in non-COPD or non-bronchospasm presentation (see Dyspnea Protocol)
- Adult heart rate ≥ 100

- Developing hypotension or relative hypotension (SBP < 105 with history of hypertension)

Notes

Reference:

Circulation 2010;122:S787-S817

CHEST October 2011;140(4_MeetingAbstracts):594A-594A. doi:10.1378/chest.1112163

CHEST August 2011;140(2):509-518. doi:10.1378/chest.10-2468

CARDIAC DYSRHYTHMIA PROTOCOL

When using any protocol, always follow the Guidelines of Proper Use (page 16).

Definition

- Disorders of cardiac rhythm

Differential Diagnosis

- Sinus tachycardia
- Atrial tachycardia
- Multifocal atrial tachycardia
- Atrial fibrillation
- Atrial flutter
- Sinus bradycardia
- Junctional bradycardia
- Atrioventricular blocks
- Premature atrial contractions
- Premature ventricular contractions

Considerations

- Unifocal premature ventricular contractions (PVCs) without associated symptoms of acute ischemic disease are usually benign and typically do not warrant treatment
- Premature atrial contractions (PACs) are usually benign
- Sinus bradycardia without hypotension usually does not warrant acute treatment
- Prolonged QTc interval on the EKG can lead to a serious arrhythmia
- PVCs with R wave on the T wave of preceding beat on the EKG or monitor can lead to ventricular tachycardia

General evaluation options

- Cardiac history
- Complete physical exam

- Associated symptoms
- Medication history
- EKG; consider monitor if heart rate ≥ 130 (adults) or ≤ 50
- CBC (depending on clinical situation)
- BMP (depending on clinical situation)
- Chest x-ray (depending on clinical situation)
- Troponin for anginal complaints or dyspnea
- BNP for dyspnea
- Consider D-dimer if PE suspected

Atrial Dysrhythmias

Sinus tachycardia

Definition

- Tachycardia in adults arising from the sinus node with a rate in adults > 100 beats/minute. Sinus tachycardia rates in pediatrics dependent on age

Considerations

- Significant sinus tachycardia (ST) that is unexplained can represent a high risk disease process
- Sinus tachycardia context is important: ST at 120 with influenza may be less concerning than ST at 105 with GI bleeding

Causes

Physiologic

- Pain or exertion

Pharmacologic

- Sympathetic agents; caffeine; bronchodilators

Pathologic

- Fever
- Dehydration
- Anemia
- Hemorrhage
- Pulmonary embolism
- Hypoxemia

- Infarction
- Ischemia
- Hyperthyroidism

Evaluation and treatment are aimed at underlying condition

Discharge instructions

- Sinus tachycardia aftercare instructions
- Follow up with PCP within 1-2 days if tachycardia persists
- Return if no improvement or worsening

Consult criteria

- Consult physician for unexplained adult ST ≥ 110 unless otherwise specified in other protocols

Premature atrial contractions

- Commonly benign; can be anxiety provoking
- Fatigue, stress or high adrenergic state can be the cause
- Evaluation is for associated disorders and not for PACs per se
- Usually no treatment needed
- If treatment desired, atenolol 50 mg PO qday or lopressor 100 mg PO qday can be used (follow up with primary care provider)

Discharge instructions

- Premature atrial contractions aftercare instructions

Atrial fibrillation

Definition

- Lack of organized atrial electrical activity and contractions. An irregularly irregular rhythm on EKG and cardiac auscultation or pulse palpation

Differential diagnosis

- Multifocal atrial tachycardia
- Wolf-Parkinson-White Syndrome (WPW)

- Atrial flutter
- Atrial tachycardia
- Supraventricular tachycardia

Considerations

- Most common cause of dysrhythmia
- Up to 9% of patients ≥ 80 years of age are affected
- CVA risk increased (do not acutely convert if present > 48 hours without therapeutic anticoagulation)
- BNP can be elevated without CHF
- Recent onset of atrial fibrillation converts spontaneously to normal sinus rhythm in 2–3 days in 2/3 of patients
- Increases mortality 1.5–2 times more than general population without atrial fibrillation
- Risk of stroke 1.5% in age 50–59 years and nearly 30% in age 80–89 years
- Commonly heart rates are 110–140 per minute

Causes

- Hypertension
- CHF
- Coronary artery disease
- Carditis
- Sick sinus syndrome
- Alcohol
- Pulmonary embolism
- Hyperthyroidism
- Sympathetic drugs
- Pneumonia
- Hyperthermia
- Hypothermia
- Postoperative
- Hypokalemia, hypomagnesemia and hypocalcemia

Management options

- Medication management to maintain normal sinus rhythm

- Medication management to achieve rate control of atrial fibrillation
- Catheter ablation
- Anticoagulation to prevent thromboembolic disease

Signs and symptoms

- Altered mental status
- Weakness
- Hypotension
- Syncope
- Angina
- CHF
- Emboli
  - Digit ischemia
  - Neurologic deficits
  - Mesenteric ischemia

Evaluation options

- EKG
- CBC
- BMP
- Chest x-ray
- Troponin for anginal complaints or dyspnea
- BNP for dyspnea or suspected CHF
- Thyroid function tests if hyperthyroidism suspected
- D-dimer if pulmonary embolism suspected
- Digoxin (digitalis) level if currently prescribed

Treatment options

- No treatment may be needed if heart rate ≤ 110 per minute
- IV NS KVO
- Oxygen if dyspneic; O2 saturation < 95% room air
- Treatment of fever or hypovolemia if contributing to rapid ventricular response > 110
- Cardizem (diltiazem) 0.25 mg/kg IV over 2 minutes (usually 20 mg initial dose)

    - May be repeated at 0.35 mg/kg IV over 2 minutes after 15 minutes of initial dose if needed (usually 25 mg)
    - Maintenance is 5–10 mg/hour IV
- Metoprolol 5 mg IV, may repeat q5 minutes prn × 2
- Cardioversion with 200J with biphasic waveform device for hypotension with rapid ventricular response (notify physician immediately for cardioversion if available)
- Wide complex atrial fibrillation is potentially a life threatening rhythm — Notify physician immediately

Anticoagulation

- Aspirin 81 mg or 325 mg PO qday in low risk patients
    - Age 60–74 years
    - Female
- Coumadin (warfarin) 5–10 mg PO qday — (INR target of 2–3) with moderate or high risk factors
    - Age > 75 years
    - CAD
    - CHF
    - Hypertension
    - Diabetes mellitus
    - Mitral stenosis
    - Prior TIA/CVA
    - Mechanical valve
- Lovenox 1 mg/kg SQ q12hr

Discharge criteria

- Stable chronic atrial fibrillation with rate ≤ 110 and pre-existing history of atrial fibrillation
- No other concerning symptoms

Discharge instructions

- Atrial fibrillation aftercare instructions
- Prescribe aspirin 81–325 mg PO qday
- See treatment options above

  - Adjust Digoxin (digitalis) if needed
  - Follow up with primary care provider within 7 days

Consult criteria

- Adult heart rate ≥ 110
- Chest discomfort
- Dyspnea
- Hypotension
- Suspected hyperthyroidism
- Acute neurologic complaints or findings
- New onset atrial fibrillation
- Age > 55
- Digoxin (digitalis) toxicity
- PT/INR not therapeutic if on Coumadin (warfarin)
  (INR < 2)

Supraventricular tachycardia

Definition

- Tachycardia not involving the sinus node that is maintained by the atria or atrioventricular node

Differential diagnosis

- Atrial fibrillation
- Atrial flutter
- Multifocal atrial tachycardia (commonly in COPD patients)
- Ventricular tachycardia
- Sinus tachycardia

Considerations

- Usually narrow complexes on EKG with rapid and regular rhythm
- Episodic most commonly
- Can have wide complexes with aberrant or retrograde conduction
- Heart rate usually 150–200/minute in adults
- Higher rates may be present in WPW
- Wide complex SVT can be ventricular tachycardia — notify physician immediately

- Treatment of wide complex SVT with calcium channel blockers, beta-blockers or Digoxin (digitalis) may result in deterioration of rhythm to ventricular fibrillation if antidromic (retrograde conduction) WPW — notify physician immediately prior to antiarrhythmia drug treatment

Presenting complaints

- Palpitations
- Dizziness
- Chest pain
- Shortness of breath
- Diaphoresis

Evaluation options

- EKG (may be all that is needed in young healthy patient)
- CBC
- BMP
- Chest x-ray if respiratory complaints or findings present
- Troponin for anginal complaints
- BNP for dyspnea or suspected CHF
- Digoxin (digitalis) level if taking digoxin

Treatment options

- IV NS KVO or INT
- Oxygen if dyspneic or O2 saturation < 95% room air
- Vagal maneuvers in stable patient
    - Breath holding
    - Bearing down like in having a bowel movement
    - Unilateral carotid massage for 10 seconds at a time in young healthy patients
    - Face immersion in cold water

Medication treatment options (discuss with physician initially)

- Adenosine 6 mg rapid IVP followed by 10–20 ml of saline — may repeat with 12 mg if needed
- Diltiazem 0.25 mg/kg over 2 minutes (usually 20 mg in adults — may be repeated with 0.35 mg/kg IV over 2 minutes (usually 25 mg in adults)

- Wide complex tachycardia notify physician immediately

Discharge criteria

- SVT conversion in stable patient without cardiac or other concerning comorbidities

Discharge instructions

- Supraventricular tachycardia aftercare instructions
- Follow up with PCP or cardiologist within 1–7 days

Recommended consult criteria

- Discuss all cases with physician before treatment and prior to discharge

Junctional rhythm

Definition

- Heart rhythm arising from AV node

Differential diagnosis

- Second and third degree AV block
- Digoxin (digitalis) toxicity
- Sinus node dysfunction
- AV nodal reentry tachycardia
- Idioventricular rhythm

Evaluation options

- EKG
- CBC
- BMP
- Chest x-ray
- Troponin for anginal complaints

- BNP for dyspnea or suspected CHF

Treatment options
- IV NS KVO or INT
- Oxygen if dyspneic or O2 saturation < 95% room air
- Dependant on cause of the rhythm

Recommended consult criteria
- Discuss all cases with physician

Sinus bradycardia

Definition
- Sinus rhythm < 60 beats per minute

Causes

Physiologic
- Vagal tone

Pharmacologic
- Calcium channel blockers; beta-blockers; Digoxin (digitalis)

Pathologic
- AMI
- Hypothyroidism
- Sick sinus syndrome
- Carotid hypersensitivity
- High intracranial pressure
- Hypoglycemia

Evaluation
- EKG
- Per other complaints or findings

Treatment
- Usually no treatment needed if heart rate ≥ 40 in healthy patient
- IV NS bolus if hypotensive and not in CHF

Discharge criteria
- Asymptomatic sinus bradycardia ≥ 50 beats/minute

Discharge instructions

- Sinus bradycardia aftercare instructions
- Follow up with PCP or cardiologist within 7 days if new onset

Consult criteria

- Heart rate < 50
- Hypotension
- Dyspnea
- Anginal complaints

Second and third degree AV block

Definition

- Second degree heart block has some atrial electrical impulses not conducted to the ventricles
- Third degree heart block has no atrial electrical impulses conducted to the ventricles

Considerations

- Can be caused by AMI or myocarditis
- Can be seen with Lyme disease
- Can occur with structural heart disease

Mobitz type 1 second degree heart block (Wenkebach)

- PR interval progressively lengthens before dropping a ventricular beat
- Can be seen in healthy athletes
- Usually asymptomatic
- May have chest pain if ischemia or myocarditis present
- Rarely have syncope
- May be drug induced — beta-blocker, calcium channel blockers, Digoxin (digitalis), amiodarone

Mobitz type 2 second degree heart block

- Intermittent dropped ventricular beats without progressive lengthening of the PR interval
- Syncope may occur

- AMI or myocarditis more common than mobitz type 1
- May be drug induced
- More serious type of heart block than mobitz type 1

Third degree heart block

- Most patients are asymptomatic
- May be hypotensive or have syncope
- Sudden death can occur
- May be caused by AMI
- Confusion can occur in elderly

Evaluation

- Cardiac monitor
- EKG
- CBC
- BMP
- Chest x-ray
- Troponin
- BNP for dyspnea or suspected CHF

Treatment

- IV NS KVO
- Oxygen if dyspneic; O2 saturation < 95% room air
- External pacing if hypotensive and heart rate < 60 (apply external pacing pads to mobitz type 2 and third degree heart block)
- Atropine 0.3–1 mg IV – discuss with physician

Consult criteria

- Notify physician promptly on all heart block patients

Ventricular Dysrhythmias

Premature ventricular contractions

Definition

- A premature ventricular contraction caused by an ectopic cardiac pacemaker in the ventricle usually > 120 msec on EKG

Consideration

- Usually benign and stable
- Usually unifocal and needs no acute treatment

Causes

- Frequently normal finding
- Digoxin (digitalis) toxicity
- Cardiac ischemia
- Cardiomyopathy
- Hypoxemia
- Mitral valve prolapse
- Myocarditis
- Cardiac contusion
- Stimulant medications or drugs (caffeine, cocaine, methamphetamines, tobacco)
- Hypokalemia
- Hypomagnesemia
- Hypercalcemia
- CHF
- Alkalosis

Evaluation

- EKG
- BMP if comorbid conditions present or on diuretics
- Other tests as dictated by symptoms or other findings

Treatment options

- Usually none
- Correction of potassium and magnesium levels if checked and significantly abnormal
- Treat underlying condition causing PVCs if present
- If antiarrhythmia treatment desired, atenolol 50 mg PO qday or metoprolol (Lopressor) 100 mg PO qday can be used (follow up with primary care provider)

Discharge criteria

- If a benign incidental finding without concerning comorbid conditions

Discharge instructions

- PVC aftercare instructions
- Follow up with primary care provider or cardiologist as needed

Consult criteria

- EKG shows R on T phenomenon
- Comorbid conditions of concern: chest pain; dyspnea; syncope; etc.
- Potassium ≤ 2.5 mEq/L
- Digoxin (digitalis) toxicity
- Prolonged QTc interval
- New onset renal insufficiency

PVC couplets or multifocal PVCs

- Consult physician
- Usually needs no treatment
    - Treating the cause may be indicated unless benign
    - If antiarrhythmia treatment desired, atenolol 50 mg PO qday or metoprolol (Lopressor) 100 mg PO qday can be used (follow up with primary care provider)

Accelerated idioventricular rhythm (AIVR)

Definition

- Wide complex ventricular rhythm
- Rate 40–120 per minute

Considerations

- Associated with reperfusion in AMI

Treatment

- Observe
    - Treating with antiarrhythmia drugs can cause asystole — do not treat patient with these drugs

Consult criteria

- Discuss all cases of AIVR with physician promptly

Ventricular tachycardia

Definition

- Tachycardia originating from the ventricles that is ≥ 120/minute and is wide complexed of ≥ 140 msec on EKG

Causes

- Cardiac ischemia
- Hypokalemia, hypomagnesemia, or hypocalcemia
- QT prolonging drugs
- Digoxin (digitalis) toxicity

Symptoms or findings

- May be asymptomatic, especially in nonsustained ventricular tachycardia (30 beat run or less)
- Chest pain
- CHF
- Hypotension
- Altered mental status

Evaluation

- Order EKG; CBC; BMP; chest x-ray; troponin
- Cardiac monitor

Treatment per physician if available

- IV NS KVO
- Oxygen to keep O2 saturation > 94%
- Lidocaine 1 mg/kg IV up to 100mg — may repeat × 2 up to 3 mg/kg followed by drip of 2–4 mg/min IV

  or
- Amiodarone 150 mg IV over 10 minutes followed by drip of 1 mg/min
- Have nurse deploy cardiac defibrillation pads on patient

- Activate cardiac code and start CPR and ACLS if no pulse present and patient unconscious

Warning

- Treating **"slow ventricular tachycardia"** (rate ≤120 beats/minute) with an antiarrhythmia drug, may actually be treating accelerated idioventricular rhythm (a life sustaining ventricular escape rhythm), resulting in asystole and death

Notes

HYPERTENSION PROTOCOL

When using any protocol, always follow the Guidelines of Proper Use (page 16).

Definition

- Adult SBP > 140 or DBP > 90
- Age 1 ≥ 104/58
- Age 6 ≥ 115/75
- Age 12 ≥ 125/82
- Age 17 ≥ 138/87

Considerations

- Most hypertension is acutely asymptomatic
- Care should be exercised in too aggressively over-treating asymptomatic hypertension acutely
- Blood pressure usually comes down with repeated measurements only. Repeat q15 min. prn
- Poor outcomes possible from lowering blood pressure too much acutely

Hypertensive categories

- Hypertensive urgency*:* SBP ≥ 180 or DBP ≥ 115 with cardiac risk factors
- Severe uncontrolled hypertension: SBP ≥ 180 or DBP ≥ 115 without cardiac risk factors
- Hypertensive emergency*:* elevated blood pressure with acute end organ compromise or injury

Evaluation

- Complete history and physical exam
- Detailed cardiopulmonary exam
- Check for peripheral edema
- Asymptomatic hypertension in above hypertensive categories, excluding hypertensive emergency, by itself may require no further acute tests
- BMP and U/A (for protein/blood) can be considered, especially if starting new hypertensive medications or in pregnancy
- Add CBC if pregnant to check platelet count

- EKG, CXR, BNP and troponin for acute signs/symptoms of cardiac disease
- Hypertensive urgency — lab appropriate to address existing risk factor screening

Treatment Options

- Hypertensive urgency — begin treatment within 24–48 hours per primary care provider
- Severe asymptomatic hypertension — begin treatment within 1–7 days per primary care provider
- SBP > 200 or DBP > 120 at discharge can begin treatment as indicated; May need 2 medications or combination medication
- Hypertensive emergency consult physician for treatment options
- Hypertensive emergency blood pressure should not be lowered more than 25% acutely
- IV therapy safer in hypertensive emergency: better control
- See CVA/TIA Protocol for CVA/TIA presentation

Discharge Criteria

- Asymptomatic SBP < 220 or DBP < 120 mm Hg
- No concerning comorbidities

Discharge instructions

- Hypertension aftercare instructions
- Follow up with PCP within 1–2 days if SBP ≥ 200 mm Hg or DBP ≥ 110
- Patient to notify PCP of visit and blood pressure readings within 1–2 days

Consult Criteria

- SBP ≥ 240 or DBP ≥ 140 at presentation (asymptomatic) with preexisting hypertension history
- Asymptomatic SBP > 220 or DBP > 120 at time of disposition with history of hypertension
- Asymptomatic SBP > 195 or DBP > 115 at time of disposition without history of hypertension
- Hypertension in pregnancy or within 6 weeks postpartum

- Hypertensive emergency
- Acute cardiac, neurologic or renal disorder suspected
    - Intracranial hemorrhage, TIA, CVA, CHF, angina, MI, acute renal failure
- New onset renal insufficiency or worsening renal insufficiency
- See General Patient Criteria Protocol (page 20)

Initiation of Outpatient Treatment Options (if desired)

SBP 140–159 or DBP 90–99

- HCTZ 25 mg PO qday

SBP 160–199 or DBP 100–115

- Lisinopril 5–10 mg PO qday (chronic renal insufficiency use 5 mg PO qday)
- HCTZ 25 mg PO qday

SBP > 200 or DBP > 115

- Clonidine 0.2 mg PO tid
- HCTZ 25 mg PO qday

Stable angina

- Atenolol 50 mg PO qday

Congestive heart failure

- Lisinopril 5–10 mg PO qday
- Lasix (furosemide) 20–40 mg PO qday

Other medications than listed above are acceptable as indicated

Notes

CONGESTIVE HEART FAILURE PROTOCOL

When using any protocol, always follow the Guidelines of Proper Use (page 16).

Definition

- Cardiac dysfunction secondary to decreased ability of the left ventricle (LV) to eject or fill with blood

Systolic dysfunction

- Decreased left ventricular ejection fraction (LVEF) < 50%

Diastolic dysfunction

- Abnormal left ventricular filling
- LVEF > 50%

Differential Diagnosis

- Pneumonia
- COPD
- Bronchitis
- Pulmonary embolism
- Noncardiac pulmonary edema
- Adult respiratory distress syndrome

Considerations

- Main treatment is vasodilatation in nonhypotensive patients
- Isolated right heart failure is without dyspnea or pulmonary congestion
- Troponin can be mildly elevated with CHF alone

BNP

- BNP < 100 rules out CHF if not obese (lower in obese patients: < 50 is cutoff)
- Elevated in renal insufficiency or renal failure (sometimes markedly)
- BNP > 200 CHF likely

- BNP > 500 : acute exacerbation likely

BNP level cutoffs dependent on assays used

Classification of heart failure

- Class 1 – no limitation of normal physical activity
- Class 2 – slight limitation of activity (fatigue, dyspnea)
- Class 3 – marked limitation of activity
- Class 4 – symptoms at rest

Findings

- Fatigue
- Malaise
- Dyspnea
- Peripheral pitting edema
- Orthopnea and paroxysmal nocturnal dyspnea
- Rales
- Cough
- Hepatomegaly
- Ascites
- Jugular venous distension
- Hypotension
- Cardiac gallop sounds

Chest x-ray

- Cephalization of flow
- Cardiomegaly
- Pleural effusion
- Accurate in diagnosis
- Can have delayed findings

Evaluation

- EKG
- Chest x-ray (upright if possible)
- CBC
- BMP
- Troponin
- BNP

Treatment Options (Non-hypotensive Patients)

- Oxygen
- IV KVO
- Nitroglycerin (NTG) SL — may repeat to decrease SBP 15–20% (if SBP ≥ 110)
- Nitroglycerin paste ½–1 inch (if SBP ≥ 110)
- Captopril 25 mg PO (or SL) if NTG not decreasing SBP adequately
    - If SBP ≥ 110 (effects start in 10 minutes and peaks in 30–40 minutes)
    - ACE inhibitors prolong survival
- Lasix (furosemide) 40–80 mg IV bolus (match home single dose) or 1 hour infusion (infusion appears to work better)
- Preferable to use vasodilators initially if possible
- Avoid morphine

Discharge Criteria

- Good response to treatment for mild chronic CHF
- Back to baseline respiratory function on room air

Discharge instructions

- CHF aftercare instructions
- Follow up with PCP or cardiologist within 1 day
- Return immediately if worse

Consult Criteria

- CHF exacerbation including
    - Inadequate response to treatment
    - New onset congestive heart failure
    - Preferable to discuss all cases with physician prior to discharge
- Normotensive (contact physician for treatment options if SBP < 120)
- Hypotension (notify physician)
- Elevated troponin
- Chest pain or anginal symptoms
- Presyncope or syncope

Notes

SYNCOPE/PRESYNCOPE PROTOCOL

When using any protocol, always follow the Guidelines of Proper Use (page 16).

Definitions

- Transient loss of consciousness or near loss of consciousness secondary to decreased perfusion of brain

Differential Diagnosis

- Cardiac arrhythmia
- Pulmonary embolism
- TIA
- CVA
- Seizures
- Dehydration
- Aortic stenosis
- Hypoglycemia
- Subarachnoid hemorrhage
- Hemorrhage
    - GI bleeding
    - Ectopic pregnancy
- Adrenal insufficiency
- Sepsis

Causes

- Neurally mediated
    - Vasovagal
    - Situational
    - Carotid sinus
- Psychiatric
- Orthostatic
    - Volume depletion or hemorrhage
    - Advanced age
- Medications
- Neurologic

- Cardiac
- Unknown

Considerations

- EKG recommended in all patients
- Testing for unexplained syncope is based on risk factors
- Vasovagal episode is the most common cause
- Medication can cause syncope or presyncope

Clinical important features suggestive of specific cause

Exertion

- Aortic stenosis
- Mitral stenosis
- Coronary artery disease

Head rotation

- Carotid-sinus syncope

Arm exercise

- Subclavian steal

Red Flags

- Exertional onset: ischemic coronary disease or aortic stenosis
- Chest pain: ischemic coronary disease
- Severe headache: subarachnoid or cerebral hemorrhage
- Low back pain: aortic dissection or aneurysm
- Dyspnea: pulmonary embolism or CHF
- Palpitations: symptomatic arrhythmia
- Neurologic deficits

Evaluation

- Syncope/presyncope lasting < 20 seconds in healthy patients get an EKG, but may not need further testing if all the following exist:
  - Age < 50
  - Normal physical exam

    - Normal vital signs and O2 sat on room air
    - No comorbidities
    - Clinically had a vasovagal episode
    - No other complaints
- Perform orthostatic vital signs
- Blood pressure measurements in both arms for comparison
- Apply Well's pulmonary embolism and DVT criteria and chart Well's score as indicated
- Record positive or negative calf tenderness and Homan's sign

All other patients order options

- CBC
- BMP
- Chest x-ray
- EKG
- UCG if pregnancy possible
- Check stool hemoccult if any of the following
    - Acutely anemic
    - Tachycardic
    - Orthostatic vital signs
    - Melena or rectal bleeding history
- Chest pain: order troponin (angina) and D-dimer
- Consider CT head for neurologic complaints, findings or headache (low yield otherwise)

Evaluation with D-dimer

D-dimer (LIA method) — some methods currently in use not reliable

- Useful if negative at cutoff value to rule out DVT or PE
- Negative D-dimer with low to moderate probability Well's DVT score largely excludes venous thromboembolic disease
- Well's DVT criteria high probability: order ultrasound scan regardless of D-dimer result
- If positive — not as useful as a negative result which usually rules out VTE (venous thromboembolic) disease

- Frequently positive with
  - Hospitalization in past month
  - Chronic bedridden or low activity state
  - Increasingly positive with age without significant acute disease process
  - CHF
  - Chronic disease processes
  - Edematous states

Well's DVT criteria

- One point each:
  - Active cancer
  - Paralysis/recent cast immobilization
  - Recently bedridden > 3 days or surgery < 4 weeks
  - Deep vein tenderness
  - Entire leg edema
  - Calf swelling > 3 cm over other leg
  - Pitting edema > other calf
  - Collateral superficial veins
- Two points — alternative diagnosis less likely

High probability: ≥ 3 points

Moderate probability: 1–2 points

Low probability: 0 points

Well's PE criteria score 3 or greater consider D-dimer and CT chest PE protocol

- Suspected DVT = 3
- Alternative diagnosis less likely than PE = 3
- Heart rate > 100 = 1.5
- Immobilization/surgery past 4 wks = 1.5
- Previous DVT/PE = 1.5
- Hemoptysis = 1
- Cancer past 6 months = 1

Well's score ≥ 6: order CTA chest PE protocol

Document positive or negative Homan's sign or calf tenderness regardless of Well's scores

Document PERC and/or Well's scores when appropriate

Pulmonary Embolism Rule-out Criteria (PERC Rule)

(Reportedly decreases significantly the likelihood of pulmonary embolism if all 8 criteria met)

- Age < 50
- Pulse oximetry > 94%
- Heart rate < 100
- No history of DVT or VTE
- No hemoptysis
- No estrogen use
- No unilateral leg swelling
- No recent surgery or trauma hospitalization past 4 weeks

Treatment Options

- Dehydration give oral rehydration in nontoxic pediatric or adult patients (see Gastroenteritis protocols)
- IV NS rehydration in all others as needed
- Blood transfusion for bleeding with anemia and symptomatic volume loss prn
- Anti-emetics prn
- Treatment aimed at cause of syncope or presyncope

Discharge Criteria

- Benign cause of syncope or presyncope in healthy patient age < 50 years

Discharge instructions

- Syncope or presyncope aftercare instructions
- Follow up with PCP within 1–2 days
- Consider ambulatory holter monitor
- Return if symptoms recur

Consult Criteria

- Syncope or presyncope > 30 seconds
- Age ≥ 50 (elderly will usually need hospital admission)
- GI bleeding
- Acute anemia, or chronic anemia with hemoglobin < 8 gms or a decrease in hemoglobin > 1 gm from previous levels
- Hypotension or tachycardia
- O2 sat < 95 on room air or acute dyspnea
- Relative hypotension (SBP < 105 with history of hypertension)
- Abnormal EKG
- Cardiac dysrhythmia
- Positive orthostatics (a normal finding occasionally in elderly)
- Unclear cause of syncope or presyncope
- Chest pain or arrhythmia

Comorbid conditions present

- Hypertension
- Diabetes
- Cardiac
- Pulmonary disease
- Pregnancy
- Pulmonary embolism
- DVT
- Neurologic complaints or findings
- Toxic ingestion
- Dehydration
- Fever

Lab and x-ray consult criteria

- New onset renal insufficiency or worsening chronic renal insufficiency
- Metabolic acidosis (increased anion gap)
- Hemoglobin decrease > 1 gm or creatinine increased > 0.5 from baseline
- Elevated LFT's
- Elevated amylase or lipase
- WBC ≥ 15,000

- Bandemia ≥ 15%
- Significant electrolyte abnormally
- Glucose ≥ 400 mg/dL in diabetic patient
- Glucose ≥ 200 mg/dL in non-diabetic patient
- Hyperglycemia with metabolic acidosis (decreased serum CO2 or elevated anion gap)
- Acute thrombocytopenia

Notes

Reference:

CHEST August 2011;140(2):509-518.
doi:10.1378/chest.10-2468

Respiratory

Section Contents

Dyspnea Protocol

Pneumonia Protocol

Adult Asthma/Acute Bronchitis Protocol

Allergy Protocol

When using any protocol, always follow the Guidelines of Proper Use (page 16).

DYSPNEA PROTOCOL

When using any protocol, always follow the Guidelines of Proper Use (page 16).

Definition

- Subjective perception of shortness of breath

Differential Diagnosis

- COPD
- Asthma
- Bronchitis
- Pneumonia
- CHF
- Angina
- Pulmonary embolism
- Pleural effusion
- Cardiac tamponade
- Pulmonary hypertension

Dyspnea of Uncertain Cause

Evaluation

If CHF suspected order:

- BNP
- BMP
- CBC
- Troponin
- EKG
- Chest x-ray

Consider pulmonary embolism if Well's PE criteria score 3 or greater

- Order D-dimer (can be frequently positive without DVT/PE in elderly, with history of hospitalization within past month, cancer history, edematous conditions, bedridden — see Chest Pain or Syncope Protocols)

Well's Pulmonary Embolism Criteria

- Suspected DVT = 3
- Alternate diagnosis less likely than pulmonary embolism = 3
- Heart rate > 100 = 1.5
- Immobilization/surgery past 4 wks = 1.5
- Previous DVT = 1.5
- Hemoptysis = 1
- Cancer past 6 months = 1

Well's PE score > 6

- Order CTA chest PE protocol
- Document positive/negative Homan's sign or calf tenderness

- If anginal equivalent suspected as complaint in elderly, refer to Chest Pain Protocol

Discharge criteria

- Panic disorder or benign hyperventilation
- Benign cause of dyspnea (i.e., mild to moderate asthma or bronchitis responding well to treatment)

Consult physician

- If angina equivalent suspected
- CHF suspected or diagnosed
- Pulmonary embolism suspected
- Uncertain diagnosis as cause of symptoms
- Discuss with physician if D-dimer positive or Well's PE criteria ≥ 3 and DVT and/or PE is considered as possible cause of dyspnea

Principles of Asthma and COPD Management

- Recognizing severity of exacerbation
- Using correct therapy
- Identify and treat any precipitants
- Make correct disposition

COPD Exacerbation

Evaluation options

- Monitor cardiac and pulse oximetry
- EKG
- Troponin
- CBC
- BMP
- Chest x-ray (heck radiology report if and when available)) and view x-ray and compare to prior films
- Consider ABG if severely dyspneic or significant respiratory fatigue
- BNP if CHF is a consideration

Initial Treatment options

- Albuterol with or without atrovent, up to 3 treatments prn 10–20 minutes apart
- Oxygen therapy to keep O2 Sat ≥ 92%

Steroid treatment options useful for moderate to severe exacerbations (caution with diabetes)

- Effectiveness starts around 6 hours after dosing
    - Prednisone 40–60 mg PO

      OR
    - Depomedrol (methylprednisolone acetate) 80–160 mg IM

      OR
    - Decadron (dexamethasone) 10 mg IV

      OR
    - Solumedrol (methylprednisolone) 80–120 mg IV

Discharge treatment options

- Albuterol or Combivent inhaler with or without spacer q4hr prn
- Rx PO zithromax or doxycycline × 5 days, or per Sanford Guide

Systemic steroid treatment options (caution with diabetes)

- Prednisone 40-60 mg qday PO for 5 days

  OR

- Depomedrol (methylprednisolone acetate) 80-120 IM

  OR

- Decadron (dexamethasone) 10 mg IV

Inhaled steroid treatment options for COPD

- Consider inhaled steroid Rx to start only after acute exacerbation has resolved
  - Prescribe double dose if already on single strength dose

    OR

  - Advair discus bid (combination of long acting beta-agonist and steroid) to be used only after acute exacerbation has resolved

Discharge criteria

- If patient returns to near baseline function with respiratory effort and O2 saturation level
- Follow up with primary care provider in 1-5 days depending on severity of presentation and response to therapy

Discharge instructions

- Follow up with primary care provider in 1-5 days depending on severity of illness and response to treatments
- Provide COPD exacerbation aftercare instructions
- Return if worse

Consult physician on

- Work of breathing is moderate to severe post-treatment
- Wheezing not resolving satisfactorily
- Patient feels they are too dyspneic to go home

- WBC ≥ 15,000 or < 3,000; Neutrophil count < 1,000
- Acute thrombocytopenia
- Bandemia ≥ 15%
- Anion gap > 18
- Significant electrolyte abnormality
- Glucose ≥ 400 mg/dL in diabetic patient
- Glucose ≥ 300 mg/dL new onset diabetic patient
- Hyperglycemia with metabolic acidosis (decreased serum CO2 or elevated anion gap)
- Heart rate ≥ 110 after all treatment is completed

Acute Asthma and Bronchitis

Peak flow % of predicted

- Mild disease > 70%
- Moderate disease 40–69%
- Severe disease < 40%

Initial Treatment Options

- Albuterol with or without atrovent up to 3 treatments prn: 15–20 minutes apart
- Oxygen therapy to keep O2 Sat ≥ 92%; Monitor pulse oximetry

Steroid treatment options useful for moderate to severe exacerbations in adults (caution with diabetes)

- Effectiveness starts around 6 hours after dosing
  - Prednisone 40–60 mg PO

    OR
  - Depomedrol (methylprednisolone acetate) 80–160 mg IM

    OR
  - Decadron (dexamethasone) 10 mg IV

    OR
  - Solumedrol (methylprednisolone) 80–120 mg IV

Steroid treatment options useful for moderate to severe exacerbations in children (caution with diabetes)

- Effectiveness starts around 6 hours after dosing
  - Prednisolone 0.5–1 mg/kg PO (NMT 60 mg)

    OR
  - Decadron (dexamethasone) 0.6 mg/kg IV or IM (NMT 10 mg)

Additional treatment options for severe exacerbations

- Terbutaline 0.25 mg SQ prn q15–20 minutes up to 3 as needed for age ≥ 12 years
  - Caution if history of coronary artery disease
- Terbutaline 0.005–0.01 mg/kg SQ q15–20 minutes up to 3 — age < 12 years (NMT 0.4 mg per dose)
- Epinephrine 0.3 mg SQ for adults
  - Caution if history of coronary artery disease
- Epinephrine 0.01 mg/kg in children not to exceed adult dose
- MgSO4 (magnesium sulfate) 1–2 gms IV over 20 minutes in adults per physician
- MgSO4 (magnesium sulfate) 25–50 mg/kg IV over 10–20 minutes per physician (NMT 2 gm) for children
- Heliox 70:30 — do not use if > 30% oxygen needed to maintain O2 saturation

Discharge treatment options

- Albuterol or Combivent inhaler with or without spacer q4hr prn
- If bacterial infection suspected: Rx PO Zithromax (azithromycin) or doxycycline (age > 8 years) × 5 days, or per Sanford Guide
- Viral infection (most healthy patients) = no antibiotics

Discharge systemic steroid treatment options (caution with diabetes)

- Prednisone 20–60 mg qday for 5 days (no taper needed) age ≥ 12 yrs

  OR
- Depomedrol (methylprednisolone acetate) 80–120 mg IM age ≥ 12 yrs

  OR
- Decadron (dexamethasone) 10 mg IV for adults or 0.6 mg IV for children not to exceed adult dose
- Pediatrics: prednisolone 1–2 mg/kg PO qday for 5 days (NMT 60 mg per day)

Discharge inhaled steroid options

- Consider inhaled steroid Rx to start only after acute exacerbation has resolved
  - Prescribe double dose if already on single strength dose

    OR
  - Advair discus bid – age > 3 years (combination of long acting beta-agonist and steroid) to be used only after acute exacerbation has resolved

Discharge Criteria

- Good response to therapy
- If patient returns to near baseline function with respiratory effort and O2 saturation level
- Wheezing resolution and no significant respiratory distress
- Peak flow ≥ 70% predicted if checked
- O2 saturation > 93% on room air
- Good follow up and compliance
- Primary care provider to follow up within 1–3 days if symptoms persist

Discharge instructions

- Follow up with primary care provider in 1–5 days depending on severity of illness and response to treatments
- Provide asthma or bronchitis aftercare instructions

Consult Criteria

- Severe respiratory distress on presentation (notify physician immediately)
- Insufficient response to treatment
- Wheezing not resolving adequately
- Patient or family feels they are too dyspneic to go home
- Cardiac cause of dyspnea suspected or confirmed
- Immunosuppression
- Peak flow < 70% predicted if measured after treatment is finished
- O2 saturation < 94% on room air post treatments
- O2 Sat < 92% in COPD patient on room air or at home O2 concentrations if on home O2 therapy
- Significant comorbid conditions
- Heart rate ≥ 110 post treatment in adults
- Hypotension develops or relative hypotension SBP < 105 with history of hypertension
- Return visit for same acute dyspnea episode
- Immunosuppression
- Age ≥ 60

Vital signs and age consult criteria

- Age < 6 months
- Adult heart rate ≥ 110
- Pediatric heart rate
    - 0–4 months ≥ 180
    - 5–7 months ≥ 175
    - 6–12 months ≥ 170
    - 1–3 years ≥ 160
    - 4–5 years ≥ 145
    - 6–8 years ≥ 130
    - 7–12 years ≥ 125
    - 12–15 years ≥ 115
    - 16 years or older ≥ 110
- Developing hypotension or relative hypotension (SBP < 105 with history of hypertension)

- O2 Sat < 94% on room air in non-COPD patient

Notes

Reference:

CHEST August 2011;140(2):509-518.
doi:10.1378/chest.10-2468

PNEUMONIA PROTOCOL

When using any protocol, always follow the Guidelines of Proper Use (page 16).

Definition

- Infection of pulmonary parenchymal tissue

Differential Diagnosis

- Pulmonary embolism
- COPD
- Asthma
- CHF
- Bronchitis
- Adult Respiratory Distress Syndrome
- Fluid overload from ESRD
- Bronchopulmonary dysplasia in children with history of prematurity

Considerations

- Number one leading cause of death from infectious disease
- Community acquired causes
    - Strep pneumoniae
    - Mycoplasma pneumoniae
    - H. influenzae
    - Legionella pneumophilia
    - Klebsiella pneumoniae
    - Influenza
- Comorbid conditions
    - Advanced age
    - Smoking
    - COPD
    - Diabetes
    - Alcoholism
    - CHF
    - HIV
    - Immunosuppression
- Signs and Symptoms

    - Cough
    - Sputum production
    - Fever
    - Chills
    - Rigors
    - Dyspnea
    - Chest pain
- WBC ≥ 15,000 suggests bacteria infection
- Very high or very low WBC predicts increased mortality

Evaluation

- CBC
- Chest x-ray (may be negative even if pneumonia is present)
- ABG if moderate to severe respiratory distress or fatigue
- See Dyspnea Protocol
- Blood cultures if toxic or hypotensive and/or patient is to be admitted

Treatment Options

- Oxygen for O2 saturation < 95% (in COPD patient < 92%) or respiratory distress
- Viral pneumonia needs no treatment unless immunosuppressed
- IV NS or oral rehydration if dehydrated (see Gastroenteritis Protocols for rehydration therapy)

Nontoxic patient treatment that is to be discharged

No chronic cardiopulmonary disease

- Zithromax PO

  OR

- Doxycycline PO x 10 days

Chronic cardiopulmonary disease present

- Second or third generation cephalosporin PO x 10 days

  OR

- Augmentin (amoxicillin/clavulanate) x 10 days PO PLUS Zithromax PO

OR

- Levaquin (levofloxacin) PO as a single agent x 10 days
- May use Sanford Guide

For patients with significant respiratory distress, hypoxemia, toxicity, or are to be admitted:

- IV NS
- IV Zithromax and Rocephin (ceftriaxone) (non-ICU)
- IV piperacillin/tazobactam (Zosyn) 4.5 gms — ICU or nursing home patient
- Consult physician

Discharge Criteria

- Nontoxic patient
- No respiratory distress
- O2 saturation >93%

Discharge instructions

- Pneumonia aftercare instructions
- Follow up with primary care provider within 1–3 days
- Return if worse

Consult Criteria

- Significant pneumonia
- Patients that the Provider feels need admission
- Significant respiratory distress
- High fever ≥ 104°F (40°C)
- Temperature < 96°F (35.5°C)
- Appears ill or toxic
- Metabolic or respiratory acidosis
- Immunosuppression
- See Dyspnea Protocol

Vital signs and age consult criteria

- Age > 65 or < 6 months
- Adult heart rate ≥ 110
- Pediatric heart rate

  - 0–4 months ≥ 180
  - 5–7 months ≥ 175
  - 6–12 months ≥ 170
  - 1–3 years ≥ 160
  - 4–5 years ≥ 145
  - 6–8 years ≥ 130
  - 7–12 years ≥ 125
  - 12–15 years ≥ 115
  - 16 years or older ≥ 110
- Developing hypotension or relative hypotension (SBP < 105 with history of hypertension)
- O2 Sat < 94% on room air in non-COPD patient; O2 Sat < 92% in COPD patient on room air or home O2 Rx

Lab and x-ray consult criteria

- New onset renal insufficiency or worsening renal insufficiency
- WBC ≥ 15,000 or < 3,000; Neutrophil count < 1,000
- Bandemia ≥ 15%
- Acute thrombocytopenia
- Anion gap > 18
- Significant electrolyte abnormally
- Glucose ≥ 300 mg/dL in diabetic patient
- Glucose ≥ 200 mg/dL in new onset diabetic patient
- Hyperglycemia with metabolic acidosis (decreased serum CO2 or elevated anion gap)
- Pleural effusion

ADULT ASTHMA/ACUTE BRONCHITIS PROTOCOL

When using any protocol, always follow the Guidelines of Proper Use (page 16).

Definition

- Reversible acute bronchospasm and airway resistance secondary to infectious, allergic, environmental or internal causes

Differential Diagnosis

- Panic disorder
- Pneumonia
- Bronchitis
- CHF
- COPD
- Pulmonary embolism
- Anaphylaxis
- URI
- Vocal cord dysfunction
- Laryngospasm
- Epiglottis
- Croup
- Retropharyngeal abscess

Considerations

- Cough is commonly the first symptom
- Viral URI, allergens or environmental factors are the precipitants frequently
- Severe episode may have decreased breath sounds without wheezing
- Inability to speak more than 2–3 words at a time indicates a severe episode
- Steroids very useful — both PO and inhaled (inhaled steroids are for prophylaxis)
- Usually there is pre-existing asthma or bronchitis history

Peak flow % of predicted

- Mild disease > 70%
- Moderate disease 40–69%
- Severe disease < 40%

Risk Factors

- Prior intubation
- Visit in the last month
- Hospitalization > 1 time
- Two emergency visits past year
- Current or recent systemic steroid use
- Concomitant disease
- Illicit drug use

Evaluation

- Complete history and physical exam
- Assess respiratory effort
- O2 saturation
- Consider peak flows before and after aerosols
- CBC and/or BMP for significant tachycardia and fever
- Check radiology interpretations prior to discharge if available

Chest x-ray

- If pneumonia suspected
- Significant respiratory distress
- CHF considered as possible cause of dyspnea
- Respiratory distress not responsive to aerosols
- Age ≥ 50
- Cardiac history

If CHF suspected

- BNP
- Troponin
- EKG

Treatment Options

- Supplemental oxygen for O2 Sat < 95% room air or significant respiratory distress

- Albuterol with or without atrovent aerosol every 15–20 minutes prn — up to 3 treatments total

Steroid treatment options useful for moderate to severe exacerbations in adults (caution with diabetes)

Effectiveness starts around 6 hours after dosing

- Prednisone 40−60 mg PO

  OR
- May give Decadron (dexamethasone) 0.6 mg/kg IM instead (NMT 10 mg) if PO route not usable (caution with diabetes)

  OR
- Depomedrol (methylprednisolone acetate) 120−160 mg IM (caution with diabetes)

Additional treatment options if needed for severe exacerbations

- Epinephrine 0.3 mg SQ (caution with coronary artery disease history)
- Terbutaline 0.25 mg SQ prn q15–20 minutes up to 3 treatments as needed (caution with coronary artery disease history)
- MgSO4 (magnesium sulfate) 1–2 gms IV over 20 minutes in adults per physician
- MgSO4 (magnesium sulfate) 25–50 mg/kg IV over 10–20 minutes per physician (NMT 2 gm) for children
- Heliox 70:30 — do not use if > 30% oxygen needed

Discharge medications

- Albuterol MDI with or without spacer prn
- Antibiotics are not usually needed
  - Consider antibiotics in smokers
  - If bacteria infection suspected, may use Sanford Guide
    - Zithromax PO

Discharge systemic steroid treatment (caution with diabetes)

- Prednisone 40–60 mg PO × 5 days (NMT 60 mg qday)

  OR

- Decadron (dexamethasone) 0.6 mg/kg IM instead (NMT 10 mg) if PO route not usable

Discharge inhaled steroids for asthma only

- Consider inhaled steroid Rx only after the acute exacerbation has resolved
  - Prescribe double dose if already on single strength dose

    OR

  - Advair discus bid for asthma or COPD only (combination long acting beta-agonist and steroid) to be used only after acute exacerbation has resolved

Discharge Criteria

- Good response to therapy
- Wheezing resolution and no significant respiratory distress
- Peak flow ≥ 70% predicted if checked
- O2 saturation > 93% on room air
- Good follow up and compliance
- Primary care provider to follow up within 1–3 days if symptoms persist

Discharge instructions

- Follow up with primary care provider in 1–5 days depending on severity of illness and response to treatments
- Provide asthma or bronchitis aftercare instructions

Consult Criteria

- Severe respiratory distress on presentation (notify physician immediately)
- Insufficient response to treatment
- Family feels patient is too ill to go home

- Peak flow < 70% predicted if measured after treatment is finished
- Moderate or severe respiratory distress post treatment
- O2 saturation < 94% on room air post treatments
- Significant comorbid conditions
- Heart rate ≥ 110 post treatment
- Hypotension develops or relative hypotension SBP < 105 with history of hypertension
- Return visit for same acute episode
- Immunosuppression
- Age ≥ 60

Lab and x-ray consult criteria

- New onset renal insufficiency or worsening renal insufficiency
- WBC ≥ 15,000 or < 3,000; Neutrophil count < 1,000
- Bandemia ≥ 15%
- Acute thrombocytopenia
- Anion gap > 18
- Significant electrolyte abnormally
- Glucose ≥ 400 mg/dL in diabetic patient
- Glucose ≥ 200 mg/dL in new onset diabetic patient
- Hyperglycemia with metabolic acidosis (decreased serum CO2 or elevated anion gap)
- Pleural effusion

Notes

ALLERGY PROTOCOL

When using any protocol, always follow the Guidelines of Proper Use (page 16).

Definition

- Systemic reaction to chemical mediator release secondary to IgE sensitization from allergen

Considerations

- Most reactions are minor with itching and localized or generalized urticaria
- Anaphylaxis is due to IgE antibody release of histamine and vasoactive mediators
- Symptom presentation possibilities
    - Occurs within 30 minutes usually
    - Can be mild
    - Wheezing
    - Dyspnea
    - Shock
    - Airway obstruction
    - Death
    - Can occur on long-term medication
- Urticaria
    - Etiology unknown usually
    - Usually self-limited
- True opioid allergy rare — usually GI upset or pseudoallergy
- Anaphylactoid reactions to contrast
    - Direct stimulation of mast cells and basophils
    - Seafood allergic patients are not allergic to radiographic contrast material
    - Related to high osmolarity of contrast materials
    - Narcotics can also cause anaphylactoid reactions
- Angioedema (may appear with urticaria)
    - Bradykinin mediated
    - Commonly from ACE inhibitors
        - Decreased metabolism of bradykinin
    - Hereditary C1 esterase deficiency

  - Leads to increased bradykinin
  - Positive family history
- Caution using steroids in diabetic patients
- Caution using epinephrine in patients with coronary disease risk factors

Evaluation

- Vital signs
- Oropharyngeal and respiratory distress assessment
- Pulmonary and cardiac exam
- Skin exam
- Chest x-ray for significant respiratory distress or O2 saturation < 93% on room air
- Soft tissue neck films for hoarseness or complaints/findings of throat swelling
- CBC and BMP for moderate to severe systemic reactions

Urticaria

- Vascular reaction of the skin with transient wheals, soft papules and plaques usually with pruritus

Treatment options

Benadryl (diphenhydramine)

- Adult: 50 mg PO or IM
- Pediatrics: 1–2 mg/kg PO or IM (NMT 50 mg)
- May continue for 5–7 days PO

Pepcid (famotidine)

- Adult: 20 mg IV or 40 mg PO
- Pediatric: 0.25 mg/kg IV or 0.5 mg/kg PO (not to exceed maximum adult dose)

Epinephrine

- Do not use if history of coronary artery disease
- Adult: 0.3 mg SQ
- Pediatrics: 0.01 mg/kg SQ not to exceed adult dose

Consider steroids (caution if diabetic)

- Prednisone 40–60 mg PO qday for 5–7 days (> 40 kg)
- Prednisone/prednisolone 1 mg/kg PO qday for 5–7 days (< 40 kg)

Discharge criteria

- Discharge with good resolution of rash and itching

Discharge instructions

- Follow up with primary care provider within 7 days
- Avoid offending agent if known
- Provide urticaria aftercare instructions

Angioedema

- Non-life threatening presentation treated same as urticaria
- Less responsive to treatment than urticaria
- Evaluate for airway compromise or significant oropharyngeal swelling
- Oxygen prn
- Consult promptly for posterior oropharyngeal angioedema
- Discharge mild lip or non-oropharyngeal angioedema with normal vital signs and no distress
- Stop ACE inhibitors if currently taking

Additional treatment if needed

Epinephrine (per physician)

- Caution if history of coronary artery disease
- Adult: 0.3–0.5 mg SQ; (if respiratory distress notify physician promptly)
- Pediatrics: 0.01 mg/kg SQ not to exceed adult dose; give IV or IM (anterior thigh) if respiratory distress (notify physician promptly)

- Responds to fresh frozen plasma or C1 esterase inhibitor concentrate

Mild Anaphylaxis

- Urticaria/angioedema

- O2 saturation > 94% room air
- No respiratory distress
- Normotensive
- No tachycardia

Treatment options

Benadryl (diphenhydramine)

- Adult: 50 mg PO or IM
- Pediatric: 1–2 mg/kg PO or IM (NMT 50 mg)
- Continue for 5–7 days PO

Pepcid (famotidine)

- Adult: 20–40 mg IV/PO
- Pediatric: 0.25 mg/kg IV/PO (NMT 40 mg)

Consider steroids

- Prednisone 40–60 mg PO qday for 5–7 days (> 40 kg)
- Prednisone/prednisolone 1 mg/kg PO qday for 5–7 days (< 40 kg)

Additional treatment if needed

Epinephrine

- Do not use if history of coronary artery disease
- Adult: 0.3 mg SQ
- Pediatrics: 0.01 mg/kg SQ not to exceed adult dose

Moderate Anaphylaxis

(Notify physician)

- Urticaria/angioedema
- Wheezing
- O2 saturation 90–94% room air
- Moderate respiratory distress
- No hypotension

Treatment options

Oxygen: nasal or mask (≥ 5 liters/minute if mask used)

Benadryl (diphenhydramine)

- Adult: 50 mg IV or IM

- Pediatric: 1–2 mg/kg IV or IM (NMT 50 mg)

Pepcid (famotidine)

- Adult: 20–40 mg IV
- Pediatric: 0.25 mg/kg IV (NMT 40 mg)

Albuterol aerosol

- With or without atrovent
- Repeat q15 min × 2 additional treatments prn
- Continuous prn (for severe dyspnea)

Additional treatment if needed

Epinephrine

- Caution if history of coronary artery disease
- Adult: 0.3 mg SQ (notify physician promptly)
- Pediatric: 0.01 mg/kg SQ not to exceed adult dose (notify physician promptly)

Glucagon

- 1–2 mg IV if on beta-blocker or resistant to epinephrine

Steroids

- Adult: Solumedrol (methylprednisolone) 125 mg IV
- Pediatric: 1–2 mg/kg IV
- Prednisone 40–60 mg PO qday for 5–7 days (> 40 kg) if discharged
- Prednisone/prednisolone 1 mg/kg (NMT 60 mg) PO qday for 5–7 days if discharged (pediatrics)
- May give Decadron (dexamethasone) 0.6 mg/kg IM instead (NMT 10 mg)

Severe Anaphylaxis

(Notify physician immediately)

- Urticaria/angioedema
- Wheezing
- O2 saturation < 90% room air
- Severe respiratory distress
- Oropharyngeal airway swelling or compromise

- Hypotension
- Intubation if impending respiratory failure — notify physician immediately
- Observation for 6 hours if to be discharged by physician
- Usually admitted

Treatment options

Oxygen: nasal or mask (> 5 liters/minute if mask used)

For shock

- IV NS 1–2 liters rapidly if hypotensive adult
- 20 cc/kg IV NS if hypotensive pediatric patient — may repeat × 2 prn

Benadryl (diphenhydramine)

- Adult: Benadryl (diphenhydramine) 50 mg IV (preferred) or IM
- Pediatric: 1–2 mg/kg IV (preferred) or IM (NMT 50 mg)

Pepcid (famotidine)

- Adult: 20–40 mg IV
- Pediatric: 0.25 mg/kg IV (NMT 40 mg)

Albuterol aerosol

- With or without atrovent
- Repeat q15 min × 2 prn
- Continuous prn for severe dyspnea

Steroids

- Adult
  - Solumedrol (methylprednisolone) 125 mg IV
  - Prednisone 40–60 mg PO qday for 5–7 days (> 40 kg) if discharged
- Pediatric
  - Solumedrol (methylprednisolone) 1–2 mg/kg IV (NMT 125 mg)
  - Prednisone/prednisolone 1 mg/kg (NMT 60 mg) PO qday for 5–7 days if discharged (pediatrics)

- May give Decadron (dexamethasone) 0.6 mg/kg IM/IV instead (NMT 10 mg)

Additional treatment if needed

Epinephrine (consult physician before administering if possible)

- Adult: 0.3–0.5 mg IV (if in shock) or IM anterior thigh
    - 1 mg IV if no pulse
        - Activate ACLS and call a code
- Pediatric: 0.01 mg/kg IV (if in shock) or IM anterior thigh (do not exceed adult doses)
- Caution with history of coronary artery disease

Glucagon

- 1–2 mg IV if on beta-blocker or resistant to epinephrine (consult physician if possible)

Discharge Criteria

- Good resolution of rash and itching in urticaria
- Discharge patients presenting with mild symptoms that have observation post-treatment for 2–4 hours without symptoms

Discharge instructions

- Follow up with primary care provider within 7 days
- Avoid offending agent if known
- Provide allergy aftercare instructions
- Return if worse

Consult Criteria

- Hypotension
- O2 saturation < 95% on room air after treatments
- Moderate to severe anaphylaxis or respiratory distress on presentation or during stay
- Altered mental status
- Oropharyngeal or throat swelling or complaints of throat swelling or dyspnea
- Wheezing not resolved

- Adult heart rate ≥ 110 post treatment
- Pediatric heart rate post treatment
    - 0–4 months ≥ 180
    - 5–7 months ≥ 175
    - 6–12 months ≥ 170
    - 1–3 years ≥ 160
    - 4–5 years ≥ 145
    - 6–8 years ≥ 130
    - 7–12 years ≥ 125
    - 12–15 years ≥ 115
    - 16 years or older ≥ 110

Notes

Endocrine

Section Contents

Diabetes and Hypoglycemia Protocol

Hypothyroidism Protocol

Hyperthyroidism Protocol

When using any protocol, always follow the Guidelines of Proper Use (page 16).

DIABETES AND HYPOGLYCEMIA PROTOCOL

When using any protocol, always follow the Guidelines of Proper Use (page 16).

Definition

- Defect in glucose regulation secondary to inadequate secretion of insulin or resistance to insulin

Considerations

Types

- Type 1: dependent on exogenous insulin to live
- Type 2: does not need insulin to live (peripheral insulin resistance and insulin-secretory defect)
- Type 2 can present initially as DKA (diabetic ketoacidosis) in African-Americans or Hispanic descent patients
- Gestational — appears with pregnancy only

Complications

- Increased infections
- Peripheral arterial insufficiency
- Skin ulcers and gangrene of lower legs and feet
- Hyperglycemic and hypoglycemic emergencies
- Pediatric cerebral edema with hyperglycemic emergencies

Vascular

- Retinopathy
- Renal insufficiency and failure
- Coronary arteries occlusion
- Aortic atherosclerosis
- Stroke

DKA

- Definition

- Plasma glucose > 250 mg/dL (usually is > 350 mg/dL)
- Serum bicarbonate < 15 mEq/L
- Arterial pH <7.3 with moderate ketonemia

- Secondary to stress
  - Infection most common
  - AMI
  - Pregnancy
  - Surgery
- Average adult fluid deficit is 6–10 liters (osmotic diuresis)
- Adjustment to serum Na (sodium) levels — each additional 100 mg% over plasma glucose of 100 add 1.6 mEq/L to serum Na levels
- Potassium body deficit can be severe despite initial normal serum level (a decrease of 0.3–0.7 mEq/L for each decrease of pH of 0.1)
  - Total body potassium deficit is 3–5 mEq/kg
- IV PO4 (phosphorous) may be needed if respiratory failure occurs
- Venous pH add 0.03 — if used instead of ABG to measure pH
- Serum osmolarity > 320 mOsm/L

Symptoms and findings (some or all)

- Weakness
- Weight loss
- Mental status changes
- Dry mucous membranes
- Tachycardia
- Nausea and vomiting
- Abdominal pain
- Kussmaul respirations (deep rapid breathing)
- Peripheral vasodilatation can cause normothermia or hypothermia despite infection

Evaluation

- CBC
- BMP
- Accucheck
- Chest x-ray

- U/A
- ABG or venous pH (add 0.03 to adjust to arterial pH)
- Blood, urine or infected site cultures if infection suspected

Serum osmolality

- If < 320mOsm/L, look for another cause of altered mental status
- Osmolol gap > 10–20; suspect substance ingestion (normal < 10)
    - Gap = Osmolality measured – Osmolality calculated (Osmolality calculation equation: 2(Na+K) + glucose/18 + BUN/2.8; normal 280–300mOsm/L)
    - Ethanol mg%/4.6 is added to osmolol gap equation if present
    - Gap > 50 carries high specificity for toxic alcohol such as methanol, ethylene glycol, or isopropyl alcohol
    - Normal gap < 10

Fluid therapy

Adult

- IV NS infused 15–20 cc/kg/hour (1–1.5 liters average)
- Continue NS if corrected Na is low
- 0.45% NS at 4–14 cc/kg/hour after bolus infusion if "corrected" Na is normal or high
- Add potassium 20–30 mEq/L when serum K reaches < 5.3 mEq/L (if urine output 0.5–1 cc/kg/hour)

Pediatric (< 16 years of age)

- IV NS 10–20 cc/kg/hour; may repeat prn; should not exceed 50 cc/kg total over 4 hours
- Continued IV with 0.45% or NS at 5 cc/kg/hour after initial fluid therapy
- If altered mental status acutely occurs, suspect cerebral edema (treatment 1–2 gms/kg mannitol IV — per physician)

Insulin therapy

- Start after IV fluids given for one hour
- Check K+ level first (can cause K+ to drop; can be dangerous if already low; should be at least 3.3 mEq/L)

Adults

- Bolus 0.15 units/kg IV and/or continuous infusion 0.1 unit/kg/hour (up to 5-7 units/hour)
- Should decrease plasma glucose 50-75 mg%/hour (if not, check hydration status)

Pediatrics

- Insulin bolus not recommended
- Continuous infusion same as adult

Potassium

- Add potassium 20-40 mEq to each liter of IV fluids when serum K+ < 5.3 if urine output 0.5-1 cc/kg/hour or initial potassium < 3.3 mEq/L
  - Serum K+ 4.5-5.2 mEq/L give 10 mEq/hour IV
  - Serum K+ 3.0-4.5 mEq/L give 20 mEq/hour IV
  - Serum K+ initially < 3.0 mEq/L hold off starting insulin and give potassium IV

Consult criteria

- All DKA patients after initial assessment

Hyperglycemic Hyperosmolar Syndrome (HHS)

- Develops over days or weeks
- Plasma glucose > 600
- Serum osmolality > 320 mOsm
- Profound dehydration: adult 8-12 liters fluid deficit
- Small amount of ketonuria; small or absent ketonemia
- Serum bicarbonate > 15
- Arterial pH > 7.3
- Some alteration of consciousness

- Higher mortality than DKA

Associated medications contributing to HHS

- Diuretics
- Propranolol
- Calcium channel blockers
- Dilantin
- Cimetidine
- Corticosteroids

Evaluation

- Same as for DKA

Treatment options

- IV NS 10–20 cc/kg/hour; may repeat prn; should not exceed 50 cc/kg total over 4 hours
- Continued IV with 0.45% or NS at 5 cc/kg/hour after initial fluid therapy
- Add D51/2NS or D5NS when plasma glucose reaches 300 mg/dL
- Start insulin infusion 0.1 unit/kg/hour (up to 5–7 units/hour) after first hour of IV fluid therapy
    - Insulin doses often lower than used in DKA

Potassium treatment

- Add potassium 20–40 mEq to each liter of IV fluids when serum K+ < 5.3 mEq/L if urine output 0.5–1 cc/kg/hour or initial potassium < 3.3 mEq/L
    - Serum K+ 4.5–5.2 mEq/L give 10 mEq/hour IV
    - Serum K+ 3.0–4.5 mEq/L give 20 mEq/hour IV
    - Serum K+ initially < 3.0 mEq/L hold off starting insulin and give potassium IV

Consult criteria

- Notify physician on all HHS patients

Hypoglycemia

Differential diagnosis

- CVA
- TIA
- Epilepsy
- Multiple sclerosis
- Psychosis

Considerations

Caused by:

- Accidental or intentional overdose of diabetic medications
- Sepsis
- Alcohol use
- Decreased caloric intake

Symptoms

- Severity symptoms depends on glucose level and rate of glucose decline
- Symptoms may be masked by beta-blockers
- Altered and decrease mental status
- Sweating
- Shaking
- Anxiety

Evaluation

- History and physical exam
- Medication and food intake history
- Accucheck every 30 minutes × 2 hours or longer until stable glucose levels achieved
- BMP
- CBC if infection suspected
- Chest x-ray if pneumonia or aspiration suspected, or hypoxic
- U/A if infection suspected

Treatment options

- Awake and alert: complex calorie intake PO
- Altered mental status: IV D50W 1 amp adults (100 calories)

- D25W — 1 gm/kg in pediatrics not to exceed adult dose
- D12.5W for neonates (1 gm/kg)
- D10W drip at 75–100 cc/hour (adult) if repeat D50W boluses needed for recurrent hypoglycemia or hypoglycemic agent overdose
- Glucagon 1 mg IM if no IV access
    - May not work with depleted glycogen stores in malnutrition
        - Liver disease
        - Alcoholics
        - Neonates
- Octreotide can be used in sulfonylurea refractory hypoglycemia
- Hydrocortisone IV for adrenal insufficiency

Discharge criteria

- Stable glucose levels in diabetic patients on preexisting insulin therapy
- Good home support
- Reliable patient

Discharge instructions

- Hypoglycemia aftercare instructions
- Follow up with primary care provider within 12–24 hours

Consult criteria

- Oral hypoglycemia therapy (usually need admission)
- Fasting hypoglycemia on no diabetic medication
- Intentional insulin overdose
- Poor home situation
- Abnormal vital signs
- Continued altered mental status
- Significant comorbidities (cancer, hepatic disease, malnutrition, etc.)

Hyperglycemia without DKA or HHS

Considerations

- Most diabetic patients with elevated glucose levels are asymptomatic
- High glucose levels can affect body water balance
- Acute treatment for levels up to 400 mg/dL usually not needed unless there is a concurrent disease process

Evaluation

- Glucose < 400 mg/dL without other disease processes or symptoms may not need further testing acutely in patient with history of poor control (if vital signs normal and mentation changes or comorbidities absent)
- Tests are directed to disease processes that may be elevating glucose levels
- BMP
- CBC if infection or inflammatory process suspected
- U/A if UTI suspected

Discharge criteria

- If new onset obese adult patient with DM without DKA or HHS and glucose ≤ 300
- Diabetic history with glucose < 400 mg/dL
- No metabolic acidosis
- No dehydration
- Normal vital signs and no mentation changes

Discharge instructions

- Hyperglycemia aftercare instructions
- Follow up with primary care provider within 1-5 days
- Return if patient develops symptoms

Consult criteria

New onset

- New adult onset DM with glucose ≥ 300 mg/dL

- New onset pediatric DM with glucose ≥ 200 mg/dL
- Hyperglycemia with metabolic acidosis (decreased serum CO2 or elevated anion gap)

Diabetic patient with

- Significant comorbid symptoms
- Metabolic acidosis
- Vomiting
- Dehydration
- Tachycardia
- Hypotension
- Relative hypotension SBP < 105 with history of hypertension
- Orthostatic vital sign changes
- Progressive renal insufficiency creatinine increase > 0.5
- Adult heart rate ≥ 110
- Pediatric heart rate
    - 12–15 years ≥ 115
    - 16 years or older ≥ 110

Glucose ≥ 400 mg/dL in asymptomatic diabetic patient

Treatment for Type 2 Adult Diabetes If Desired

Obese

Monotherapy

- Metformin 500 mg PO bid with or after meals × 1 week, increase weekly by 500 mg to achieve 1000 mg PO bid
- Decreases HbA1c approximated 1.5%

Second drug if needed

- Glyburide (Micronase) 2.5 mg PO qday after breakfast (elderly 1.25 mg PO)—may need to decrease metformin to prevent hypoglycemia (warn patient about possibility of hypoglycemia

Third drug if needed

- Exenatide (Byetta) 5 mcg SQ bid x 1 month and then may increase as needed to 10 mcg SQ bid
  - Give 1 hr. before AM and PM meals

OR

- Insulin glargine 10 units SQ–adjust by 1 unit/day to achieve fasting glucose < 100 mg/dL

Non-obese

Monotherapy

- Metformin 500 mg PO bid with or after meals × 1 week, increase weekly by 500 mg to achieve 1000 mg PO bid
  - Decreases HbA1c approximated 1.5%

OR

- Glyburide (Micronase) 2.5 mg PO qday after breakfast (elderly 1.25 mg PO)

Second drug if needed

- Metformin 500 mg PO bid with or after meals × 1 week, increase weekly by 500 mg to achieve 1000 mg PO bid

OR

- Glyburide (Micronase) 2.5 mg PO qday after breakfast (elderly 1.25 mg PO)

Third drug if needed

- Exenatide (Byetta) 5 mcg SQ bid x 1 month and then may increase as needed to 10 mcg SQ bid
  - Give 1 hr. before AM and PM meals

OR

- Insulin glargine 10 units SQ–adjust by 1 unit/day to achieve fasting glucose < 100 mg/dL

Elderly

Monotherapy

- Prandin 0.5–4 mg PO up to qid ac (not to exceed 16 mg qday)

Monotherapy failure

- Consider switch to NPH insulin 10 units SQ bedtime

Asians

Monotherapy

- Pioglitazone (Actos) 30 mg PO qday — do not use in bladder cancer, history of bladder cancer, moderate to severe hepatic impairment or symptomatic heart failure (NYHA class 3 or 4)

Second drug if needed

- Metformin 500 mg PO bid with or after meals × 1 week, increase weekly by 500 mg to achieve 1000 mg PO bid

Third drug if needed

- Micronase 2.5 mg PO qday after breakfast (elderly 1.25 mg PO)

  OR
- Exenatide (Byetta) 5 mcg SQ bid x 1 month and then may increase as needed to 10 mcg SQ bid (not FDA approved with Actos)
  - Give 1 hr. before AM and PM meals

  OR
- Insulin glargine 10 units SQ–adjust by 1 unit/day to achieve fasting glucose < 100 mg/dL

Symptomatic patients

- Prandin 0.5–4 mg PO up to qid ac (not to exceed 16 mg qday) or insulin to decrease glucose at start of monotherapy initiation

Notes

HYPOTHYROIDISM PROTOCOL

When using any protocol, always follow the Guidelines of Proper Use (page 16).

Definition

- Deficiency or lack of thyroid hormone that causes slowing of metabolic progresses

Differential Diagnosis

- Hypothermia
- Sepsis
- Depression
- Constipation
- Addison's disease
- Chronic fatigue syndrome
- Dysmenorrhea
- Goiter — lithium induced
- Nontoxic goiter
- Hypopituitarism
- Subacute thyroiditis
- Iodine deficiency
- Ovarian insufficiency
- Prolactin deficiency

Considerations

- Deficiency of thyroid hormone
- Develops over months to years
- Primary hypothyroidism 95% of cases
- Secondary hypothyroidism 5% of cases
- Postpartum thyroiditis is 5% and usually occurs 3–6 months after delivery
- Myxedema coma is a rare, life threatening condition usually of elderly women
    - Precipitated by environmental stress, infection and medications
    - Frequently a clinical diagnosis initially

Signs and symptoms

- Goiter
- Cold intolerance
- Hypothermia
- Bradycardia
- Lethargy
- Depression
- Hair loss
- Dry coarse skin
- Weight gain
- Constipation
- Headache
- Husky voice
- Deep tendon ankle jerk reflex with prolonged recovery phase
- Ataxia

Causes

- Idiopathic
- Hashimoto's thyroiditis
- Radioiodine treatment for hyperthyroidism (Grave's disease)
- Thyroid resection
- Lithium
- Amiodarone
- Dilantin
- Carbamazepine
- Iodides
- Pituitary or hypothalamic disorders: tumor, radiation, surgery, sarcoidosis
- Postpartum

Evaluation

- Complete history and physical examination

Testing options depending on history and findings

- CBC
- BMP
- Chest x-ray for pericardial effusions and cardiomegaly

- ABG if respiratory insufficiency
- EKG
- U/A
- Thyroid stimulation hormone (TSH)
- Thyroid function tests if available

Treatment Options

- Mild symptoms or subclinical disease refer to primary care provider or endocrinologist
- Preferable for primary care provider to start thyroid hormone replacement
    - Synthroid 0.1 mg PO qday — age ≤ 60 years
    - Synthroid 0.025–0.05 mg PO qday — age > 60 years (1/2 of this dose if history of heart disease) — discuss with physician

Myxedema coma — notify physician immediately

- End of spectrum of hypothyroidism
- IV NS as needed for hypotension
- Levothyroxine 400 mcg IV slow infusion
- May need intubation
- Hydrocortisone sodium succinate (Solu–Cortef) 100 mg IV
- Treat any infection
- Passive rewarming

Discharge Criteria

- Mild disease

Discharge instructions

- Hypothyroidism aftercare instructions
- Follow up with primary care provider within 7 days
- Return if worse

Consult Criteria

- Unstable patient
- Altered mental status
- Hypothermia
- Metabolic or respiratory acidosis

- Respiratory insufficiency
- Refer to General Patient Criteria Protocol (page 20)

Notes

HYPERTHYROIDISM PROTOCOL

When using any protocol, always follow the Guidelines of Proper Use (page 16).

Definition

- Conditions from excess thyroid hormone

Differential Diagnosis

- Panic disorder
- Septic shock
- Delirium tremens
- Neuroleptic malignant syndrome
- Serotonin syndrome
- Withdrawal syndromes
- Heat illness
- Cocaine toxicity
- Sympathomimetic drug overdose
- Congestive heart failure
- Pheochromocytoma
- Pregnancy

Considerations

- Grave's disease most common form — autoimmune disease
- 1–2% of patients progress to thyroid storm
- Thyroid storm is potentially fatal

Signs and Symptoms

- Tachycardia
- Weight loss
- Heat intolerance
- Fever
- Diaphoresis
- Dehydration
- Diarrhea
- Goiter
- Hypotension
- Atrial fibrillation

- Exophthalmos and lid lag (Grave's disease only)
- Fine tremor

Causes

- Grave's disease — most common
- Idiopathic — second most common (toxic multinodular goiter)
- Subacute thyroiditis
- Postpartum thyroiditis
- Overdose of thyroid hormone
- Iodine induced
- Amiodarone

Thyroid storm

Severe symptoms

- Shock
- Fever
- Altered mental status
- Psychosis
- CHF
- Jaundice

Precipitated by

- Stress
- Infection
- Surgery
- Cardiovascular events
- Preeclampsia
- DKA or HHS
- Stopping antithyroid medication
- Vigorous palpation of thyroid

Evaluation

- Complete history and physical examination

Testing

- CBC
- BMP
- Calcium
- LFT's

- EKG
- Thyroid function tests
- TSH

Treatment Options

- O2 supplemental
- Tylenol for fever (no aspirin)

Moderate thyrotoxicosis

- PTU 150–450 mg/day PO or NG tube
- Propranolol 20–40 mg PO q4hr until tachycardia controlled
- Decadron (dexamethasone) 2 mg PO or IV q6hr in adults
- Decadron (dexamethasone) 0.15 mg/kg/dose PO or IV q6hr in pediatrics (not to exceed adult dose)

Thyroid storm treatment options

- IV NS 100–200 cc/hr in adults or higher if needed for vital sign findings
- IV NS 1–3 × daily fluid maintenance prn for pediatrics

Propylthiouracil (PTU)

- Adult: 600–1,000 mg IV
- Pediatric: 5–7 mg/kg/day

SSKI

- 1–5 drops PO 1 hour after PTU

Decadron (dexamethasone)

- Adult: 2 mg IV q6hr
- Pediatric: 0.15 mg/kg IV

Propranolol

- 1–2 mg IV; repeat q 10–15 min. prn (caution with CHF and DKA)

Outpatient treatment

- Initiate PTU 150 mg PO qday as outpatient

Discharge Criteria

- Mildly symptomatic patients that respond to therapy

Discharge instructions

- Hyperthyroidism aftercare instructions
- Follow up with primary care provider or endocrinologist within 1–2 days

Consult Criteria

- Moderate thyrotoxicosis
- Fever
- Thyroid storm — notify physician immediately
- Adult heart rate ≥ 110
- Pediatric heart rate
    - 0–4 months ≥ 180
    - 5–7 months ≥ 175
    - 6–12 months ≥ 170
    - 1–3 years ≥ 160
    - 4–5 years ≥ 145
    - 6–8 years ≥ 130
    - 7–12 years ≥ 125
    - 12–15 years ≥ 115
    - 16 years or older ≥ 110

Notes

Toxic Ingestions

Section Contents — one protocol

Toxicology Protocol

When using any protocol, always follow the Guidelines of Proper Use (page 16).

TOXICOLOGY PROTOCOL

When using any protocol, always follow the Guidelines of Proper Use (page 16).

Considerations

Principles of toxicology

- Reduce exposure (remove from skin and environment)
- Reduce absorption
- Increase elimination
- Supportive care
- Give specific therapy and antidotes when appropriate

Pearls

- Most pediatric accidental ingestions of common OTC medications are of low dose and may require only observation for 2–4 hours
- Intentional ingestions require acute psychiatric intervention
- Ascertain types and amount of ingestion

Syrup of Ipecac not usually recommended

Activated charcoal

- Usually of no benefit
- Can be used if no aspiration risk < 1 hour post ingestion with serious ingestions
- May be considered > 1 hour post serious ingestion with agents that delay absorption or GI transit

Orogastric lavage use indications

- Presentations approximately within one hour post-ingestion
- No known antidote
- Substance does not bind activated charcoal

Whole bowel irrigation indications and considerations

- With lithium and iron ingestion

- In "body stuffers"
- Beware of aspiration risk
- Avoid with decreased bowel sounds, surgical abdomen, hypotension

Toxidromes (causes and symptoms)

Opioids

Agents

- Narcotics

Findings

- CNS depression
- Respiratory depression
- Miosis

Sympathomimetics

Agents

- Cocaine
- Amphetamine

Findings

- Agitation
- Pupil dilation
- Diaphoresis
- Tachycardia
- Hypertension
- Hyperthermia

Cholinergic

Agents

- Insecticides

Findings

- Salivation
- Lacrimation
- Diaphoresis
- Nausea
- Vomiting
- Urination
- Defecation

- Muscle fasciculations
- Weakness
- Bronchorrhea

Anticholinergic

Agents

- Antihistamines
- Atropine
- Scopolamine

Findings

- Altered mental status
- Dilated pupils
- Dry/flushed skin and mucous membranes
- Urinary retention
- Decreased bowel sounds
- Hyperthermia

Salicylates

Agents

- Aspirin
- Oil of wintergreen (1 tsp lethal in child weighing < 10 kg; 1 cc has 14 gms of salicylate)

Findings

- Tachypnea
- Respiratory alkalosis
- Metabolic acidosis
- Altered mental status
- Tinnitus
- Tachycardia
- Nausea
- Vomiting
- Diaphoresis

Hypoglycemia

Agents

- Oral hypoglycemia agents
- Insulin

Findings

- Altered mental status
- Diaphoresis
- Tachycardia
- Hypertension

Serotonin syndrome

Agents

- Meperidine or dextromethorphan + MAOI
- SSRI (selective serotonin reuptake inhibitor) + tricyclic antidepressant
- SSRI + amphetamine
- Tricyclic antidepressant + amphetamine
- MAOI + amphetamine
- SSRI overdose

Findings

- Altered mental status
- Increased muscle tone
- Hyperreflexia
- Hyperthermia

Evaluation

- Complete history and physical exam
- Contact Poison Control Center or consult physician
- Monitoring and EKG with potentially toxic ingestions
- Send someone to patient's home to obtain ingestants if necessary
- BMP
- Specific drugs levels if available
- Calculate anion gap: Na – Cl – HCO3
- CT head for altered mental status not clearly attributable to toxin
- Evaluate for comorbid conditions
- ASA and acetaminophen nomograms as indicated

Anion gap mnemonic — A CAT MUDPILES

A – Alcoholic ketoacidosis
C – Cyanide; carbon monoxide
A – Aspirin; other salicylates
T – Toluene
M – Methanol; metformin
U – Uremia
D – DKA
P – Paraldehyde; phenformin
I – Iron; INH
L – Lactic acidosis
E – Ethylene glycol
S – Starvation

Osmolol gap > 10–20 suspect substance ingestion (Normal < 10)

- Gap = Osmolality measured – Osmolality calculated (calculation equation: 2(Na+K) + glucose/18 + BUN/2.8; normal 280–300mOsm/L)
- Ethanol mg%/4.6 is added to osmolol gap equation if present
- Gap > 50 carries high specificity for toxic alcohol such as methanol, ethylene glycol, or isopropyl alcohol
- Normal gap < 10

Treatment Options

- Nontoxic ingestions: observation and discharge with instructions and follow up
- Suspected toxic ingestions: refer to previous Considerations section and contact Poison Control Center or consult physician
- IV NS
- Hypotension
    - Adult IV NS 500–1000 cc bolus if hypotensive (consult physician)
    - Pediatrics 20 cc/kg IV NS bolus, may repeat × 2 prn (consult physician)
- Specific antidotes per physician (or poison control center)
- Coma cocktail

- Dextrose
- Naloxone (Narcan)
- Thiamine
- Flumazenil (**do not use if known, suspected or possible chronic benzodiazepine user**)

Hemodialysis indications for severe ingestions

- Ethylene glycol or methanol (fomepizole should be given also as treatment)
- Salicylate
    - Level > 90 in acute ingestion
    - Level > 60 in chronic ingestion
    - Severe symptoms
    - Unable to alkalinize urine in a less severe ingestion
    - Massive ingestion (death may result if not hemodialyzed promptly)
- Phenobarbital
- Theophylline
- Lithium
- Valproic acid level > 750 or severe symptoms
- Diethylene glycol
- Massive acetaminophen > 1000 mcg/ml if early post-ingestion

Seizures

- Adult: lorazepam 2–6 mg IV; may repeat q10–15 minutes prn
- Pediatric: lorazepam 0.05–0.1 mg/kg IV; may repeat q10–15 minutes prn (NMT 10 mg)
- If no IV available in children, use Diastat (diazepam rectal gel)
    - Age up to 5 years: 0.5 mg/kg
    - Age 6–11 years: 0.3 mg/kg
    - Age > 12 years: 0.2 mg/kg
    - Round up to available dose: 2.5, 5, 7.5, 10, 12.5, 15, 17.5, 20 mg/dose
- Midazolam IV/IM/PR/ET/intranasal 0.1–0.2 mg/kg/dose; not to exceed a cumulative dose of 10 mg)

Antidotes (if clinically indicated)

- Acetaminophen: N-acetylcysteine
    - Give if ingestion suspected with elevated ALT
    - Give even if acetaminophen induced hepatic failure present and acetaminophen no longer measurable
- Anticholinergic: physostigmine
- Benzodiazepines: flumazenil (thought to increase seizure potential — controversial)
- Beta-blockers: glucagon
- Calcium channel blockers: calcium chloride, insulin
- Calcium channel blocker severe toxicity
    - CaCl 1–3 gms (10–30 mg/kg) q30 min. prn up to 8 doses
    - High dose insulin therapy
        - Bolus of 0.5–1 Unit/kg, followed by a drip with a rate of 0.5–1 Unit/kg/hr
        - If blood glucose < 250 give supplemental IV glucose (D10)
        - Accucheck q15 min. to avoid hypoglycemia
    - Levophed IV if hypotensive per physician
- Carbon monoxide: 100% O2; consider hyperbaric chamber
- Coumadin (warfarin): vitamin K, FFP
- Cyanide: cyanide antidote kit
- Digoxin (digitalis): digibind
- Ethylene glycol and methanol: fomepizole
- Iron: deferoxamine
- INH: pyridoxine (vitamin B6)
- Methemoglobinemia: methylene blue
- Organophosphates: atropine and/or PAM, atrovent aerosol for bronchospasm
- Tricyclic antidepressants: NaHCO3
- Opiates: narcan (naloxone) for toxic narcotic overdose
    - For adults: 0.4–2 mg IV or IM
    - For pediatrics: narcan (naloxone) 0.1 mg/kg IV or IM (NMT 2 mg)

Lipid antidote — local anesthetic overdose or intra-arterial injection with cardiac arrest (consult physician immediately to assume care of patient)

- Start ACLS
- Give Intralipid 20% 1 cc/kg over 1 minute; repeat twice more at 3–5 minute intervals
    - Convert to an infusion at a rate of 0.25 mL/kg/min, continuing until hemodynamic stability is restored; do not exceed 8 cc/kg
    - May be useful for fat soluble agent toxicity such as verapamil
- No human trials performed
- Anecdotal reports and animal data available only
- Lipidrescue.org recommended as reading for those interested in this therapy

Discharge Criteria

- Psychiatrically cleared
- No toxicity present or is totally detoxified
- Hemodynamically stable
- Good follow up and home situation

Discharge instructions

- Drug or substance ingestion aftercare instructions
- Refer for substance abuse treatment as indicated
- Follow up with PCP within 1 days as needed
- Return if worse

Consult Criteria

- Notify physician immediately for potentially dangerous ingestions or toxicity
    - Unstable vital signs
    - Metabolic acidosis
    - Altered mental status
- Acetaminophen ingestion
    - Pre-school child of 200 mg/kg or greater
    - Older child and adult > 150 mg/kg or total dose of 7.5 gms
    - Nomogram positive for toxicity

    - Liver function abnormalities
    - Delayed presentation
- Aspirin 150 mg/kg or serum level > 40 mg%
    - Lethal dose 300 mg/kg
- Discuss toxic ingestions with physician

Notes

Neurology

Section Contents

Headache Protocol

Dizziness Protocol

CVA/TIA Protocol

Bell's Palsy Protocol

Adult Seizure Protocol

Pediatric Seizure Protocol

Delirium Protocol

When using any protocol, always follow the Guidelines of Proper Use (page 16).

HEADACHE PROTOCOL

When using any protocol, always follow the Guidelines of Proper Use (page 16).

Definition

- Cephalic pain disorder

Differential Diagnosis

- Tension headache
- Migraine headache
- Cluster headache
- Sinusitis
- Otitis media
- Trigeminal neuralgia
- Brain tumor
- Subarachnoid hemorrhage
- Subdural hematoma
- Epidural hematoma
- Temporal arteritis
- Chronic daily headache
- Thunderclap headache
- Analgesic rebound headache
- CVA
- Meningitis
- Encephalitis
- Normal pressure hydrocephalus
- Ventricular peritoneal shunt malfunction
- Temporal mandibular joint disorder

Considerations

- "Functional" or "Primary" headache
    - No detectable cause (not uncommon)
    - Migraine
    - Cluster
    - Headache tension type
- "Organic" or "Secondary"

  - From pain sensitive structures; vessels; periosteum
  - Post concussion headaches
  - Spinal tap headaches
- History is one of the more important tools in headache evaluation
- New headache type in elderly suggestive of a higher risk process
- Do not use response to therapy to judge seriousness of headache
- Subarachnoid hemorrhage (SAH) 1% of all headaches in ED
  - Sudden onset and reaching maximal intensity in seconds to minutes
  - 1/3 not exertional
  - May awake with SAH
  - Sentinel leak in SAH headache may improve over time

Historical red flags

- Sudden onset or onset with exertion
- New, progressive, frequent headaches
- Trauma
- Cancer history
- Immunosuppression/HIV
- Clotting disorders
- First headache
- Worst headache
- Fever

Evaluation

- Complete history and physical exam
- Check gait, motor and sensory exam
- Funduscopic exam

Lab *(usually not needed in most headaches)*

- CBC
- ESR (age > 50 years: temporal arteritis) — not needed with no changes in chronic headache pattern
- Carbon monoxide level prn

- UCG prn

Benign Headaches — Tension, Migraine, Cluster

General treatment options for all types of benign headaches

- Decadron (dexamethasone) 10 mg IV or IM for adults may be ordered, when not contraindicated, to decrease return visits for same headache
- O2 therapy can be given for all types of headaches

Tension headache

- Pressing or tightening (nonpulsatile quality)
- Frontal-occipital location
- Bilateral: mild/moderate intensity
- Not aggravated by physical activity

Treatment

- NSAID's PO prn
- Tylenol prn
- Fiorinal 1–2 PO q4hr prn not to exceed 6 per 24 hour period
- Midrin 1–2 caps qid PO prn

Migraine

Associated with:

- Photophobia
- Phonophobia
- Nausea and vomiting
- May be unilateral or bilateral
- Aura occurs 20%
    - Scotoma (blind spots)
    - Fortification (zigzag patterns)
    - Scintilla (flashing lights)
    - Unilateral paresthesia/weakness
    - Hallucinations
    - Hemianopsia

Treatment options

- Compazine (prochlorperazine) 5–10 mg IV or IM
- Thorazine (chlorpromazine) 75 mg with Benadryl (diphenhydramine) 25 mg IM
- Ergots DHE 1 mg IV or IM
- Reglan (metoclopramide) 10 mg IV or IM
- Sumatriptan 6 mg SQ (do not use with history of coronary artery disease) — read drug information
- Maxalt (rizatriptan) 5–10 mg PO q2h prn for headache not to exceed 30 mg/d (do not use with history of coronary artery disease) — read drug information
- Midrin 2 caps PO initially then 1 cap PO q1hr prn not to exceed 5 caps/day
- Toradol (ketorolac) 30–60 mg IM (do not use if creatinine is elevated)
- Compazine suppository (prochlorperazine) 25 mg PR bid prn
- Narcotic prn (not as preferred)

Cluster

- Lancinating and severe
- Sudden onset — peaks in 10–15 minutes
- Unilateral facial
- Duration: 10 minutes to 3 hours per episode
- Character: boring and lancinating to eye
- Distribution: first and second divisions of the trigeminal nerve (approximately 18–20% of patients complain of pain in extratrigeminal regions)
- Frequency: may occur several times a day for 1–4 months (often nocturnal)
- Periodicity: circadian regularity in 47%
- Remission: long symptom-free intervals occur in some patients 2 months to 20 years

Treatment options

- O2 8 LPM face mask or 100% nonrebreather mask

- Sumatriptan 6 mg SQ (do not use with history of coronary artery disease) — read drug information
- Lidocaine 1 cc of a 10% solution placed on a swab in each nostril for 5 minutes is potentially helpful
- Capsaicin applied intranasally (has a burning sensation side effect)

Trigeminal neuralgia

- Commonly idiopathic
- Shock like severe pains in the distribution of trigeminal nerve
- Onset usually around age 60–70 years of age
- Pains last seconds to less than 2 minutes
- Can be triggered by specific activities such as eating, talking, brushing teeth, etc.
- No associated neurologic deficits
    - A sensory deficit excludes the diagnosis

Glossopharyngeal neuralgia

- Pain is over the distribution of glossopharyngeal nerve triggered by coughing, yawing, swallowing cold liquids

Occipital neuralgia

- Pain is in the posterior scalp region

Treatment options of cranial neuralgias

- Carbamazepine 200 mg PO bid to start (DOC)
    - Titrate increasing dose every 3 days by 200 mg
    - Effective dose is usually 600–1200 mg qday
    - Instruct patient they will need monitoring for aplastic anemia and severe leucopenia
- Dilantin (phenytoin) for carbamazepine failures (lower rate of success in treating neuralgia
    - Dose of 300–600 mg PO qday (levels need monitoring)

    - Cerebyx (fosphenytoin) 250 mg IV for severe attack
- Lamictal (lamotrigine) 100–400 mg PO qday (NMT 250 mg PO qday in children)

Discharge criteria

- Uncomplicated cases

Discharge instructions

- Trigeminal neuralgia aftercare instructions
- Follow up with PCP or neurologist in 7–10 days

Consult criteria

- Complicated cranial neuralgias

Temporal arteritis

- True emergency of the elderly
    - Age of onset 50–70 years of age
    - Six times more common in females than in males
- Headache localized over eye or to scalp
- Fever, malaise and weight loss are associated symptoms
- Jaw claudication is important associated symptom
- Frequently associated with polymyalgia rheumatica (joint and muscles aches)
- ESR 50–100
- C-reactive protein elevated usually
- Vision loss can occur early in course of disease

Treatment

- Prednisone 40–80 mg PO bid for several months to one year

Discharge criteria

- Minimal symptoms can be treated as outpatient
- Severe symptoms or question of eye involvement should be admitted with IV high dose steroid treatment and ophthalmology consultation obtained

- Discuss all temporal arteritis cases with physician

Discharge instructions

- Temporal arteritis aftercare instructions
- Follow up with PCP within 1 day
- Return for visual changes

Consult criteria

- Discuss all temporal arteritis cases with physician

Headaches Prompting CT Brain Scan Consideration

- Worst headache of life — Consider lumbar puncture if CT negative
- Change in headache from previous headache symptoms/patterns
- Neurologic complaints
- New onset seizure with headache
- Complaints of altered mental status
- Migraine aura that is sensory or motor
- Change in migraine aura
- Focal deficits
- Headache > 24 hours
- Thunderclap headache
- Headache in elderly
- Historical Red Flag Headaches
- Recommend that all CT brain scan patients prior to discharge should be discussed with physician

Consider Following "Don't Miss Diagnoses"

(Perform testing for possible diagnoses when suspected)

- Subarachnoid hemorrhage
- Meningitis and encephalitis
- Temporal arteritis
- Acute narrow angle closure glaucoma
- Hypertensive emergencies
- Carbon monoxide poisoning

- Cerebral venous sinus thrombosis (seen, for example, with OCP use or with women with coagulopathy)
- Trigeminal neuralgia
- Pseudotumor cerebri
- Acute strokes
- Mass lesions

Discharge Criteria

- Benign headache diagnosis and prognosis
- Trigeminal or cranial neuralgias refer to neurologist (website tna.support.org)

Discharge instructions

- Headache aftercare instructions
- Refer to PCP or neurologist within 7–10 days as needed
- Return if headache persists > 24 hours

Consult Criteria

- Headache with fever unless consistent with a benign process
- Neck/nuchal rigidity
- Headaches where CT brain scan performed
- Follow General Patient Criteria Protocol (page 20) for care/evaluation not covered in this protocol
- Possible High Risk Headache
- Acute neurologic complaints or findings
- Above diagnosis suspected in the "Don't miss diagnosis" section
- Return visit for same headache
- Age ≥ 60 unless known chronic headache patient without pattern change
- Questionable diagnosis
- Status migrainosus (> 24 hours; dehydration)
- "Historical Red Flags" headache

Lab consult criteria

- Adult WBC ≥ 14,000 or < 1,000 neutrophils
- Pediatric WBC ≥ 15,000 or < 1,000 neutrophils
- Bandemia
- Thrombocytopenia — acute

- Metabolic acidosis
- Significant electrolyte abnormality
- Glucose ≥ 400 mg/dL in diabetic patient
- Glucose ≥ 300 mg/dL in new onset diabetes
- Hyperglycemia with metabolic acidosis (decreased serum CO_2 or elevated anion gap)

Notes

DIZZINESS PROTOCOL

When using any protocol, always follow the Guidelines of Proper Use (page 16).

Definitions

- Sensation of being off balance or of movement of body or surrounding environment

Differential Diagnosis

- Vestibular disorder of inner ear
- Cardiac arrhythmia
- Pulmonary embolism
- TIA
- CVA
- Seizures
- Dehydration
- Aortic stenosis
- Hypoglycemia
- Subarachnoid hemorrhage
- Hemorrhage
    - GI bleeding
    - Ectopic pregnancy
- Adrenal insufficiency
- Sepsis
- Hypotension

Considerations

- Vertigo: peripheral ("inner ear") or central
- Disequilibrium: suggests CNS disorder

Can be:

- Presyncope
- Generalized weakness
- Cardiopulmonary
- Metabolic
- Emotional disorder

Peripheral Vertigo

- Sensation of movement worsened with head movement or position change
- Horizontal nystagmus; rotary nystagmus
- Nausea and vomiting
- No vital sign abnormalities
- No focal neurologic deficits, neurologic complaints or other significant comorbidities
- No further testing may be needed

Central vertigo

- Not worse on movement
- Vertical nystagmus
- Infrequent nausea and vomiting
- Central nervous system findings present

Evaluation

- Complete history and physical examination
    - Check for nystagmus, gait abnormalities
    - Hallpike maneuver prn
- For benign peripheral vertigo no further testing may be needed
- Consider CT brain scan for
    - Ataxia
    - Vertical nystagmus
    - Neurologic deficits or complaints
    - Headache
    - Consult physician
- CBC, BMP, EKG, CXR as indicated for patients that may have a disorder besides peripheral vertigo causing symptoms
- Toxicology screen and medication levels as indicated
- Follow Chest Pain, Dyspnea, TIA, Syncope/Presyncope or other Protocols as indicated

Treatment Options

- Benign Paroxysmal Positional Vertigo: Epley maneuver
- Peripheral benign vertigo: meclizine, or Phenergan (promethazine), or benzodiazepines can be considered

- Consider steroids and/or acyclovir (or valacyclovir — Valtrex) — or other herpes medication for vestibular neuronitis or labyrinthitis
- Avoid antihistamines if not peripheral vertigo

Discharge Criteria

- Peripheral vertigo with normal vital signs and O2 saturation
- Not ataxic
- Acute central nervous system or metabolic disorder not suspected

Discharge instructions

- Provide dizziness aftercare instructions
- Refer to primary care provider, neurologist or ENT within 10 days as needed

Consult Criteria

- Neurologic abnormalities or complaints
- If CT brain scan needed or performed
- Cardiogenic, pulmonary, toxicology cause of dizziness
- Age ≥ 70
- Uncertain or unknown cause of dizziness
- Syncope or presyncope > 30 seconds
- Refer to General Patient Criteria Protocol (page 20)

Lab and x-ray consult criteria

- New onset renal insufficiency or worsening renal insufficiency
- WBC ≥ 15,000 or < 3,000; Neutrophil count < 1,000
- Bandemia ≥ 15%
- Acute thrombocytopenia
- Increased anion gap
- Metabolic acidosis
- Significant electrolyte abnormally
- Glucose ≥ 400 mg/dL in diabetic patient
- Glucose ≥ 300 mg/dL in non-diabetic patient
- Pleural effusion
- New onset renal insufficiency or worsening renal insufficiency

Notes

CVA/TIA PROTOCOL

When using any protocol, always follow the Guidelines of Proper Use (page 16).

Definition

- TIA — An acute and temporary neurologic dysfunction caused by a focal decrease in blood flow to the central nervous system
- CVA — A neurologic dysfunction caused by a focal decrease in blood flow to the central nervous system that causes death in the affected area

Differential Diagnosis

- CVA
- Bell's palsy
- Migraine
- Subarachnoid hemorrhage
- Brain tumor
- Multiple sclerosis
- Intracerebral hemorrhage
- Seizure disorder
- Transient global amnesia (TGA)
- Hypoglycemia

Considerations

- TIA always lasts less than 24 hours
    - They usually last 15 minutes to 1 hour in duration
- Up to 40% of patients with TIA have actually had small infarctions by MRI criteria
    - 10.5% of TIA's will have a CVA within 90 days
        - Half of these will occur within 2 days
    - Up to 21 % of CVA's will die or have major cardiac event
- Up to 16% of TIA patients will have a headache
- Most TIA patients should be hospitalized; especially cardiogenic etiology and crescendo TIA's
- Syncope is seldom a TIA

Symptoms

- Acute in onset
- Focal
- Reaching intensity within seconds
- Begin at the same time
- Most common symptoms and signs are
    - Motor and/or sensory deficit on one side of the body
    - Loss of speech or comprehension
    - Loss of vision in one eye or one hemifield
- Vertebrobasilar CVA/TIA presenting as syncope is typically associated with other brainstem signs:
    - Diplopia
    - Ataxia

Most common symptoms and signs

- Hemiparesis
- Hemiataxia
- Hemisensory loss
- Speech difficulty
- Visual difficulty — diplopia or visual loss

High risk factors to develop CVA following TIA

- Age > 60
- Diabetes
- TIA lasting > 10 minutes
- Motor weakness
- Speech impairment

0 factors = 0% CVA; 5 factors = 34% CVA occurrence

TIA mimics

Migraines

- Migraines symptoms usually migrate and grow, without the abrupt symptoms of TIA

Syncope

- Hypoperfusion usually produces loss of consciousness, but focal deficits can occasionally be seen, especially after an episode of true syncope

Vertigo

- True vertigo without other findings is seldom central. Look especially for other brainstem signs

Epilepsy

- Focal paralysis without motor activity occurs rarely

TGA

- Transient global amnesia without any other neurologic deficit

Intracerebral hemorrhage

- Symptoms rarely are transient

Multiple sclerosis

- Onset is typically much slower than TIA

Hypoglycemia

- Some alteration in consciousness usually present

Nondescript complaints

- Acute onset of focal symptoms is occasionally a conversion reaction, but be aware of the possibility of embellishment of a real deficit

Evaluation Options

- CBC
- CMP
- EKG
- CT brain scan at time of initial presentation
- Chest x-ray
- C-RP
- ESR
- PT/INR
- Assess for focal neurologic deficits in addition to cardiac and general exam
- Check gait as needed

Assess for other causes

- Migraines

- Seizures
- Vertigo
- TGA
- Medication side effect/toxins
- Multiple sclerosis
- Intracerebral hemorrhage
- Lumbar puncture if subarachnoid hemorrhage is suspected
- Blood cultures if infected emboli are suspected (e.g., SBE)

Acute CVA presentations less than 4.5 hours from onset (notify physician)

- Rapidly perform NIHSS (NIH Stroke Scale) and examine patient
- Order stat CT brain without contrast
- Consult physician and neurologist immediately after ordering CT brain scan
    - If available and appropriate to the specific institution and the patient's clinical situation, order contrast CT brain after plain CT brain completed per physician (renal patients discuss with physician or radiologist prior to contrast)
- Determine patient eligibility for t-PA with physician and a course of action if possible
- Repeat NIHSS immediately when patient returns from CT brain scan and discuss with physician
    - To give thrombolysis treatment, blood pressure targets initially are:
        - SBP ≤ 185 mm Hg
        - DBP ≤ 110 mm Hg
- Follow established specific institution's acute stroke policies if present instead of this section

Time targets for t-PA candidates

- Door to Provider: 10 min
- Access to neurologic expertise: 15 min
- Door to CT scan completion: 25 min
- Door to CT scan interpretation: 45 min
- Door to treatment: 60 min
- Admission to monitored bed: 6 hr

TIA Treatment Options

- Aspirin 325 mg per day (if no cerebral hemorrhage)
- Consider Plavix (clopidogrel) for ASA failure or ASA allergy (if no cerebral hemorrhage)
- Aggrenox can be used instead of aspirin or Plavix (clopidogrel)
- Coumadin (warfarin) is most effective if atrial fibrillation present
- Lower head of bed to flat position to improve cerebral circulation
- Avoid hypotonic IV fluids

Hypertension treatment for TIA and CVA nonthrombolysis candidates

- Consult physician for treatment preferred
    - Treat SBP ≥ 220 mm Hg or MAP ≥ 130 mm Hg carefully (avoid rapid or large decreases in BP > 15%)
        - Labetalol 10–20 mg IV over 1–2 minutes — may repeat q10min and double as needed to maximum dose of 150 mg

          or
        - Nicardipine 5mg/hr IV and titrate as needed
    - Avoid treating SBP < 220 mm Hg or MAP < 130 mm Hg
        - Unless AMI, severe CHF, aortic dissection or hypertensive encephalopathy or ICH (intracranial hemorrhage) is present
    - Notify physician promptly if intracranial hemorrhage present
        - SBP > 180 mm Hg is treatable

Admission Criteria

- Acute CVA
- Most TIA's
    - High risk criteria
    - Crescendo/recurrent TIA's
    - Cardiogenic etiology of TIA

- Recent single TIA's are often offered admission because of the high risk of subsequent stroke and to facilitate rapid work-up
- Septic emboli diagnosis is possible
- Likelihood that patient would not return for outpatient work-up

Discharge Criteria

- Not surgical or anticoagulation candidate
- Patient declines admission for evaluation
- Fully worked up in recent past
- Neurologically stable

Discharge instructions

- TIA aftercare instructions
- Discharge instructions should include early follow-up along what signs and symptoms to watch for, and to return immediately for further symptoms

Consult Criteria

- All TIA or CVA patients
- CT brain scan with acute findings
- Unclear diagnosis
- Refer to General Patient Criteria Protocol (page 20)

Lab and x-ray consult criteria

- New onset renal insufficiency or worsening renal insufficiency
- WBC ≥ 15,000 or < 3,000; Neutrophil count < 1,000
- Bandemia
- Acute thrombocytopenia
- Increased anion gap
- Metabolic acidosis
- Significant electrolyte abnormally
- Glucose ≥ 400 mg/dL in diabetic patient
- Glucose ≥ 300 mg/dL in non-diabetic patient
- Hyperglycemia with metabolic acidosis (decreased serum CO2 or elevated anion gap)
- Pleural effusion

- New onset renal insufficiency or worsening renal insufficiency

Current inclusion guidelines for the administration of t-PA are:

- Diagnosis of ischemic stroke causing measurable neurologic deficit
- Neurologic signs should not be clearing
- Neurologic signs not be minor and isolated
- Caution should be exercised in treating patients with major deficits (higher risk of hemorrhagic conversion)
- Symptoms not be suggestive of subarachnoid hemorrhage
- Onset of symptoms < 4.5 hours before beginning treatment
- No head trauma or prior stroke in past 3 months
- No MI in prior 3 months
- No GI/GU hemorrhage in previous 21 days
- No arterial puncture in noncompressible site during prior 7 days
- No major surgery in prior 14 days
- No history of prior intracranial bleed
- SBP < 185 mm Hg and DBP < 110 mm Hg
- No evidence of acute trauma or bleeding
- Not taking an oral anticoagulant, or if so INR < 1.7
- If taking heparin within 48 hours must have a normal activated prothrombin time (aPT)
- Platelet count > 100,000 µL
- Blood glucose level greater than 50 mg/dL (2.7 mmol)
- No seizure with residual postictal impairments
- CT scan does not show evidence of multilobar infarction (hypodensity > 1/3 hemisphere) — increased risk of hemorrhagic conversion
- The patient and family understand the potential risks and benefits of therapy

References:

- Stroke. May 2007;38(5):1655-711

- Stroke. 2010;41;2108

NIH stroke scale

Do not augment or interpret patient's responses on what you think the patient can do. Only record what the patient exactly does.

1a – Level of consciousness (LOC)

- 0 = **Alert;** keenly responsive
- 1 = **Not alert;** arousable by minor stimulation to obey, answer, or respond
- 2 = **Not alert;** requires repeated stimulation to attend, or is obtunded and requires strong or painful stimulation to make movements (not stereotyped)
- 3 = **Responds only** with reflex motor or autonomic effects or is totally unresponsive, flaccid, and areflexic

1b – LOC questions — asked month and age (must be exact)

- 0 = **Answers** both questions correctly
- 1 = **Answers** one question correctly
- 2 = **Answers** neither question correctly

1c – LOC commands — asked to open and close eyes and then to grip and release non-paretic hand

- 0 = **Performs** both tasks correctly
- 1 = **Performs** one task correctly
- 2 = **Performs** neither task correctly

2 – Best gaze

- 0 = **Normal**
- 1 = **Partial gaze palsy;** gaze is abnormal in one or both eyes, but forced deviation or total gaze paresis is not present
- 2 = **Forced deviation,** or total gaze paresis not overcome by the oculocephalic (doll's eyes) maneuver

3 – Visual

- 0 = **No visual loss**
- 1 = **Partial hemianopsia**
- 2 = **Complete hemianopsia**

- 3 = **Bilateral hemianopsia** (blind including cortical blindness)

4 – Facial palsy

- 0 = **Normal symmetrical movements**
- 1 = **Minor paralysis** (flattened nasolabial fold, asymmetry on smiling)
- 2 = **Partial paralysis** (total or near-total paralysis of lower face)
- 3 = **Complete paralysis** of one or both sides (absence of facial movement in the upper and lower face)

5 – Motor arm (score for each arm)

- 0 = **No drift;** limb holds 90 (or 45) degrees for full 10 seconds
- 1 = **Drift;** limb hold 90 (or 45) degrees, but drifts down before full 10 seconds; does not hit bed or other support
- 2 = **Some effort against gravity;** limb cannot get to or maintain (if cued) 90 (or 45) degrees, drifts down to bed, but has some effort against gravity
- 3 = **No effort against gravity;** limb falls
- 4 = **No movement**
- UN = **Amputation** or joint fusion, explain: ____________________________________

6 – Motor leg (score for each leg)

- 0 = **No drift;** leg holds 30-degree position for full 5 seconds
- 1 = **Drift;** leg falls by the end of the 5-second period but does not hit bed
- 2 = **Some effort against gravity;** leg falls to bed by 5 seconds, but has some effort against gravity
- 3 = **No effort against gravity;** leg falls to bed immediately
- 4 = **No movement**
- UN = **Amputation** or joint fusion, explain: ____________________________________

7 – Limb ataxia

- 0 = Absent

- 1 = Present in one limb
- 2 = Present in two limbs
- UN = **Amputation** or joint fusion, explain: ___________________________

8 – Sensory

- 0 = **Normal;** no sensory loss
- 1 = **Mild-to-moderate sensory loss;** patient feels pinprick is less sharp or is dull on the affected side; or there is a loss of superficial pain with pinprick, but patient is aware of being touched.
- 2 = **Severe to total sensory loss;** patient is not aware of being touched in the face, arm, and leg

9 – Best Language

- 0 = **No aphasia;** normal
- 1 = **Mild-to-moderate aphasia;** some obvious loss of fluency or facility of comprehension, without significant limitation on ideas expressed or form of expression. Reduction of speech and/or comprehension; however, makes conversation about provided materials difficult or impossible. For example, in conversation about provided materials, examiner can identify picture or naming card content from patient's response.
- 2 = **Severe aphasia;** all communication is through fragmentary expression; great need for inference, questioning, and guessing by the listener. Range of information that can be exchanged is limited; listener carries burden of communication. Examiner cannot identify materials provided from patient response.
- 3 = **Mute, global aphasia;** no usable speech or auditory comprehension

10 – Dysarthria

- 0 = **Normal**
- 1 = **Mild-to-moderate dysarthria;** patient slurs at least some words and, at worst, can be understood with some difficulty.
- 2 = **Severe dysarthria;** patient's speech is so slurred as to be unintelligible in the

absence of or out of proportion to any dysphasia, or is mute.

- UN = **Intubated** or other physical barrier, explain:________________________________

11 – Extinction and Inattention (Neglect)

- 0 = **No abnormality**
- 1 = **Visual, tactile, auditory, spatial, or personal inattention** or extinction to bilateral simultaneous stimulation in one of the sensory modalities.
- 2 = **Profound hemi-inattention or extinction to more than one modality**; does not recognize own hand or orients to only one side of space.

NOTE: If the patient in 1a has a score of 3, then the rest of the exams usually are scored a 3 for each category

Reference:
http://www.ninds.nih.gov/doctors/NIH_Stroke_Scale.pdf

Notes

Bell's Palsy Protocol

When using any protocol, always follow the Guidelines of Proper Use (page 16).

Definition

- Dysfunction or paralysis of the 7th cranial nerve unilaterally of acute onset and usually idiopathic etiology

Differential Diagnosis

- Vascular
  - TIA
  - CVA
  - Aneurysm
- Infectious
  - Lyme disease
  - Herpes zoster
  - Mononucleosis
- Neoplastic
  - Tumor of pons or cerebellopontine angle or acoustic nerve
  - Skull based tumor, cholesteatoma
- Multiple sclerosis

Considerations

- 7th cranial nerve dysfunction
- Affects 1 in 65 persons in a lifetime
- Complete recovery in 65% of patients at 3 months and 85% at 9 months
- Steroids and Valtrex (valacyclovir) or acyclovir recommended only in the initial 72 hours of symptoms with complete or nearly complete paralysis — not useful otherwise
- Slowly progressive facial paralysis suggestive of cancer
- Recurrent paralysis can be seen with Bell's palsy or more commonly with tumor

- Bilateral 7th nerve weakness excludes Bell's palsy and is suggestive of infectious causes such as Lyme disease or VZV (varicella zoster virus)
- Forehead sparing of motor function usually indicates upper motor neuron lesion (CVA)
- Lyme disease should be considered as a cause in endemic areas
- Bell's palsy can be mimicked by pontine brainstem lesion
- Other associated signs and symptoms:
    - Vestibular signs
    - Diabetes and hypertension higher risk for pontine lesions

Signs and Symptoms

- Typical presentation is subacute weakness of one side of the face
- Often associated with pain near the ear
- No sensory loss although patient may complain of vague sensation on the face
- Hyperacusis due to paralysis of the stapedius sometimes occurs
- Distortion of taste sometimes occurs although this is seldom a presenting complaint
- Weakness of eye closure is helpful to differentiate from stroke where eye opening may be impaired
- Asymmetry of mouth movement is most obvious with grimacing and smiling
- Maximal defect is 5 days from onset
- Forehead and lower facial muscles both weak
    - If forehead spared of weakness, suspect central lesion (CVA, tumor)
- Increased tear flow
- Dry eyes
- Rash or vesicles around ear on affected side suggests herpes zoster (Ramsey-Hunt syndrome). Usually significant pain near the ear

Causes

- Idiopathic usually
- Infectious causes

  - Most cases of Bell's palsy are thought to be due to virus infections
    - HSV 1 or 2
    - VZV
  - EBV
  - Lyme disease is a rare cause of Bell's palsy
- Sarcoidosis can present with facial palsy
- Other infections such as osteomyelitis, primary ear infections, and meningitis are less likely
- Neoplasm of local tissues near the ear and skull base or neoplastic meningitis
- Pontine (brainstem) lesion, including cerebellopontine angle lesion
- Aneurysm of the basilar artery or branch with resultant neural compression

Evaluation Options

- Usually no testing except history and physical exam
- Testing driven by suspected processes
  - CBC
  - ESR or C-reactive
  - Lyme titer
  - HIV test
  - Serum glucose
  - CT brain if suspected central lesion (usually not needed)

Treatment Options

- Artificial tears
- Tape eyelids closed on affected side at night only
- Steroids are commonly used unless specifically contraindicated
  - Prednisone 1 mg/kg/day up to 60 mg/day × 7 days without rapid taper
- Antivirals are commonly used although data are conflicting
  - Valtrex (valacyclovir) 1000 mg PO tid × 5 days

    OR
  - Acyclovir 400 mg PO 5 ×/day × 7–10 days

    OR

    - Famciclovir 500 mg tid × 5–10 days
- Physical therapy may be used for patients with moderate to severe deficits

Discharge Criteria

- Isolated 7th nerve palsy

Discharge instructions

- Bell's palsy aftercare instructions
- Follow up with primary care provider or neurologist within 7 days
- Discharge precautions noted:
    - Return if additional symptoms or significant worsening
    - Complete administration of medications
- Ensure follow-up after discharge

Consult Criteria

- Suspected other causes of palsy
- Central nervous system findings or complaints
- Refer to General Patient Criteria Protocol (page 20) as needed

Notes

Adult Seizure Protocol

When using any protocol, always follow the Guidelines of Proper Use (page 16).

Definition

- Focal or generalized electrical depolarizations of the brain resulting in focal or generalized neurologic and motor findings with or without loss of consciousness

Differential Diagnosis

- Pseudoseizures
- Migraines
- Encephalitis
- Meningitis
- Transient global amnesia (TGA)
- Psychogenic unresponsiveness
- TIA (rare TIA's can present with focal motor activity or unresponsiveness)
- Syncope
- Hypoglycemia
- Conversion reaction

Considerations

Generalized seizures (most common)

Classic tonic-clonic (grand mal)

- Sustained generalized muscle contractions followed by loss of consciousness

Absence seizures (petit mal)

- Brief episodes of sudden immobility and blank stares

Partial seizures

Simple

- Brief sensory or motor symptoms without loss of consciousness
    - Focal motor seizures is an example

Complex

- Mental or psychiatric symptoms
- Affect changes
- Confusion
- Automatisms
- Hallucinations
- Impaired consciousness

Status epilepticus (SE)

- Newly defined as seizure > 5 minutes or 2 or more seizures in which patient does not recover consciousness
- Older definition > 30 minutes or 2 or more seizures in which patient does not recover consciousness (controversy exists about definition)
- Mortality of 10–12%
- Failure to recognize nonconvulsive SE increases poor outcomes
- Prolonged SE leads to electromechanical dissociation
    - Exhibit minor movements: twitching of eyes, face, hands, feet; coma

Prolactin level

- Helpful if drawn within 10–20 minutes of seizure and elevated 2 times normal
    - Syncope can also elevate prolactin levels
- Normal prolactin level favors pseudoseizure but cannot differentiate seizure from syncope
- Normal prolactin does not rule out seizure however

Pseudoseizures

- Closed eyes during seizure: 96% sensitive; 98% specific in indicating pseudoseizure
- Open eyes during seizure: 98% sensitive; 96% specific in indicating true seizure

First time seizure has 25% recurrence in 2 years

Epilepsy defined as 2 of more seizures not provoked by other illness or causations

Causes

- Idiopathic
- Genetic
- Hypoglycemia or hyperglycemia
- Hypernatremia and hyponatremia
- CVA
- Cerebral mass
- Intracranial hemorrhage — especially subarachnoid or intraparenchymal
- Traumatic brain injury
- Cocaine
- Meningitis
- Encephalitis
- Eclampsia
- Fever
- Prescribed drugs (lowered seizure threshold especially with some antibiotics and analgesics)
- Withdrawal syndromes (drugs and alcohol)

Evaluation

- Assess airway and breathing
- Cardiac and O2 saturation monitoring
- Complete history and physical
- Obtain seizure history and treatment
- Obtain history of associated symptoms
- Drug abuse history

Patients with chronic seizures and no change in typical seizure pattern, without comorbid findings or symptoms

- BMP
- Seizure drug levels if acutely measurable

All other seizures with comorbid considerations and new onset seizures

- CMP, Mg^{++}, prolactin level in select patients
- Pregnancy test in childbearing age women
- Consider lumbar puncture (LP) in immunocompromised patient or with meningitis signs
- Consider LP in patients with seizure and fever
- CBC; U/A; chest x-ray as indicated by associated symptoms or findings
- Blood alcohol and drug screen as indicated
- Serum anticonvulsant levels for anticonvulsant therapy that are acutely measurable
- CT brain scan on first time seizures if available
- CT brain scan on elderly or patients taking Coumadin
- CT brain scan for head trauma
- Consider stat EEG for suspected nonconvulsive SE

Treatment Options

- Notify physician promptly of seizures occurring in the department or clinic
- Intubation if airway not secure
- IV NS KVO
- Nasal oxygen

Initial treatment

- Lorazepam 2–6 mg IV if actively seizing
  - May repeat q10–15 minutes for recurrent seizures prn (NMT 10 mg)

Adjunctive treatments as needed

- Thiamine 100 mg IM/IV for alcoholism history (or if not known)
- Glucose D50W 1 amp if hypoglycemic
- Prophylactic lorazepam can be given in the first 12 hours of alcoholic withdrawal
- Magnesium sulfate 4 gms IV over 5–10 minutes for eclampsia

Status epilepticus (beware of "too slow and too low" treatment)

- Lorazepam 0.1 mg/kg IV (NMT 10 mg)
- Cerebyx (fosphenytoin) 15–20 mg/kg IV at 100 mg/minute if no response in 5 minutes to lorazepam

Drugs that can be used if lorazepam and Cerebyx (fosphenytoin) fail

- Propofol per physician (intubate patient)
- Lidocaine 1 mg/kg up to 100 mg; may be repeated (NMT 3 mg/kg)
- Valproic acid 15 mg/kg over 1–5 minutes; (NMT 40 mg/kg)
    - 5 mg/kg/hr drip
- Phenobarbital 10 mg/kg IV at 100 mg/hr per physician (seldom used in adults)
- Pentobarbital or thiopental per physician (rarely used)

Management of refractory status epilepticus (consult physician immediately)

- Referral to an intensive care unit
- Anesthetic agents such as midazolam, propofol or barbiturates (thiopental, pentobarbital) for generalized convulsive status epilepticus
- Non-anesthetic anticonvulsants such as phenobarbital or valproic acid for nonconvulsive status epilepticus

Discharge Criteria

- Patient with normal neurologic exam and no concerning comorbidities
- No known structural brain disease
- Patients usually do not need to be started on seizure outpatient treatment at that time if patient had single brief seizure without previous seizure history, and has a normal exam, normal imaging and no further seizures
- With treatment, after oral or parenteral load with anticonvulsant

- Without treatment if risk of recurrent seizure is judged to be low

Discharge instructions

- Seizure aftercare instructions
- Advise of seizure precautions/safety issues prior to discharge (for example – no driving)

Consult Criteria

- Notify physician promptly on all actively seizing patients
- Discuss all seizure patients with prior to discharge
- Notify physician of any other neurologic abnormalities
- Abnormal imaging studies
- Significant abnormal lab tests
- Abnormal vital signs and O2 saturation < 95% on room air (<92% O2 saturation in COPD patients)

Notes

PEDIATRIC SEIZURE PROTOCOL

When using any protocol, always follow the Guidelines of Proper Use (page 16).

Definition

- Focal or generalized electrical depolarizations of the brain resulting in focal or generalized neurologic and motor findings with or without loss of consciousness

Differential Diagnosis

- Pseudoseizures
- Migraines
- Encephalitis
- Meningitis

Considerations

Generalized seizures (most common)

Classic tonic-clonic (grand mal)

- Sustained generalized muscle contractions followed by loss of consciousness

Absence seizures (petit mal)

- Brief episodes of sudden immobility and blank stares

Partial seizures

Simple

- Brief sensory or motor symptoms without loss of consciousness
  - Focal motor seizures is an example

Complex

- Mental or psychiatric symptoms
- Affect changes
- Confusion
- Automatisms
- Hallucinations
- Impaired consciousness

Status epilepticus (SE)

- Newly defined as seizure > 5 minutes or 2 or more seizures in which patient does not recover consciousness
- Older definition > 30 minutes or 2 or more seizures in which patient does not recover consciousness (controversy exists about definition)
- Mortality of 10–12%
- Failure to recognize nonconvulsive SE increases poor outcomes
- Prolonged SE leads to electromechanical dissociation
    - Exhibit minor movements: twitching of eyes, face, hands, feet; coma

Prolactin level

- Helpful if drawn within 10–20 minutes of seizure and elevated 2 times normal
    - Syncope can also elevate prolactin levels
- Normal prolactin level favors pseudoseizure but cannot differentiate seizure from syncope
- Normal prolactin does not rule out seizure however

Pseudoseizures

- Closed eyes during seizure: 96% sensitive; 98% specific in indicating pseudoseizure
- Open eyes during seizure: 98% sensitive; 96% specific in indicating true seizure

First time seizure has 25% recurrence in 2 years

Epilepsy defined as 2 or more seizures not provoked by other illness or causations

Causes of Seizures Amenable to Treatment

- Hypoglycemia
- Hyponatremia
- Hypocalcemia
- Hypomagnesemia
- Isoniazid ingestion treated with pyridoxine
- Hypertension

Evaluation

- Assess airway and breathing
- Cardiac and O2 saturation monitoring
- Complete history and physical
- Obtain seizure history and treatment
- Obtain associated symptoms
- Drug abuse history

Patients with chronic seizures and no change in typical seizure pattern, without comorbid findings or symptoms

- BMP
- Seizure drug levels if acutely measurable

All other seizures with comorbid considerations and new onset seizures

- CMP, prolactin level in select patients
- Pregnancy test in childbearing age females
- Consider lumbar puncture on the immunocompromised patient or patient that has meningitis signs
- Consider LP in patients with seizure and fever
- CBC; U/A; chest x-ray as indicated by associated symptoms or findings
- Blood alcohol and drug screen as indicated
- Serum anticonvulsant levels for anticonvulsant therapy that are acutely measurable
- CT brain scan on first time seizures if available
- CT brain scan for head trauma
- Consider stat EEG if no resolution of post-ictal lethargy and for suspected nonconvulsive SE

Treatment Options

- Intubation if airway not secure
- IV NS KVO
- Nasal oxygen

Initial treatment options

- Lorazepam 0.05–0.1 mg/kg IV; may repeat q10–15 minutes prn
- Diastat (diazepam rectal gel) if no IV available

    - Age up to 5 years: 0.5 mg/kg
    - Age 6–11 years: 0.3 mg/kg
    - Age > 12 years: 0.2 mg/kg
    - Round up to available dose: 2.5, 5, 7.5, 10, 12.5, 15, 17.5, 20 mg/dose
- Midazolam IV/IM/PR/ET/intranasal 0.1–0.2 mg/kg/dose; not to exceed a cumulative dose of 10 mg

Adjunctive treatments as needed

- Dextrose: 0.25–0.5 g/kg/dose (1–2 cc of 25% dextrose) intravenously for hypoglycemia; not to exceed 25 gm/dose
- Naloxone (Narcan): 0.1 mg/kg/dose intravenously preferable (if needed may administer intramuscularly or subcutaneously) for narcotic overdose (do not exceed 2 mg)
- Thiamine: 100 mg intramuscularly for possible deficiency
- Pyridoxine (vitamin B6): 50–100 mg intravenously/intramuscularly for possible deficiency
- Rocephin (ceftriaxone) 50–100 mg/kg IV or IM not to exceed 2 grams if meningitis suspected (may use Sanford Guide), initiate treatment with antibiotics prior to cerebrospinal fluid (CSF) analysis or brain imaging
    - Give Decadron (dexamethasone) 15 minutes before antibiotics or with antibiotics

Status epilepticus (beware of "too slow and too low" treatment)

- Lorazepam 0.1 mg/kg IV (NMT 10 mg)
- Cerebyx (fosphenytoin) 15–20 mg/kg IV at 100 mg/minute if no response in 5 minutes to lorazepam or midazolam (Versed)
- Keppra (Levetiracetam) 20 mg/kg IV

Drugs that can be used if above medications fail

- Pentobarbital 1 mg/kg boluses IV to maximum 5 mg/kg per physician
- Valproic acid 15 mg/kg over 1–5 minutes (NMT 40 mg/kg)

  - 5 mg/kg/hr drip
- Phenobarbital 20 mg/kg IV at 100 mg/hr per physician

Management of refractory status epilepticus (consult physician immediately)

- Referral to an intensive care unit
- Anesthetic agents such as midazolam, propofol or barbiturates (thiopental, pentobarbital) for generalized convulsive status epilepticus
- Non-anesthetic anticonvulsants such as phenobarbital or valproic acid for nonconvulsive status epilepticus

Discharge Criteria

- Patient with normal neurologic exam and no concerning comorbidities
- No known structural brain disease
- Most patients usually do not need to be started on seizure outpatient treatment at time of discharge
- No further seizures
- With treatment, after oral or parenteral load with anticonvulsant
- Without treatment if risk of recurrent seizure is judged to be low

Discharge instructions

- Seizure aftercare instructions
- Advise of seizure precautions/safety issues prior to discharge (for example – no driving)
- Contact primary care physician or provider to alert of ED visit and arrange follow up

Consult Criteria

- Notify physician promptly on all actively seizing patients
- Discuss all seizure patients with prior to discharge
- Notify physician of any neurologic abnormalities
- Abnormal imaging studies
- Significant abnormal lab tests

- Abnormal vital signs and O_2 saturation < 95% on room air

Notes

DELIRIUM PROTOCOL

When using any protocol, always follow the Guidelines of Proper Use (page 16).

Definition

- Acute organic brain syndrome manifested by impaired thinking, confusion, deficits in attention, fluctuating course, impaired speech and other symptoms and signs of impaired cognition

Causes of delirium

Medications and substances

- Ethanol
- Anticholinergics
- Antihistamines
- Sedatives
- Narcotics
- Antidepressants
- Lithium
- Neuroleptics
- Tagamet (cimetidine)

Withdrawal

- Ethanol
- Benzodiazepines
- Narcotics

Metabolic

- Electrolyte abnormalities (Na and Ca)
- Hypoglycemia and hyperglycemia
- Acid-base disturbance
- Dehydration
- Hypoxia
- End organ insufficiency – liver, kidney and lungs
- Vitamin deficiency – thiamine, folate
- Fever or hypothermia

Infectious

- Urinary tract infection – especially in elderly
- Encephalitis or meningitis
- Pneumonia
- Sepsis
- Influenza

Neurologic

- Brain tumor
- Subdural hematoma
- Intracerebral hemorrhage
- Seizure disorder
- CVA

Endocrine

- Hyperthyroidism
- Hypothyroidism
- Parathyroid – hyper and hypoparathyroidism

Cardiovascular

- Congestive heart failure
- Arrhythmia
- Acute myocardial infarction

Conditions that mimic delirium

- Dementia
- Depression
- Schizophrenia
- Mania
- Wernicke's aphasia

Evaluation of delirium

Mental status examination

OMI HAT (OMI = organic disease; HAT = psychiatric or functional)

- O – Orientation
- M – Memory
- I – Intellect
- H – Hallucinations
- A – Affect disorder
- T – Thought disorder

Functional Disorder

- Age 15–40 years old
- Onset gradual
- Not confused
- Appears depressed

Organic disorder

- Middle age or elderly
- Non-adolescent children
- Labile course
- Confused
- Visual hallucinations
- Vital signs frequently abnormal

Testing Options

- CBC
- BMP
- LFT's
- U/A
- Chest x-ray
- EKG

Tested as indicated

- Drug levels
- Thyroid studies
- Urine drug screen
- Blood alcohol
- Blood cultures
- CT brain
- Lumbar puncture for CSF analysis
- Urine culture

Treatment of delirium

- Treat underlying illness
- Restore any fluid or electrolyte imbalances
- Discontinue any unnecessary medication that is contributing to delirium (discuss with physician)

Consult criteria for delirium

- Discuss all cases with physician

- Physician should examine all delirium or acute altered mental status patients unless from ethanol or drug abuse

Notes

Back

Section Contents

Back Pain Protocol

Flank Pain Protocol

When using any protocol, always follow the Guidelines of Proper Use (page 16).

BACK PAIN PROTOCOL

When using any protocol, always follow the Guidelines of Proper Use (page 16).

Differential Diagnosis

- Muscular pain
- Aortic aneurysm
- Vertebral infection
- Epidural hematoma
- Epidural abscess
- Herniated nucleus pulposus (HNP)
- Renal colic
- Pyelonephritis
- Cancer

Considerations

- Most back pain is benign
- Usually is without acute neurologic signs
- Radiculopathy is frequently an associated complaint or finding
- Fever may be harbinger of spinal or vertebral infection in patients with IV drug abuse or recent instrumentation
- Elderly have increased risk of vertebral fractures with or without injury

Spinal cord compression signs

- Urinary retention with overflow incontinence or voiding
- Fecal incontinence
- Decreased rectal tone
- Decreased perineal sensation
- Cauda equina syndrome
    - Urinary retention is most common finding in cauda equina syndrome
    - Patients without urinary retention have an approximately 1/10,000 chance of having cauda equina syndrome

Warning flags in back pain

- Cancer history (Pain not relieved by rest)
- Chronic infections or fever history
- Night pain
- Prolonged pain
- Depression
- HIV history
- Unexplained weight loss
- Substance abuse
- Disability pursuit
- Urinary retention

Evaluation

- Complete history and physical examination
- Check reflexes, SLR, and neurovascular exam
- Check rectal tone; perineal sensation; urinary bladder retention in suspected cauda equina syndrome
- Healthy non-elderly patients without direct blunt trauma usually need no tests
- Elderly frequently need spine films due to higher incidence of vertebral fractures
- Plain back/pelvic films may be needed in falls, MVC's, direct blunt trauma, depending on severity of injury mechanism
- U/A if renal disease suspected or significant injury mechanism
- D-dimer if aortic dissection considered
- CBC, C-RP (or ESR) for fever with vertebral back pain as only other symptom or finding

CT spine

- Acute neurologic complaints or findings
- Compression fracture > 30%
- Burst fracture (goes through entire vertebral body – unstable)
- Posterior vertebral involvement
- Traumatic back pain out of proportion to expectation

MRI for spinal cord findings or symptoms

Treatment Options

- NSAID's
- Short narcotic course prn for severe pain
- Avoid Demerol (meperidine)
- Preferably no prolonged bed rest unless fracture present
- Limit bed rest to no more than 1-2 days if possible (unless compression fracture)
- Muscle relaxants of questionable usefulness
- Salmon calcitonin for compression fractures that can be discharged

Discharge Criteria

- Uncomplicated presentation and findings
- Ability to control pain and ambulate
- Orthopedic referral for fractures

Discharge instructions

- Refer to primary care provider within 10 days as needed
- If HNP suspected refer to neurosurgeon or orthopedic surgeon within 10 days
- Back pain aftercare instructions

Consult Criteria

- Severe pain with inability to ambulate
- Progressive neurologic deficits
- Signs of cauda equina syndrome
- Signs of spinal cord compression or injury
- Evidence of infectious, vascular, or neoplastic etiologies
- Nontraumatic pediatric back pain
- Fracture
- Suspected aortic disease as cause of pain

Lab and x-ray consult criteria

- New onset renal insufficiency or worsening renal insufficiency

- WBC > 15,000 or < 3,000; Neutrophil count < 1,000
- Bandemia ≥ 15%
- Acute thrombocytopenia
- Metabolic acidosis
- Significant electrolyte abnormally
- Glucose ≥ 400 mg/dL in diabetic patient
- Glucose ≥ 300 mg/dL in non-diabetic patient
- Hyperglycemia with metabolic acidosis (decreased serum CO_2 or elevated anion gap)
- Pleural effusion
- New onset renal insufficiency or worsening renal insufficiency
- Refer to General Patient Criteria Protocol as needed (page 20).

Notes

Flank Pain Protocol

When using any protocol, always follow the Guidelines of Proper Use (page 16).

Differential Diagnosis

- Renal colic
- Biliary colic
- Aortic aneurysm
- Mechanical back pain
- Herpes zoster
- Pyelonephritis
- Renal vein thrombosis
- Retroperitoneal bleeding
- Appendicitis

Considerations

- Renal colic is most common misdiagnosis of ruptured abdominal aortic aneurysm
- Aortic disease cause more frequent in elderly
- No hematuria on U/A with 10–15% of kidney stones
- Flank ecchymosis indicative of intra-abdominal bleeding

Evaluation

- Detailed abdomen, back, flank, and neurovascular exam

Musculoskeletal suspected as cause

- No tests unless blunt injury occurred
- Blunt trauma consider x-ray
- CBC and U/A as indicated

Kidney stone suspected

- KUB
- UA

CT abdominal/pelvis scan considered

- In elderly
- Unclear diagnosis

- Aortic cause suspected
- Inadequate response to pain medications

D-dimer

- Can be used as screening test to rule out aortic disease if negative (98% specific)
- Coumadin (warfarin) can cause false negative D-dimer
- Elderly have a positive D-dimer > 50% of the time without acute process

U/A

- UTI symptoms
- Obtain urine C&S if pyelonephritis suspected or a diabetic with UTI

Treatment Options

- Toradol (ketorolac) 30 mg IV with or without Dilaudid (hydromorphone) 0.5–1 mg IV (or other equipotent narcotic) and Phenergan (promethazine) 6.25 mg or Zofran (ondansetron) 4 mg IV for suspected renal colic
    - Do not use Toradol (ketorolac) if creatinine is elevated
- Musculoskeletal can be treated with Tylenol, OTC medication, NSAID or short narcotic course
- Narcotic short course prn on discharge for renal colic pain, with or without Toradol (ketorolac)
- Phenergan (promethazine) prn
- Flomax (tamsulosin) 0.4 mg PO every day for 2-4 weeks days for ureteral calculus
- Simple UTI: Septra DS, cephalosporin or quinolone for 3 days — consider single dose therapy
- Pyridium: 200 mg TID prn urinary symptoms — do not dispense more than 6 for acute cystitis
- Pyelonephritis: 10–14 days of simple UTI antibiotic regimen
    - IV Rocephin (ceftriaxone) or Levaquin (levofloxacin) × 1 can be given initially
- Herpes zoster Rx as indicated

Discharge Criteria

- Renal colic controlled
- Simple cystitis
- Pyelonephritis in nontoxic patient and able to hold down medication at home
- Benign musculoskeletal disorder

Discharge instructions

- Flank pain aftercare instructions
- Refer to primary care provider or urologist as indicated within 1–7 days

Consult Criteria

- Unknown cause of moderate to severe flank pain
- Unable to hold oral fluids down at home
- Heart rate ≥ 110, hypotension or relative hypotension (SBP < 105 with history of hypertension)
- Suspected vascular cause of flank pain
- Toxic UTI patient
- Unable to hold down medications at home
- WBC ≥ 14,000
- New onset anemia
- Inadequate renal colic relief
- Age ≥ 60 without firm diagnosis
- New onset renal insufficiency or worsening renal insufficiency
- Solitary kidney with ureteral calculus
- Pyelonephritis with ureteral calculus

Notes

Gastrointestinal

Section Contents

Abdominal Pain Protocol

CT Abdominal Scan Issues

Adult Gastroenteritis Protocol

Irritable Bowel Syndrome Protocol

Appendicitis Protocol

Antibiotic-associated Colitis Protocol

Inflammatory Bowel Disease Protocol

Gastroesophageal Reflux Disease (GERD)

Peptic Ulcer Disease and Gastritis Protocol

Gallbladder Disease Protocol

Hepatitis Protocol

Gastrointestinal Bleeding Protocol

Gastrointestinal Foreign Body Protocol

Anorectal Disorder Protocol

Constipation Protocol

When using any protocol, always follow the Guidelines of Proper Use (page 16).

ABDOMINAL PAIN PROTOCOL

When using any protocol, always follow the Guidelines of Proper Use (page 16).

Differential Diagnosis

- See below locations of pain

Considerations

- Appendicitis may have normal WBC
    - WBC ≥ 10,000 with left shift in 80–90% of patients
- WBC is a poor predictor of surgical disease
- Consider EKG in epigastric pain with CAD risk factors and a benign exam
- Constitutional history important

Diagnostic pitfall

- Diagnosing UTI with mildly elevated WBC's in the general range of 7–15 WBC's on U/A as the cause of moderate to severe abdominal pain and/or tenderness, especially in females and those without infectious urinary complaints

Locations of pain

RUQ

- Gallbladder disease
- Liver disease
- Peptic ulcer disease

Epigastric

- Peptic ulcer
- Cardiac ischemia
- Gallbladder disease
- Pancreatitis
- Aortic aneurysm
- Mesenteric ischemia
- Small bowel disorder

LUQ

- Colon disorder
- Spleen disorder
- Liver disease
- Constipation

Right and left flanks

- Renal colic
- Pyelonephritis
- Aortic aneurysm

Periumbilical

- Pancreatitis
- Peptic ulcer
- Mesenteric ischemia
- Aortic aneurysm
- Intussusception

RLQ

- Appendicitis
- Mesenteric adenitis
- Diverticulitis
- Renal colic
- Ectopic pregnancy
- Ovarian cyst rupture
- Colitis
- Constipation
- Intussusception

LLQ

- Diverticulitis (most common area)
- Renal colic
- Ectopic pregnancy
- Ovarian cyst rupture
- Colitis
- Intussusception
- Constipation

Suprapubic

- Cystitis
- Prostatitis

- Proctitis
- Perirectal abscess

Groin

- Inguinal hernia
- Femoral hernia
- Inguinal ligament strain
- Femoral pseudoaneursym post cardiac catheterization

Appendicitis

- See Appendicitis Protocol

Diverticulitis

- Prevalence increases with age
- Usually pain and tenderness in LLQ of abdomen
- Fever may occur
- WBC may not be elevated in 60% of patients
- CT abdominal/pelvis imaging study of choice
- Patients with mild to moderate diverticulitis without systemic signs of infection or peritoneal signs may be discharged home on antibiotics and a clear liquid diet for 2–3 days and advanced as tolerated
    - Flagyl (metronidazole) 500 mg PO qid for 10 days
    - Cipro (ciprofloxacin) 500 mg PO bid or Levaquin (levofloxacin) 500–750 mg PO qday with Flagyl (metronidazole) for 10 days
    - Septra DS PO bid can be used instead of Cipro (ciprofloxacin) or Levofloxacin if needed
    - May use Sanford guide also

Biliary colic and cholecystitis

- See Gallbladder Disease Protocol

Pancreatitis

- Major causes are gallstones lodged in pancreas and ethanol consumption
- Severe pain usually in central abdomen and vomiting very common
- Chronic pancreatitis may develop

- Fever may occur
- Obtain CBC, amylase, lipase, LFT's and U/A
- Ultrasound if cholecystitis suspected
- Treatment options
  - IV fluids 100–1,000 cc/hour for adults as clinically indicated
  - Phenergan (promethazine) 6.25 mg IV or 25–50 mg IM

    OR
  - Zofran (ondansetron) 4–8 mg IM or IV
  - Stadol (butorphanol) 0.25–1 mg IV or 2 mg IM

    OR
  - Dilaudid (hydromorphone) 0.25–1 mg IV or 1–2 mg IM
  - Small narcotic doses for very elderly

Mesenteric ischemia

- Mortality high – 70–90%, especially with low flow circulatory states such as CHF
- Order CBC, BMP, lactate level, amylase, lipase and CT abdomen/pelvis
- Severe pain with less than expected tenderness on exam (may only have mild tenderness)
- Vomiting and diarrhea frequently present
- Risk factors are CHF, atrial fibrillation, and athero-sclerotic disease
- May have metabolic acidosis secondary to bowel infarction
- Intestinal angina may occur after a meal

Small bowel obstruction (SBO)

- Usually from postsurgical adhesions
- Pain is usually severe if obstruction is complete
- Vomiting is very common
- Hyperactive bowels sounds seen early in process
- Abdominal distension common
- Check for hernias
- Order CBC, amylase, lipase and BMP
- Obtain flat and upright plain abdominal films — may be negative in 30%

    - Consider CT abdomen/pelvis if SBO suspected and plain films nondiagnostic

Large bowel obstruction

- 60% from malignancy, 20% from diverticulitis and 5% from cecal volvulus
- Abdominal distension is significant
- Abdomen is hyperresonant on percussion
- Fever, rebound tenderness and rigidity suggest perforation
- Order CBC, BMP, lactate level if acidotic, and flat and upright abdominal films
- Ogilvie syndrome is acute colonic pseudoobstruction
    - Needs to be decompressed to avoid perforation

Hernia

Differential diagnosis

- Epididymitis
- Hydrocele
- Lymphogranuloma Venereum
- Testicular torsion
- Pseudoaneurym of femoral artery
- Varicocele
- Groin abscess

Considerations

- Reducible hernia can have contents returned to abdominal cavity
- Incarcerated hernia cannot be reduced
    - Not strangulated
    - Bowel obstruction not uncommon
    - Painful
- Strangulated hernia
    - Blood flow compromised with possible necrosis of bowel
    - Significant pain and tenderness
    - If reduced, pain and tenderness persists

Types of hernia

- Umbilical
    - Through umbilical ring
    - Common in childhood
    - Usually resolves by age 2 years
- Inguinal
    - Indirect inguinal hernia
        - Through inguinal ring into the inguinal canal following spermatic cord to scrotum
    - Direct inguinal hernia
        - Through Hasselbach's triangle (above inguinal ligament
- Femoral
    - Through femoral canal
    - Frequently become incarcerated or strangulated
- Ventral or incisional hernia
    - Post surgical complication
    - Usually without pain or incarceration

Gastroenteritis

- See Gastroenteritis Protocols for adults and pediatrics

Flank pain or kidney stone pain (renal colic) see respective protocols

Elderly abdominal pain

- Pain perception and abdominal exam altered in elderly
- Admissions and surgery rates are higher in elderly
- Consider mesenteric and cardiac ischemia in elderly
- Elderly may have normal WBC with serious disease
- Appendicitis missed 50% of the time
- CT abdominal/pelvis commonly used as serious organic disease is more prevalent
- Diverticulitis: WBC is normal 50% of the time

- Consider ruptured aortic aneurysm especially with flank pain thought to be renal colic
- Polypharmacy and medication side effects can be a cause of abdominal complaints

Pediatric abdominal pain

- Peritonitis patient is immobile
- Colic patient is writhing
- Absence of fever does not rule out serious illness
- Discuss with physician prior to ordering CT abdomen/pelvis in children

Pediatric appendicitis

- Frequently missed age < 2 years
- With abdominal pain, fever is most useful sign in appendicitis
- CBC may be normal
- Absolute neutrophil count < 6750 significantly decreases the likelihood of appendicitis
- Less than 50% have classic presentation
- Missed appendicitis is second most common reason for pediatric malpractice suits in the emergency department
- Perforation occurs in majority of patients < 4 years of age with appendicitis
- Treatment delayed > 36 hours increases rate of perforations up to 65% of appendicitis cases
- C-reactive protein is nonspecific and not helpful if positive in determining cause of inflammation or abdominal pain
- U/A can have pyuria, bacteriuria or hematuria in 20–40% of patients

General Evaluation

History

- Pain onset and duration
- Location and migration
- Appetite
- Exacerbating factors
- Prior surgical, medical and medication history

- Vomiting and fever history
- Bowel and urinary history
- Constitutional history
- Melena or bleeding
- Last normal menstrual cycle
- Menstrual abnormalities

Physical examination

- Observe for distension
- Auscultation for bowel sounds and arterial bruits
- Gently palpate entire abdomen
- Percuss for liver size; and for ascites if present
- Perform rectal exam for masses; tenderness; prostate disease; gross blood; occult blood when indicated
- Palpation of entire abdomen and document any findings of:
    - Tenderness location and severity
    - Rebound tenderness
    - Voluntary and involuntary guarding
    - Pulsatile masses
    - Abdominal masses

Objective testing

Benign findings and complaints in nonelderly healthy patient

- Consider no tests

Moderate complaints and findings, or if diabetic

- CBC and BMP

Urine or renal disease

- U/A
- CBC and BMP if pyelonephritis suspected
- Urine culture as indicated (complicated UTI)

Pancreatitis

- Amylase and lipase
- CBC and BMP

Gallbladder disease
- Gallbladder ultrasound as needed
- CBC and BMP
- Amylase, lipase and LFT's

Hepatic or metastatic malignant disease
- Liver function tests
- CBC and BMP

Fertile female
- UCG

Constipation or obstruction
- KUB or flat/upright films

Consider CT scan in adults for
- Suspected appendicitis or diverticulitis
- Flank pain of unknown etiology
- Rebound tenderness in adults
- Suspected bowel obstruction not seen on plain flat and upright abdominal films
- Elderly with moderate to severe pain

Discuss pediatric CT scans with physician prior to ordering – ultrasound can be used for appendicitis evaluation

Outpatient Treatment Considerations
- OTC medications
- Hydrocodone or synthetic codeine derivatives as needed
- Avoid Demerol (meperidine)
- Phenergan (promethazine) or Zofran (ondansetron) prn nausea or vomiting

Parenteral Treatment Considerations
- IV NS 100–1,000 cc/hour for adults as clinically indicated
- IV NS 1–2 times maintenance in children if stable, otherwise discuss with physician
- Nausea or vomiting (adjust for children)

  - Phenergan (promethazine) 6.25 mg IV (adult or pediatrics) or 25–50 mg IM adult or 0.5 mg/kg IM for children

    OR

  - Zofran (ondansetron) 4 mg IM or IV (adults and pediatrics)
- Pain control (adjust for children)
  - Stadol (butorphanol) 0.25–1 mg IV or 1–2 mg IM for adults

    OR

  - Dilaudid (hydromorphone) 0.25–1 mg IV or 1–2 mg IM for adult or 0.015 mg/Kg IV or IM for pediatrics
  - Small narcotic and Phenergan (promethazine) doses for the very elderly

Discharge Criteria

- Mild pain and tenderness in nonelderly healthy patient with normal vital signs consider symptomatic treatment if benign disease process suspected
- Biliary colic with normal vital signs and exam that resolves with treatment may not require labs and may be discharged
- Acute and self-limited process suspected such as gastroenteritis in stable nontoxic patient
- Reducible hernia

Discharge instructions

- To primary care provider or surgeon for follow-up in 1 day if pain is moderate to severe, otherwise in 5–7 days
- To primary care provider for abnormal lab within 1 week unless chronic in nature
- Abdominal pain aftercare instructions

Consult Criteria

- Moderate pain in age ≥ 60 years
- Abdominal pain that develops hypotension or relative hypotension (SBP < 105 with history of hypertension)
- Toxic appearance
- Dehydration

- Significant GI blood loss or melena
- Acute surgical abdomen or rebound tenderness
- Moderate to severe pain of uncertain cause
- Severe pain with any diagnosis
- Intractable vomiting
- Return ED visit within 14 days for same acute abdominal pain complaint

Discuss with physician if following suspected or diagnosed

- Appendicitis
- Cholecystitis
- Pancreatitis
- Diverticulitis
- Aortic aneurysm
- Bowel obstruction
- Ectopic pregnancy
- Intra-abdominal abscess
- Mesenteric ischemia
- Incarcerated or strangulated hernia

Lab consult criteria (if checked)

- Hemoglobin decrease > 1 gm or creatinine increase> 0.5 from baseline
- Hemoglobin < 10 gms
- Elevated LFT's
- Elevated amylase or lipase
- WBC ≥ 14,000
- Bandemia
- Increased anion gap
- Metabolic acidosis
- Significant electrolyte abnormally
- Glucose ≥ 400 mg/dL in diabetic patient
- Glucose ≥ 300 mg/dL in non-diabetic patient
- Hyperglycemia with metabolic acidosis (decreased serum CO2 or elevated anion gap)
- Acute thrombocytopenia

Vital sign and age consult criteria

- Any abdominal pain age ≥ 70 years

- Adult heart rate ≥ 110
- Pediatric heart rate
    - 0–4 months ≥ 180
    - 5–7 months ≥ 175
    - 6–12 months ≥ 170
    - 1–3 years ≥ 160
    - 4–5 years ≥ 145
    - 6–8 years ≥ 130
    - 7–12 years ≥ 125
    - 12–15 years ≥ 115
    - 16 years or older ≥ 110

Notes

CT Abdominal Scan Issues

When using any protocol, always follow the Guidelines of Proper Use (page 16).

Cancer Risk from One CT Estimated

- Adults: 1/1500–2000
- Children under 1 year of age: 1/500
- Decreasing risk with increasing age

Oral contrast considerations

- Adds little if anything to interpretation
- Some radiologists uncomfortable without it
- Appendicitis diagnosed without and with contrast
    - Sensitivity 95% vs. 92%
    - Specificity 97% vs. 94%
    - Accuracy 97% vs. 89%
- Message: Non-oral contrast CT is better in diagnosing appendicitis

IV contrast considerations

- Does not improve accuracy of noncontrast studies
- In very thin patients without much body fat IV contrast is needed

There is no connection between seafood and/or shellfish allergy and IV contrast allergy

Treatment of Allergy to IV Contrast

- Benadryl (diphenhydramine) 50 mg in adult or weight based in children
- Decadron (dexamethasone) 10 mg IV in adult or 0.6 mg/kg IV in children (not to exceed 10 mg)
- May not be effective since steroid dosing should be done 12 hours before IV contrast

Prior History of Asthma

- 1/1000 chance of severe reaction to IV contrast
- No reason to withhold contrast study

Creatinine Considerations

- Majority of patients do not need a creatinine measurement
- Needed with history of risk factors
    - Renal insufficiency
    - Elderly
    - Diabetes
    - Multiple myeloma
    - Volume depletion
    - Diuretic therapy
    - NSAID's use
    - ACE inhibitor use
    - CHF
    - Anemia

Prevention of Contrast-induced Nephropathy (CIN)

- There is a lack of good data
- Considerations for 0 or 1 risk factor above
    - Before procedure: 1 liter of D5W mixed with 3 amps of $NaHCO_3$ at 3 cc/kg for 1 hour
    - During procedure: low volume iso-osmolar contrast
    - After procedure: 1 liter of D5W mixed with 3 amps $NaHCO_3$ at 1 cc/kg for 6 hours
- Considerations for 2 or more risk factors — do above

Plus

- N-acetylcysteine 150 mg/kg IV 30 minutes before procedure and 600–1200 mg PO bid × 2 doses after procedure

OR

- Vitamin C 3 gms PO 2 hours before procedure and bid PO after procedure for 1 day

Metformin and IV contrast

- No increase in lactic acidosis if creatinine normal

Notes

ADULT GASTROENTERITIS PROTOCOL

When using any protocol, always follow the Guidelines of Proper Use (page 16).

Definition

- Acute inflammatory or infectious process of the stomach and intestines
- Rheumatoid Colitis
- Appendicitis
- Cholecystitis
- Pancreatitis
- Mesenteric ischemia
- Aortic aneurysm
- Peptic ulcer disease
- GERD
- Biliary colic
- Renal colic
- Bowel obstruction
- Inflammatory bowel disease

Definitions

- Diarrhea > 3 loose bowel movements (BM's) per day
- Dysentery
    - Disorders with intestinal inflammation (usually colon)
    - Abdominal pain
    - Tenesmus
    - Frequent BM's with blood and mucus in stool
- Enteritis — small bowel inflammation
- Gastritis — stomach inflammation
- Gastroenteritis symptoms
    - Acute inflammation of stomach and intestines with abdominal pain
    - Weakness
    - Nausea
    - Diarrhea

- Anorexia
- Fever

Considerations

- Diarrhea most common manifestation (virus most common cause)
- Enteritis — often with bloating, periumbilical pain, nausea/vomiting (viral most common cause)
- Colitis — can have localized left sided pain, rectal bleeding
- Antibiotics can cause diarrhea — C. difficile (antibiotic-associated or "pseudomembranous" colitis)
- Association between antibiotic use, enterohemorrhagic Escherichia coli and hemolytic-uremic syndrome remains unproven

Invasive bacteria — frequently with occult or gross blood

- Campylobacter
- Salmonella
- Shigella
- Vibrio
- Yersinia

Food-borne disease

- Staph aureus most common: 1–6 hours post food ingestion
- Bacillus cereus: 1–36 hours post food ingestion
- Cholera: profuse rice water stools
- Ciguatera: Fish; 5 minutes–30 hours
- Traveler's diarrhea: E. coli usually
- Camping: Giardia, water ingestion, beavers

Evaluation

- Travel, food and antibiotic history
- Healthy patient without toxicity and with acute onset of symptoms and mild to no tenderness and normal vital signs may not require further testing
- Consider CBC, BMP if vital signs abnormal or with significant tenderness

- Consider stool WBC, RBC, cultures for fever; blood in stool
- Consider rectal exam
- Imaging usually not necessary unless
  - Obstruction suspected
    - Abdominal flat and upright films
    - Consider CT abdomen/pelvis if bowel obstruction suspected and plain films negative
  - Consider CT abdomen/pelvis for elderly with abnormal vital signs and significant tenderness or pain

Treatment Options

Dehydration

Oral Rehydration Therapy (ORT) for mild to moderate dehydration

- Oral rehydration formula (WHO, Rehydralyte or Pedialyte) for mild to moderate dehydration or serum CO2 13–18 mEq/L or Na+ 146–152 mEq/L — if able to take PO fluids
  - Zofran (ondansetron) 8 mg chewable tablet if vomiting or 4–8 mg IM
  - 15–30 cc every 1–2 minutes for 1–4 hours for age > 12 — start 20 minutes after Zofran (ondansetron) given
  - Hold ORT 10 minutes if vomiting occurs then resume
  - Re-assess for urine production, improved heart rate, and absence of severe vomiting
  - Recheck serum CO2 if initially < 17 mEq/L
  - Mild dehydration give 20 cc/kg in < 4 hours
  - Moderate dehydration give 20–40 cc/kg in 1–4 hours
- Severe dehydration give IV NS 200–500 cc/hour over 2–4 hours or 1000 cc/hour for 1 hour (notify physician)
  - Hypotension or signs of poor organ perfusion (lactic acid > 2) give NS at

500–1,000 cc/hour up to 2 liters or IV 500–1,000 cc bolus (consult physician promptly)

Diarrhea

- Nontoxic, non-dehydrated healthy patients with mild abdominal tenderness, benign vital signs and diarrhea may be discharged without further testing
- Pepto-Bismol — good for traveler's diarrhea
- Quinolone 1, 3 or 5 day course, especially with traveler's diarrhea
- If C. difficile colitis suspected from recent antibiotic use:
    - Mild to moderate symptoms
        - Flagyl (metronidazole) 500 mg PO tid × 10 days
        - Floristor PO bid × 10 days (OTC)
    - Severe symptoms consult physician
    - Stop offending antibiotic
    - See primary care provider within 1–2 days for follow-up

Antimotility agents

- Loperamide (most preferred due to safety profile)
- Diphenoxylate (heme negative stools only)

Vomiting

- Phenergan (promethazine) PO/PR/IM (if IV give no more than 6.25 mg/dose as single dose)
- Zofran (ondansetron) 4–8 mg PO/IM/IV

Abdominal pain treatment outpatient considerations

- OTC medications
- Hydrocodone or synthetic codeine derivatives as needed
- Avoid Demerol (meperidine)

Abdominal pain parenteral treatment considerations

- Stadol (butorphanol), Nubain (nalbuphine) or Dilaudid (hydromorphone): IV or IM — avoid Demerol (meperidine)
- Give Phenergan (promethazine) 6.25 mg (if IV) or Zofran (ondansetron) as needed for nausea
- Adjust doses for weight in pediatrics

Discharge Criteria

- Healthy nontoxic patient with stable vital signs

Discharge instructions

- Gastroenteritis aftercare instructions
- Resume regular diet as soon as possible
- To primary care provider for follow-up in 1–2 days if symptoms are moderate to severe if discharged, otherwise within 5–7 days if symptoms persist
- To primary care provider for abnormal lab within 1 week unless chronic in nature
- Return within 3 days if symptoms not improving

Consult Criteria

- Toxic appearance
- Dehydration > 5%
- Significant blood loss or melena
- Suspected or diagnosed appendicitis, cholecystitis, pancreatitis, diverticulitis, aortic aneurysm, bowel obstruction
- Acute surgical abdomen
- Moderate pain of uncertain cause
- Severe pain
- Narcotic IM/IV dosing that is given acutely
- Intractable vomiting
- Return ED visit within 14 days for same acute abdominal pain complaint

Lab consult criteria (if checked)

- Metabolic acidosis (increased anion gap)
- Hemoglobin decrease > 1 gm or creatinine increase> 0.5 from baseline

- Elevated LFT's
- Elevated amylase or lipase
- WBC ≥ 15,000
- Bandemia
- Significant electrolyte abnormally
- Glucose ≥ 400 mg/dL in diabetic patient
- Glucose ≥ 300 mg/dL in non-diabetic patient
- Hyperglycemia with metabolic acidosis (decreased serum CO2 or elevated anion gap)
- Acute thrombocytopenia

Vital sign and age consult criteria

- Age ≥ 70
- Adult heart rate > 100 post-treatment
- Hypotension or relative hypotension (SBP < 105 with history of hypertension)
- Orthostatic vital signs

Notes

IRRITABLE BOWEL SYNDROME PROTOCOL

When using any protocol, always follow the Guidelines of Proper Use (page 16).

Definition

- A functional disorder without specific pathology of abdominal pain and altered bowel habits

Differential Diagnosis

- Anxiety disorder
- Biliary colic
- Inflammatory bowel disease
- Ischemic colitis
- Antibiotic-associated colitis
- Endometriosis
- Gastroenteritis
- Food allergies
- Malabsorption
- Porphyria
- Colon carcinoma
- Thyroid disease

Considerations

- Is a disorder of exclusion of other disease processes
- Hypersensitivity to pain and symptoms
- Association with psychopathology common
- Is a chronic relapsing disorder
- Females 2–3 times more likely to have the disorder than males

Common Symptoms and Findings

- Abdominal pain
- Diarrhea
- Constipation
- Mucus in stool
- Abdominal distension

- Stress related commonly
- Fibromyalgia is frequently present

Symptoms not consistent with IBS

- Middle age or later onset
- New symptom presentations
- Fever
- Weight loss
- Nocturnal symptoms
- Progressive symptoms
- Rectal bleeding
- Painless diarrhea

Evaluation

- History and physical examination
    - Rectal examination for occult blood as indicated

Lab test options

- CBC
- BMP
- Thyroid panel as indicated
- Plain flat and upright x-rays as indicated
- Amylase and lipase as indicated
- CT abdominal and pelvis scan as indicated (usually not needed)

Treatment Options

- Add fiber to diet
- Reassurance regarding symptoms and diagnosis
- Stress management suggestions
- Consider psychiatric referral

Antispasmodic agents

- Bentyl (dicyclomine) 10–40 mg PO qid ac (before meals) or with pain onset
- Levsin (hyoscyamine) 0.125– 0.25 mg q4hr and or prn (NMT 1.5 pills/day) for adults
- Levsin (hyoscyamine) 1/2–1 pill qid PO q4hr or prn (NMT 6 tabs/day) for age 2–12 years

Antidiarrheal agents

Lomotil (diphenoxylate/atropine)

- Age > 12 years: 1–2 tabs PO qid ac prn
- Age 8–12 years: 2 mg PO 5 times qday prn
- Age 5–7 years: 2 mg PO qid prn
- Age 2–4 years: 2 mg PO tid prn

Imodium (loperamide)

- Adult: 4 mg PO after 1st loose stool, then 2 mg PO after each following loose stool prn (NMT 16 mg/day)
- Pediatric: 0.1 mg/kg PO after each loose stool not to exceed adult total daily dose

Other agents

- SSRI's
- Elavil 10–100 mg PO qday prn (start low dose)

Discharge Criteria

- No other concerning disease process diagnosed

Discharge instructions

- Irritable bowel syndrome aftercare instructions
- Follow up with PCP within 10 days or as needed

Consult Criteria

- WBC ≥ 14,000
- Severe pain
- Age ≥ 60 years
- Heart rate > 100
- Dehydration
- Patient appears toxic
- Fever
- Weight loss
- Progressive symptoms
- Rectal bleeding
- See General Patient Criteria Protocol (page 20) for items not covered in this protocol

Notes

APPENDICITIS PROTOCOL

When using any protocol, always follow the Guidelines of Proper Use (page 16).

Definition

- Inflammation of the appendix secondary to luminal obstruction

Differential Diagnosis

- Pelvic inflammatory disease
- Ruptured ovarian cyst
- Endometriosis
- Mesenteric adenitis
- Inflammatory bowel disease
- Colon carcinoma
- Mesenteric ischemia
- Ureteral colic
- Pyelonephritis
- Biliary colic
- Abdominal abscess
- Diverticulitis
- Ectopic pregnancy
- Ovarian torsion
- Constipation

Considerations

- Appendicitis missed 50% of the time in elderly

Presentations

- Migration of pain from periumbilical area to RLQ has sensitivity and specificity of 80%
- Nausea present in 61–92% of patients
- Anorexia present in 74–78% of patients
- Diarrhea or constipation noted in around 18% of patients
- Duration of symptoms less than 48 hours in 80% of adults, but may be longer in elderly and with perforation

- History of previous similar pain noted in 23% of patients and should not be used to rule out appendicitis
- Common to have low-grade fever or no fever
- High fever develops with abscess formation secondary to appendiceal rupture
- Fecaliths and lymphoid hyperplasia most common causes secondary to luminal obstruction

Physical findings

- 96% of patients with RLQ tenderness — most specific sign
- The most specific exam findings are guarding, percussion tenderness, rebound tenderness and rigidity
- Rosving, Obturator, Psoas signs present in minority of patients and their absence should not be used to rule out appendicitis

Lab findings

- Normal C-reactive protein after abdominal pain for 24 hours has a high negative predictive value ruling out appendicitis
- U/A showing WBC's and urinary complaints not uncommon in appendicitis

Pregnancy and appendicitis

- First trimester pain in RLQ
- Second trimester pain at level of umbilicus
- Third trimester pain in RUQ
- Anorexia in one-third to two-thirds of patients
- Nausea usually present

Pediatric appendicitis

- Frequently missed age < 2 years
- With abdominal pain, fever is most useful sign in appendicitis
- CBC may be normal
- Absolute neutrophil count < 6750 significantly decreases the likelihood of appendicitis
- Less than 50% have classic presentation

- Missed appendicitis is second most common reason for pediatric malpractice suits in the emergency department
- Perforation occurs in majority of patients < 4 years of age with appendicitis
- Treatment delayed > 36 hours increases rate of perforations up to 65% of appendicitis cases
- C-reactive protein is nonspecific and not helpful if positive in determining cause of inflammation or abdominal pain
- Appendicitis: U/A can have pyuria, bacteriuria or hematuria in 20–40%

Evaluation

- History and physical examination
    - Specific attention to onset and progression of symptoms

Testing

- CBC
- BMP
- U/A
- UCG in fertile females (includes those with bilateral tubal ligations)
- LFT's as indicated
- Amylase and lipase as indicated
- Plain flat and upright if obstruction suspected
- CT abdominal and pelvic scan in adults as needed
- CT abdominal and pelvic scans in pediatrics needs serious consideration of the risk potential for later cancer development — discuss with physician before ordering
    - Ultrasound has usefulness in pediatric appendicitis

Discharge Criteria

- None

Consult Criteria

- All appendicitis or suspected appendicitis patients

Notes

ANTIBIOTIC-ASSOCIATED COLITIS PROTOCOL

When using any protocol, always follow the Guidelines of Proper Use (page 16).

Definition

- Inflammation of the bowel secondary to Clostridium difficile and recent antibiotic use or hospitalization

Differential Diagnosis

- Crohn's disease
- Ulcerative colitis
- Irritable bowel syndrome
- Gastroenteritis
- Toxic megacolon
- Diverticulitis

Considerations

- 20% of hospitalized patients acquire the infection
    - Diarrhea develop in 30% of these
- Colitis is caused by a toxin produced by C. difficile
- Should be considered with antibiotic use past 2 months or hospitalization in past 3 days
- Asymptomatic colonization occurs in 1–3% of the healthy population
- A brief exposure to an antibiotic can cause C. difficile colitis
    - Symptoms usually start 3–9 days after antibiotic initiation
- Age ≥ 60 years is a risk factor
- Relapse after treatment is common
- Elevated WBC is found in 50–60% of patients

Symptoms and Findings

- Mild to moderate watery diarrhea
    - Usually not bloody
- Crampy abdominal pain

- Loss of appetite
- Fever usually in severe cases
- Lower abdominal tenderness
    - Rebound tenderness suggests bowel perforation

Evaluation

- History and physical examination
- Lab test options
    - CBC
    - BMP
    - U/A
    - Stool cultures for C. difficile and other pathogens
    - Enzyme immunoassay for C. difficile A and B toxins
        - Available in 2.5 hours
        - Sensitivity 75–80%
- Imaging options
    - Plain upright and flat x-rays if toxic megacolon suspected
    - CT abdominal and pelvis scan may be needed

Treatment Options

- Stop antibiotics (consult physician if antibiotic treatment crucial in treating previous condition)
    - May be all that is needed in mild cases without fever, abdominal pain and elevated WBC
- Mild to moderate diarrhea or colitis
    - Flagyl (metronidazole) 500 mg PO tid for 10–14 days
    - Floristor PO bid for 10–14 days (over the counter)
- More severe cases
    - Vancomycin 125 mg PO qid for 10 days
    - Floristor PO bid for 10–14 days (over the counter)
- Antidiarrheal agents should be avoided
- Analgesics
- Symptoms improve usually in 3 days on above antibiotics

Discharge Criteria

- Mild to moderate C. difficile or antibiotic-associated colitis
- See General Patient Criteria Protocol (page 20)

Discharge instructions

- Antibiotic-associated colitis aftercare instructions
- Stop current antibiotics
- Follow up with primary care provider within 3–5 days
- Return if symptoms worsen or do not improve
- Wash hands frequently with soap and water

Consult Criteria

- Fever
- WBC ≥ 15,000
- Severe pain
- Rebound tenderness
- CT scan shows colitis
- Dehydration
- See General Patient Criteria Protocol (page 20)

Notes

INFLAMMATORY BOWEL DISEASE PROTOCOL

When using any protocol, always follow the Guidelines of Proper Use (page 16).

Definition

- Inflammatory disorder of unknown cause from ulcerative colitis or Crohn's disease

Differential Diagnosis

- Appendicitis
- Diverticulitis
- Endometriosis
- Pelvic inflammatory disease
- Colon carcinoma
- Antibiotic-associated colitis
- Irritable bowel syndrome
- Ischemic colitis

Considerations

- Ulcerative colitis is limited to the large intestine
- Crohn's disease can be anywhere in the gastrointestinal tract
- Kidney stone incidence is increased in Crohn's disease
- Smoking increases the risk Crohn's flares and severity of disease

Ulcerative colitis presentations and findings

- Bloody diarrhea
- Abdominal pain and cramping
- Fever in more severe cases
- Rectal tenesmus or urgency
- Nausea and vomiting
- Dehydration
- Anemia
- Total colectomy is curative

Crohn's disease

- Insidious onset
- Usually nonbloody diarrhea
- Half of cases have perianal fistulas or abscesses
- Weight loss
- Skip regions of intestinal involvement
- Fever
- Arthritis
- Uveitis
- Hepatitis
- Anemia

Evaluation

- History and physical examination
- Lab test options
  - CBC
  - BMP
  - LFT's
  - Amylase and lipase
  - U/A
- Imaging options
  - Plain upright and flat x-rays if toxic megacolon suspected
  - CT abdominal and pelvis scan

Treatment

Crohn's disease

Mild disease

- Antidiarrheal medications qid for diarrhea without active colitis
  - Imodium (loperamide) 2 mg PO qid prn
  - Lomotil (diphenoxylate/atropine) 5 mg PO qid prn

Moderate disease

- Prednisone 30–60 mg PO qday 7–10 days
- Sulfasalazine 0.5–1.5 gms PO 2–4 times a day for mild to moderate disease
- Flagyl (metronidazole) 250–500 mg PO qid for fistula complications for 1 month

Ulcerative colitis

Mild disease

- Antidiarrheal medications qid for diarrhea without active colitis
  - Imodium (loperamide) 2 mg PO qid prn
  - Lomotil (diphenoxylate/atropine) 5 mg PO qid prn

Moderate disease

- Prednisone 30–60 mg PO for 7–14 days followed by taper of 5 mg/week (should see PCP within 1–3 days after discharge)

Discharge Criteria

- Mild to moderate disease
- Prior history of Crohn's disease or ulcerative colitis
- Heart rate ≤ 100 for age ≥ 14 years

Discharge instructions

- Crohn's disease or ulcerative colitis aftercare instructions
- Smoking cessation for Crohn's disease patients
- Follow up with PCP within 1–3 days
- Refer perianal disease to surgeon within 7–10 days

Consult Criteria

- Severe pain
- Fever
- Heart rate > 110/minute for age ≥ 14 years
- WBC ≥ 13,000
- Dehydration
- Hypotension
- Appears toxic
- Toxic megacolon
- Unable to self hydrate
- Vomiting
- Progressive anemia
- Hemoglobin < 10 gms

- See General Patient Criteria Protocol (page 20) for items not in this protocol

Notes

Reference:
Mayo Clin Proc, June 2011, pg. 557

Gastroesophageal Reflux Disease (GERD) Protocol

When using any protocol, always follow the Guidelines of Proper Use (page 16).

Definition

- When the amount of gastric juice that refluxes into the esophagus exceeds the normal limit, causing symptoms with or without associated esophageal mucosal injury

Differential Diagnosis

- Acute coronary syndrome
- Biliary colic
- Peptic ulcer disease
- Esophagitis
- Esophageal spasm
- Achalasia
- Irritable bowel syndrome
- Asthma from aspiration

Considerations

- 40% of the population experience GERD monthly
- Most patients with hiatal hernias do not experience clinically significant reflux
- Acid secretion is the same with or without GERD

Causes and effects

- Obesity
- Smoking
- Decrease in lower esophageal sphincter (LES) tone or function (most common cause)
- Erosive gastritis
- Esophageal stricture
- UGI bleeding
- Recurrent pneumonia
- Asthma

Medications that can cause:

- Calcium channel blockers
- Nitrates
- Beta-blockers
- Theophylline

Foods and beverages that can cause:

- Coffee
- Chocolate
- Tea
- Alcohol
- Tomato products
- Citrus products

Signs and Symptoms

- Heartburn (burning from epigastric up through chest to neck at times)
- Dysphagia
- Odynophagia
- Regurgitation
- Belching
- Worse bending over or lying down
- Usually transiently relieved with antacids

Evaluation

- Consider high risk differential diagnoses and test as indicated

Treatment Options

- Antacids
- Analgesics (excluding NSAID's or aspirin)
- Avoid late night or heavy meals
- Stop smoking and alcohol intake
- Avoid drugs and foods/beverages that decrease LES
- Reglan (metoclopramide) — caution with long term usage — tardive dyskinesia)
- H2 blockers prn
- Proton pump inhibitors prn
- Elevate head of bed 6-8 inches
- Fundoplication (refer to surgery as outpatient)

Discharge Criteria

- Uncomplicated GERD
- Refer to primary care provider or gastroenterologist within 1–3 weeks

Discharge instructions

- GERD aftercare instructions

Consult Criteria

- UGI bleeding
- Esophageal obstruction
- Dehydration
- Toxic appearing patients
- Uncertain diagnosis as cause of patient complaints
- Refer to General Patient Criteria Protocol (page 20) as needed

Notes

PEPTIC ULCER DISEASE AND GASTRITIS PROTOCOL

When using any protocol, always follow the Guidelines of Proper Use (page 16).

Definition

- Inflammatory changes in the gastric mucosa or discrete mucosal defect in the stomach or duodenum

Differential Diagnosis

- GERD
- Gastroenteritis
- Acute coronary syndrome
- Biliary colic
- Peptic ulcer disease
- Esophagitis
- Esophageal spasm
- Irritable bowel syndrome
- Abdominal aortic aneurysm
- Mesenteric ischemia
- Hepatitis
- Inflammatory bowel disease
- Pancreatitis
- Pulmonary embolism

Considerations

- Consider high risk differential diagnoses and test as indicated

Causes

- H. pylori responsible for 90–95% of duodenal ulcers and 80% of gastric ulcers
- NSAID's interfere with prostaglandin synthesis and lead to breakdown in mucosa
- Smoking
- Alcohol intake
- Aspirin

- Steroids

Signs and Symptoms

- Epigastric pain and burning 80–90%
- Epigastric tenderness
- Gastric ulcer pain worsened by food
- Duodenal ulcer pain improved by food
- Nausea
- Vomiting
- UGI bleeding
- Hematemesis
- Melena
- Peritonitis with perforation
- Anemia

Evaluation Options

- Mild symptoms and findings with normal vital signs treat symptomatically
- Moderate or severe symptoms or tenderness
    - CBC
    - BMP
    - Amylase
    - Lipase
    - Consider LFT's
- Peritonitis findings
    - Upright chest x-ray and abdominal films to evaluate for free air
    - CT abdominal and pelvis if diagnosis is uncertain or age ≥ 65 years
- EKG
    - Age ≥ 60 years with unimpressive abdominal exam and no cardiac risk factors
    - Age < 60 years with cardiac risk factors for coronary artery disease with unimpressive abdominal exam
    - Consider CT abdominal/pelvis scan with age ≥ 70 if diagnosis not reasonably certain

Treatment Options

- Unstable patient notify physician immediately

- Stable nonacute patient
    - Antacids prn
    - H2 blockers
    - Proton pump inhibitors × 1–2 months

Antibiotics with PPI only if H. pylori documented with testing

- Biaxin (clarithromycin) 500 mg PO × 14 days
- Flagyl (metronidazole) 500 mg PO × 14 days

OR

- Biaxin (clarithromycin) 500 mg PO bid × 14 days
- Amoxicillin 1,000 mg bid × 14 days

Discharge Criteria

- Uncomplicated exam and findings consistent with gastritis or peptic ulcer disease

Discharge instructions

- Peptic ulcer or gastritis aftercare instructions
- To primary care provider for follow-up in 1 day if pain is moderate to severe, otherwise in 5–7 days
- To primary care provider for abnormal lab within 1 week unless chronic in nature
- Return within 3 days if not improving

Consult Criteria

- GI bleeding
- Moderate pain age ≥ 65 years
- Abdominal pain that develops hypotension or relative hypotension (SBP < 105 with history of hypertension)
- Toxic appearance
- Dehydration
- Significant blood loss or melena
- Suspected or diagnosed appendicitis, cholecystitis, pancreatitis, diverticulitis, aortic aneurysm, bowel obstruction
- Acute surgical abdomen or rebound tenderness
- Moderate to severe pain of uncertain cause
- Severe pain with any diagnosis

- Intractable vomiting
- Return ED visit within 14 days for same acute abdominal pain complaint

Lab consult criteria (if checked)

- Hemoglobin decrease > 1 gm or creatinine increase> 0.5 from baseline
- Elevated LFT's
- Elevated amylase or lipase
- WBC ≥ 14,000
- Bandemia
- Increased anion gap
- Significant electrolyte abnormally
- Glucose ≥ 400 mg/dL in diabetic patient
- Glucose ≥ 300 mg/dL in non-diabetic patient
- Hyperglycemia with metabolic acidosis (decreased serum CO2 or elevated anion gap)
- Acute thrombocytopenia

Vital sign and age consult criteria

- Age ≥ 70 years
- Adult heart rate ≥ 110
- Pediatric heart rate
    - 0–4 months ≥ 180
    - 5–7 months ≥ 175
    - 6–12 months ≥ 170
    - 1–3 years ≥ 160
    - 4–5 years ≥ 145
    - 6–8 years ≥ 130
    - 7–12 years ≥ 125
    - 12–15 years ≥ 115
    - 16 years or older ≥ 110

GALLBLADDER DISEASE PROTOCOL

When using any protocol, always follow the Guidelines of Proper Use (page 16).

Definition

- Disease of gallbladder from gallstone obstruction of cystic duct or infection and inflammation of the gallbladder without gallstones

Differential Diagnosis

- Peptic ulcer disease
- Acute myocardial infarction
- Angina
- Right-sided pulmonary embolism
- Right pneumonia
- Right renal colic
- Hepatitis
- Mesenteric ischemia
- Cholangitis
- Pyelonephritis
- Gastroenteritis
- Aortic aneurysm
- Pancreatitis

Considerations

- Common in females age ≥ 40 years
- Moderate to severe pain and tenderness RUQ of abdomen
- Nausea and vomiting very common
- Charcot's triad: (1) Jaundice, (2) Fever, (3) RUQ abdominal pain
- Fever occurs with advanced disease
- Increased morbidity and mortality in diabetes
- Ascending cholangitis is a life threatening infection of common bile duct

- May increase LFT's, amylase, lipase and bilirubin with common duct gallstones
- Acalculus cholecystitis has a higher mortality than cholecystitis with gallstones
    - Seen more in elderly and diabetic patients

Evaluation

- History for
    - Onset
    - Severity
    - Duration
    - Associated symptoms
    - Previous episodes
- Abdominal exam for
    - Tenderness
    - Guarding
    - Rebound tenderness
    - Distension

Testing options

- CBC
- U/A
- UCG if fertile female
- LFT's
- Amylase
- Lipase
- Gallbladder ultrasound may be needed with elevated WBC and if amylase or lipase elevated
- If pain, tenderness and vomiting resolve with treatment, testing may not be needed

Treatment Options

- IV NS 1 liter bolus if hypotensive (notify physician promptly)
- Pain and vomiting treatment
- Dilaudid (hydromorphone) prn
- Stadol (butorphanol) prn
- Nubain (nalbuphine) prn
- Phenergan (promethazine) or Zofran (ondansetron) prn

Discharge Criteria

- Resolution of pain, tenderness, vomiting
- Gallbladder ultrasound without findings of cholecystitis or choledocholithiasis (if performed)
- No fever or chills
- Diagnosis reasonable certain for biliary colic

Discharge instructions

- Gallbladder disease aftercare instructions
- Return within 1 day if pain persists or worsens
- Refer to general surgeon or primary care provider within 7 days

Consult Criteria

- WBC ≥ 13,000
- Bandemia ≥ 15%
- Rebound tenderness
- Intractable nausea or vomiting
- Pain not resolved with treatment
- Cholecystitis
- Choledocholithiasis
- Cholangitis

Lab consult criteria

- Hemoglobin decrease > 1 gm or creatinine increase> 0.5 from baseline
- Elevated LFT's
- Elevated amylase or lipase
- Increased anion gap
- Acute thrombocytopenia
- Significant electrolyte abnormally
- Glucose ≥ 300 mg/dL in diabetic patient
- Glucose ≥ 200 mg/dL in non-diabetic patient
- Hyperglycemia with metabolic acidosis (decreased serum CO2 or elevated anion gap)

Vital sign and age consult criteria

- Age ≥ 60
- Adult HR ≥ 110 post treatment
- Hypotension or orthostatic vital signs

Notes

HEPATITIS PROTOCOL

When using any protocol, always follow the Guidelines of Proper Use (page 16).

Definition

- Inflammation of the liver

Differential Diagnosis

- Biliary colic
- Cholecystitis
- Cholangitis
- Peptic ulcer disease
- Gastritis
- Gastroenteritis
- Aortic aneurysm
- Pancreatitis

Considerations

- Frequently asymptomatic
- Ranges from asymptomatic to fulminate hepatitis and liver failure
- Misdiagnosed frequently as nonspecific viral syndrome
- Viral causes are most frequent: hepatitis A – 40%, hepatitis B – 30%, hepatitis C – 20%
    - Hepatitis A: fecal-oral transmission most common cause
    - Hepatitis B: exposure to infected blood or body fluids most common cause
    - Hepatitis C: percutaneous exposures most common cause
- Autoimmune disorders can cause hepatitis
- Toxic causes
- Acetaminophen is frequent worldwide cause (can cause liver failure)
- Ethanol (causes 50% of end-stage liver disease in U.S.)
- Isoniazid
- Ecstasy (MDMA)
- Industrial solvents and cleaning solutions

- Iron

Viral hepatitis

Risk factors

- Male homosexuality
- Hemodialysis
- IV drug abuse
- Raw seafood
- Blood product transfusion
- Tattoos or body piercing
- Foreign travel
- Sexual exposure to hepatitis B carrier

Preicteric phase

- Flu-like illness with fever, chills and malaise
- Nausea, vomiting, anorexia

Icteric phase

- Dark urine
- Light stools
- Pruritus
- Right upper quadrant tenderness
- Tender hepatomegaly

Nonalcoholic fatty liver most common cause of elevated LFT's in U.S. (ALT > AST frequently)

- Associated with obesity; Type-II DM; hyperlipidemia
- Most patients asymptomatic
- Bilirubin rarely elevated
- Can lead to hepatic cirrhosis
- Treatment is weight loss
- Usually a benign course

Evaluation

- Complete history and physical exam
- Alcohol and drug history
- Special attention to acetaminophen or acetaminophen containing medicines

- Check acetaminophen level if ALT elevated with possible history of acetaminophen containing medication usage
- CBC
- BMP
- LFT's (SGOT/AST is commonly 2 times > SGPT/ALT in alcoholic hepatitis)
- PT/PTT/INR
- Ammonia level if encephalopathic
- Rectal exam if encephalopathic for stool blood or BUN elevated out of proportion to creatinine level
- U/A
- Consider viral serology
- Monospot if pharyngitis present
- Acetaminophen level if suspected usage

Treatment Options

- IV D50W 1 amp if hypoglycemic
- Hypotension give 250-500 cc NS bolus and notify physician
- Treat ongoing hypoglycemia with D5 1/2NS drip of 100-150 cc/hour
- Usually supportive
- Acetadote for acetaminophen toxicity as indicated
    - May need treatment if ALT elevated with history of recent acetaminophen containing medication usage, even if acetaminophen level is 0
- Cessation of ethanol use
- No acetaminophen

Discharge Criteria

- Stable patient
- PT < 3 seconds elevation
- INR < 1.5
- See General Patient Criteria Protocol (page 20)

Discharge instructions

- Hepatitis aftercare instructions
- Primary care provider within 1-2 days
- Gastroenterology within 1-2 days unless chronic liver disease without acute exacerbation

Consult Criteria

- Toxic acetaminophen level on nomogram or elevated ALT regardless of level if acetaminophen containing medication usage is suspected
- Hypoglycemia
- Altered mental status
- PT prolonged > 3 seconds
- INR > 1.5
- Bilirubin > 5
- Intractable vomiting
- Significant comorbid conditions
- Significant electrolyte or fluid disturbances
- Age ≥ 70
- Ascites
- GI bleeding
- Immunosuppression
- Fever
- LFT's > 5 times normal

Notes

Gastrointestinal Bleeding Protocol

When using any protocol, always follow the Guidelines of Proper Use (page 16).

Differential Diagnosis

- Peptic ulcer disease
- Esophagitis
- Mallory-Weiss tear
- Esophageal varices
- Diverticular disease
- Colon cancer
- Colon polyps
- Arteriovenous malformation
- Aortoenteric fistula
- Hemorrhoids

Considerations

- Upper gastrointestinal (UGI) bleeding can cause melena
- UGI bleeding
  - Rapid transit can cause gross blood per rectum
  - Elevates BUN out of proportion to creatinine
  - Can lead to hepatic encephalopathy in hepatic cirrhosis patients
- Lower gastrointestinal (LGI) bleeding
  - Bright or dark red gross blood
  - Frequently painless
  - Frequently a diverticular source in elderly
- Hemorrhoidal bleeding usually bright red and not mixed with stools
- Can present with dyspnea, chest pain; syncope, altered mental status

Evaluation

- Complete history and physical exam (including rectal exam for hemoccult testing or gross bleeding)

- Medication history
- Prior GI history
- CBC
- BMP
- PT/INR
- PTT if on heparin
- Ammonia and LFT's if mental status altered
- Type and screen for history of significant bleeding
- Type and cross if
  - Hypotensive
  - Adult heart rate ≥ 120
  - Orthostatic vital signs
- Hemorrhoidal bleeding with benign bleeding history and normal vital signs may not need lab tests

Treatment Options

- IV NS 500–1000 cc bolus if hypotensive adult (notify physician promptly)
- Pediatric: 20 cc/kg IV NS bolus, may repeat × 2 prn if hypotensive (notify physician promptly)
- Proton pump inhibitors (PPI) for upper GI bleeding or peptic ulcer disease/gastritis/esophagitis
- Transfusion with PRBC's/FFP/platelets 2:1:1 ratio if hypotension persists or significant acute anemia (consult physician promptly first)
- Avoid > 2 liters of isotonic fluids for acute blood loss before transfusion of blood products started if possible
- Consider N-G tube for UGI bleeding (consult physician)

Hemorrhoids

External hemorrhoids

Medical treatment for mild to moderate painful thrombosed hemorrhoids

- Warm soaks (sitz baths) or hot towel applied in lateral decubitus position
- Stool softeners
- Anusol, Anusol HC or Protofoam HC topical preparations
- Tuck's pads prn (witch hazel)
- Analgesics

- Avoid exacerbating activities

Excisional treatment for severe painful acute thrombosed hemorrhoids (usually within 72 hours of symptoms)

- Prep area with betadine
- Spread buttocks with assistant's help or use tape
- Infiltrate base of hemorrhoid with 2–5 cc of 1% lidocaine with epinephrine (use plain lidocaine in coronary artery disease patients)
- Infiltrate into the hemorrhoid with 1–2 cc of lidocaine with epinephrine (use plain lidocaine in coronary artery disease patients)
- Elliptical incision (preferred) in roof/top of hemorrhoid 2–3 mm wide radially in line from anus
  - Avoid deeper anal verge and sphincter
- Remove clots(s) by expressing or with forceps
- May be packed with 0.25 gauze (removed in 6 hours) or have gelfoam applied as needed
- Analgesics

Internal hemorrhoids

Medical treatment similar to external hemorrhoid treatment

Discharge Criteria

- Healthy patient
- Normal vital signs
- Stable CBC if checked
- Normal coagulation studies if checked
- Good follow up
- Negative or insignificant blood on rectal exam

Discharge instructions

- GI bleeding or hemorrhoid aftercare instructions

- Refer to primary care provider or GI physician within 5–7 days

Consult Criteria

- Significant blood loss or melena present
- Hematemesis
- Suspected or diagnosed aortic aneurysm
- Acute surgical abdomen
- Moderate to severe pain of uncertain cause
- Severe pain with any diagnosis
- Return ED visit within 14 days for same complaint

Vital signs and age consult criteria

- Age ≥ 70
- SBP < 90 or relative hypotension (SBP < 110 with history of hypertension)
- Adult heart rate > 100
- Orthostatic vital signs
- Pediatric heart
  - 0–4 months ≥ 180
  - 5–7 months ≥ 175
  - 6–12 months ≥ 170
  - 1–3 years ≥ 160
  - 4–5 years ≥ 145
  - 6–8 years ≥ 130
  - 7–12 years ≥ 125
  - 12–15 years ≥ 115
  - 16 years or older ≥ 110

Lab consult criteria

- Hemoglobin < 12 gms unless chronic
- Hemoglobin decrease > 1 gm
- Bandemia ≥ 15%
- Metabolic acidosis
- Significant electrolyte abnormally
- Glucose ≥ 400 mg/dL in diabetic patient or > 200 mg/dL in non-diabetic patient
- Hyperglycemia with metabolic acidosis (decreased serum CO2 or elevated anion gap)
- Acute thrombocytopenia (common in alcoholics)

- Elevated coagulation studies
- Creatinine increase > 0.5 from baseline
- Elevated LFT's

Notes

GASTROINTESTINAL FOREIGN BODY PROTOCOL

When using any protocol, always follow the Guidelines of Proper Use (page 16).

Definition

- Ingestion of a foreign body that may or may not be impacted

Considerations

- Most pass without assistance or danger once past the pylorus
- Sharp objects > 5 cm or multiple in number may need endoscopic removal

Esophageal foreign body

Symptoms

- Foreign body sensation
- Dysphagia

Areas of narrowing

- Cricopharyngeus muscle (most common)
    - C6
- Aortic arch and tracheal carina
    - T4
    - T6
- Lower esophageal sphincter (GE junction)
    - T11

Evaluation options

Chest x-ray findings

- Coins
    - Tracheal foreign body
        - Oriented anterior–posterior
    - Esophageal foreign body
        - Oriented transversely
- Bones may be seen on chest x-ray

Gastrograffin or barium swallow

- For nonopaque foreign bodies

CT scan

- For nonopaque foreign bodies
- Superior to gastrograffin or barium swallow

Button battery

- Must be removed immediately if lodged in esophagus
  - If passed esophagus does not need immediate removal
  - If passed pylorus in 48 hours does not need removal
- Rapid burns occur within 6 hours if impacted
- Lithium batteries have worse outcomes
- Consult physician immediately for retained esophageal button battery
  - **Intranasal button batteries need immediate removal**

Esophageal food impaction

- Esophageal disease present usually
  - Esophageal stricture from GERD common
- Complete obstruction patient cannot hold saliva down

Treatment options

- Endoscopic removal
- Glucagon (not too successful)
  - Adult 1–2 mg IV may repeat in 10–20 minutes if needed
  - Pediatric 0.02–0.03 mg/kg IV (NMT 0.5 mg)
- Foley catheter removal
  - Performed by physician if available
  - Do not use
    - If esophageal disease present
    - Foreign body present more than 72 hours

Discharge Criteria

- Resolved foreign body impaction
- Benign foreign body that will likely pass
- Button battery
  - If passed esophagus
  - If passed pylorus in 48 hours

Discharge instructions

- Esophageal or gastrointestinal foreign body aftercare instructions
- Refer to GI or PCP within 48 hours to assess foreign body evacuation

Consult Criteria

- Retained esophageal foreign bodies
- Sharp foreign bodies
- Button battery in esophagus
- Unresolved esophageal food impaction
- Continued symptoms of foreign body
- Continued dysphagia
- Foreign bodies unlikely to spontaneously pass

Notes

ANORECTAL DISORDER PROTOCOL

When using any protocol, always follow the Guidelines of Proper Use (page 16).

Conditions

- Hemorrhoids
- Anal Fissure
- Perianal/perirectal abscess
- Rectal prolapse
- Pruritus ani
- Pilonidal cyst/abscess

Hemorrhoids

Definition

- Pathologic swelling of veins in the rectum

Differential diagnosis

- Rectal prolapse
- Proctitis
- Crohn's disease and ulcerative colitis
- Condyloma acuminata
- Pregnancy related vein engorgement

Considerations

- Symptoms range from none to severe pain
- External hemorrhoids develop distal to the dentate line
    - Are bluish-purplish in color
- Internal hemorrhoids are above the dentate line
    - No sensory innervation and usually painless
    - Usually cannot be felt when not prolapsed
- Bright blood that drips into toilet or as streaks on stool is commonly from internal hemorrhoids
- Commonly thought to be from constipation or straining, but this is controversial
- Blood is not mixed inside stool

Internal hemorrhoid grading

- 1st degree = projects into canal
- 2nd degree = protrudes with defection then retracts
- 3rd degree = protrudes with straining but only retracts by manual manipulation
- 4th degree = prolapsed and cannot be reduced

Evaluation options

- Usually history and physical examination with rectal exam is all that is needed
- CBC for tachycardia or history of moderate to severe bleeding
- PT/INR if on Coumadin (warfarin)

Treatment options

External hemorrhoids

Medical treatment for mild to moderately painful thrombosed hemorrhoids

- Warm soaks (sitz baths) or hot towel applied in lateral decubitus position
- Stool softeners
- Anusol, Anusol HC or Proctofoam HC topical preparations
- Tuck's pads prn (witch hazel)
- Analgesics
- Avoid exacerbating activities

Excisional treatment for severe painful acute thrombosed hemorrhoids (usually within 72 hours of symptoms)

- Prep area with betadine
- Spread buttocks with assistant's help or use tape
- Infiltrate base of hemorrhoid with 2-5 cc of 1% lidocaine with epinephrine
- Infiltrate into the hemorrhoid with 1-2 cc of lidocaine with epinephrine
- Elliptical incision (preferred) in roof/top of hemorrhoid 2-3 mm wide radially in line from anus

    - Avoid the deeper anal verge and sphincter
  - Remove clots(s) by expressing or with forceps
  - May be packed with 0.25 inch gauze (removed in 6 hours) or have gelfoam applied as needed
  - Analgesics

Internal hemorrhoids

Medical treatment similar to external hemorrhoid treatment

Surgical referral and treatment

- Failure of conservative treatment
- Excessive and/or prolonged bleeding
- Gangrenous 4th degree hemorrhoid (emergency)
- Concurrent anal fistula or fissure
- 3rd and 4th degree internal hemorrhoids with severe symptoms
- Patient requests referral

Discharge criteria

- Uncomplicated internal and external hemorrhoids

Discharge instructions

- Warm soaks (sitz baths) or hot towel applied in lateral decubitus position
- Stool softeners and bulk laxatives (psyllium fiber)
- Anusol, Anusol HC or Proctofoam HC topical preparations
- Hemorrhoid aftercare instructions

Consult criteria

- See surgical referral above

Anal fissure

Definition

- Superficial linear tear of the anus

Differential diagnosis

- Crohn's disease
- Ulcerative colitis
- Carcinoma
- Syphilis, gonorrhea and other STD
- HIV and AIDS
- Herpes simplex
- Rectal foreign bodies (as a cause)
- Pilonidal cyst or sinus
- Proctitis

Considerations

- Most common cause of painful rectal bleeding
- Distal to the dentate line
- Usually occur in posterior anal midline (90%) or anterior anal midline (10%)
    - If not in midline consider other diseases
- Most resolve in 2–4 weeks (may last several months)
- Refractory cases may require surgery
- Causes increased anal sphincter pressures

Evaluation

- Usually only need history and rectal exam

Treatment options

- WASH regimen
    - Warm water, shower or sitz bath after bowel movement
    - Analgesics
    - Stool softener
    - High-fiber diet
- Intra-anal nitroglycerin ointment 0.4% bid topically applied for 2 weeks if failure of WASH regimen
- Botulinum toxin injection locally
- Topical application of clove oil cream for chronic anal fissure
- Topical 0.5% nifedipine ointment

Discharge criteria

- Uncomplicated anal fissure

Discharge instructions

- Anal fissure aftercare instructions
- WASH regimen

Consult criteria

- Refractory anal fissure
- Other disease process suspected
- Anal fistula

Perianal abscess

Definition

- Infection and collection of pus just outside the anus

Differential diagnosis

- Perirectal abscess
- Squamous cell carcinoma
- Crohn's disease

Considerations

- May be associated with a fistula tract into rectum
- Peak incidence is third to fourth decade of life
- Males affected more than females
- Common in infants
- Arises from obstruction of the anal crypts
- Usually patient is afebrile

Evaluation

- Usually history and physical exam is all that is needed

Treatment

- Incision and drainage of abscess avoiding anal verge
  - Pack abscess for 1–2 days (patient removes pack or return visit for removal)
- Antibiotics usually are not necessary
- Analgesics prn

Discharge criteria

- Uncomplicated perianal abscess

Discharge instructions

- Sitz baths 3 times a day and after bowel movements for 3–4 days
- Stool softeners
- Perianal abscess aftercare instructions

Consult criteria

- Perirectal abscess suspected
- Anal fistula
- Other disease process suspected
- Fever
- Immunocompromised patient

Perirectal abscess

Definition

- Abscess in the deeper perirectal spaces

Differential diagnosis

- Perianal abscess
- Crohn's disease
- Inflammatory bowel disease
- Rectal carcinoma
- Foreign body
- Sexually transmitted disease
- Proctitis
- Hemorrhoids
- Necrotizing fasciitis

Considerations

- Caused by obstruction of the anal crypts
- Fever and leukocytosis common (WBC can be normal)
- Severe pain present
- Sepsis can occur
- Increased pain with sitting, coughing or bowel movement
- Rectal or perirectal drainage in ¼ of patients

- Severe tenderness in rectum on digital examination
- May or may not be palpable
- Results in fistula in 25–50% of patients
- Urinary retention in 5% of patients

Evaluation options

- History and physical examination including rectal exam
- CBC
- BMP if diabetic
- Blood cultures if toxic appearing or immunocompromised
- CT abdomen/pelvis scan if diagnosis is in doubt on history and physical examination
- If in doubt and CT not performed, an 18 or 20 gauge needle aspiration of the most tender and/or swollen area after sterile skin prep can be used to help diagnose abscess (not to be used for definitive treatment

Treatment

- Per physician and/or surgeon
- Analgesics parentally prn

Discharge criteria

- Do not discharge

Consult criteria

- All perirectal abscess patients

Rectal prolapse

Definition

- Mucosal or full thickness prolapse of rectal tissue through anus

Differential diagnosis

- Hemorrhoids
- Proctitis
- Intussusception

Considerations

- Fecal incontinence and constipation commonly develop after prolapse
- Ulceration of rectal tissue may occur
- May be caused by staining and constipation
- 90% of children with rectal prolapse will spontaneously resolve
- Peak incidence is the 4th and 7th decades of life
- Much more common in females (80–90% of total)
- Children peak incidence less 1 year of age
    - Cystitis fibrosis associated with prolapse

Findings

- Protruding rectal mucosa
- Thick concentric mucosal ring
- Gap noted between anal canal and rectum
- Decreased anal sphincter tone

Evaluation

- History and physical examination including rectal exam
- Barium enema (preferred) or colonoscopy
- Tests for any associated conditions as needed

Treatment

- Adults are treated surgically
- Children usually treated nonsurgically and underlying condition is treated
- Attempt gentle digital reduction of rectum
    - Granulated table sugar applied to the rectal tissue causes an osmotic shift of fluid out of the mucosa decreasing the swelling in a few minutes that facilitates reduction of the prolapse
- Stool softeners

Discharge criteria

- Reducible mucosal or rectal prolapse

Discharge instructions

- Rectal prolapse aftercare instructions if available

- Stool softeners

Consult criteria

- All patients should be referred to surgeon
- Emergency consultation if incarcerated, ischemic or perforated rectal tissue

Pruritus ani

Definition

- Chronic anal itching

Differential diagnosis

- Eczema
- Psoriasis
- Pinworm infestation
- Scabies
- Urticaria
- Contact dermatitis
- Hemorrhoids

Considerations

- Worse at night usually
- Can be caused by increased moisture around anus or fecal leakage
- May be from certain foods, clothing, poor rectal hygiene, or medications

Evaluation options

- Cellophane tape when waking up in morning for pinworms if suspected
- 10% KOH skin scraping for fungus

Treatment options

- Diphenhydramine or hydroxyzine prn for itching
- Hydrocortisone cream 1% course bid prn for 5–10 days
- Avoid offending foods, clothing or agents
- Treat underlying condition if known
- Clean anus completely post-defecation
- Corn starch powder to dry skin

Discharge criteria

- Uncomplicated cases

Discharge instructions

- Pruritus ani aftercare instructions

Consult criteria

- Refractory cases refer to gastroenterologist

Pilonidal cyst/abscess

Definition

- A cyst that develops in the skin of the sacrococcygeal region 4–5 cm posterior to the anus

Differential diagnosis

- Anal fistula
- Perirectal abscess
- Hidradenitis suppurativa

Considerations

- Thought to be an acquired condition for folliculitis from hair that gets impacted into the skin
- More common in males
- Affects 26 out of 100,000 persons in the U.S.
- Occurs most commonly in late teens and early twenties
- Painful when acutely infected

Evaluation

- History and physical examination is usually all that is needed

Treatment

- For abscess perform I&D off midline, angulating into abscess cavity
    - See Soft Tissue Abscess section in book
- Remove any hair and granulation tissue
- Pack with gauze (medicated ribbon gauze has no added benefit)
    - Remove packing in 1–2 days

- No I&D for asymptomatic patients without significant symptoms
- Phenol injection into cyst by experience Providers

Discharge criteria

- Uncomplicated pilonidal cyst or abscess after procedural I&D
- Asymptomatic patients

Discharge instructions

- Pilonidal cyst aftercare instructions
- Return if pain returns or fever develops
- Refer to surgeon for definitive treatment

Consult criteria

- Pilonidal abscess near anus
- Patient toxicity
- Fever ≥ 101°F (38.3°C)

Notes

Constipation Protocol

When using any protocol, always follow the Guidelines of Proper Use (page 16).

Definition

- A gastrointestinal motility disorder resulting in 2 of the following
    - Less than 3 bowels movements per week
    - Hard lumpy stools
    - Straining
    - Incomplete defecation sensation
    - Anorectal obstruction sensation
    - Manually assisting defecation

Differential diagnosis

- Large bowel obstruction

Considerations

- Most common digestive complaint
- Affects 15% of the U.S. population
- Usually treated medically with improvement in symptoms
- 30% higher incidence in nonwhite population
- May be asymptomatic or have pain with above definition symptoms

Red flag symptoms

- Unexplained weight loss
- Vomiting
- Inability to pass flatus
- Abdominal pain
- Rectal bleeding

Types

Primary or idiopathic constipation

- Normal transit constipation
- Slow transit constipation
    - Infrequent stools and decreased urgency

        - Impaired phasic colon activity
    - Pelvic floor dysfunction
        - Dysfunction of pelvic floor or anal sphincter

Secondary constipation

- Caused by
    - Low fiber diet
    - Decreased fluid intake
    - Lack of exercise
    - Anal fissures
    - Diabetes mellitus, hypothyroidism
    - Stroke, spinal cord injuries, multiple sclerosis
    - Parkinson's disease
    - Antidepressants
    - Anticholerginerics
    - Narcotics
    - Calcium channel blockers
    - Antacids
    - NSAID's
    - Depression

Evaluation options

- Usually history and examination is all that is needed
- CBC for weight loss, fever or bleeding
- BMP for diabetes mellitus or vomiting
- Abdominal flat and upright films for vomiting
- CT abdominal/pelvic scan for vomiting, weight loss or unusually severe pain

Treatment options

Prevention

- Good fluid intake
- Exercise
- High fiber diet
- Avoid constipating medications

Acute ED or office treatment

- Fleets mineral oil enema

  - Adult 1 bottle
  - Pediatric 30–60 ml (Age 2–11 years)
- Fleet bisacodyl enema
  - Adult 30 ml (1 bottle)
  - Pediatric (2–12 years) 15 ml
- Fleet enema
  - Adult 118 ml (1 bottle)
  - Pediatric 5–12 years Pedia-Lax 1 bottle 59 ml
  - Pediatric 2–5 years Pedia-Lax ½ bottle
  - Do not use in megacolon, CHF, ascites, renal failure or intestinal obstruction
- Glycerin suppository
  - Age > 6 years 1 suppository
  - Age 2–6 years Fleet's Babylax applicator (4 ml)
- Digital disimpaction

Acute home treatment

- Dulcolax suppository or tablet
- Colace
- Fleet's enema
- Prune juice

Chronic home treatment

- High fiber diet
- Psyllium (Metamucil)
  - < 6 years 1 gm PO qday-tid in water or juice
  - Age 6–11 years 1.7 gm (powder) in water or juice PO qday-tid or 1 oral wafer, increase slowly as needed
  - > 12 years 2–6 caps qday-tid or 2 wafers PO qday increasing as needed
- Magnesium hydroxide (Milk of magnesia)
  - Age 6–11 years 15–30 ml PO qday prn
  - Age > 12 years 30–60 ml PO qday prn
- Polyethylene glycol (MiraLax)
  - Age < 17 years – 0.8 gm/kg in 8 oz. of liquid PO qday prn up to 4 days
  - Age ≥ 17 years – 1 capful in 8 oz. liquid PO qday prn up to 4 days

Constipation induced by opioids with advanced illness

- Methylnaltrexone (Relistor) weight-base dosing

Discharge criteria

- Uncomplicated findings
- Normal vital signs

Discharge instructions

- Constipation aftercare instructions
- See Gastroenterologist referral criteria

Consult criteria

- Red flag symptoms
- Fever
- Vomiting
- Tachycardia
- Metabolic acidosis
- Significant gross rectal bleeding
- Melena
- Rebound abdominal tenderness
- Moderate to severe tenderness

Referral to gastroenterologist criteria

- Recent onset
- Rectal bleeding
- Weight loss
- Recent bowel habit changes

Notes

Urinary and Male Genitourinary

Section Contents

Kidney Stone Protocol

Urinary Tract Infection Protocol

Chronic Renal Failure Protocol

Male Genitourinary Protocol

When using any protocol, always follow the Guidelines of Proper Use (page 16).

KIDNEY STONE PROTOCOL

When using any protocol, always follow the Guidelines of Proper Use (page 16).

Definition

- Ureteral colic produced by passage of renal calculus from kidney into the ureter

Differential Diagnosis

- Renal colic
- Biliary colic
- Aortic aneurysm
- Mechanical back pain
- Herpes zoster
- Pyelonephritis
- Renal vein thrombosis
- Retroperitoneal bleeding
- Appendicitis

Considerations

- Sudden severe pain onset located in the lateral mid to lower back or lower quadrant with occasional radiation to the groin
- Nausea or vomiting usually occurs
- Fever usually absent
- Groin pain felt when kidney stone at ureterovesicular junction (UVJ)
  - Most common location of impaction
- Aortic aneurysm can mimic ureteral colic
  - Renal colic is most common misdiagnosis of ruptured abdominal aortic aneurysm
- Retained kidney stones in the renal calyces rarely cause pain
- Hematuria on U/A absent 10–15% of the time
- KUB reveals approximately 30% of the kidney stones
- Pelvic calcifications commonly are phleboliths (benign)
- Abdominal exam frequently benign
- Abdominal tenderness can occur with high grade ureteral obstruction

- Flomax (tamsulosin) 0.4 mg qday Rx outpatient allows larger kidney stones to pass frequently — up to 1 cm
    - Flomax (tamsulosin) may be given for 2-4 weeks to pass ureteral calculus
- Most kidney stones pass given time
- Stones up to 1 cm can be managed conservatively in the absence of fever, infection and renal failure if pain is controlled
- CT abdomen/pelvis 97% accurate
- Thrombocytosis can occur with ureteral obstruction in pyelonephritis patients

Evaluation Options

U/A and KUB

- May be all that is needed on healthy patients with typical presentation

UCG in sexually active fertile females

BMP

- Diabetic patient
- Tachycardia present
- Hypotension present
- SBP < 105 with history of hypertension

CBC

- Fever present
- Tachycardia present
- Hypotension present
- SBP < 105 with history of hypertension

Consider CT abdomen and pelvis without contrast

- Uncertain diagnosis
- Age ≥ 60
- Abdominal pulsatile mass
- Possibility of aortic aneurysm considered

Urine culture if fever or pyuria present

Treatment Options

Acute treatment

- Toradol (ketorolac) 30 mg IV with or without Dilaudid (hydromorphone) 0.5– 1 mg (or equipotent narcotic IV) and Phenergan (promethazine) 6.25 mg IV or Zofran (ondansetron) 4 mg IV; may repeat narcotics × 2 prn if stable vital signs and no significant altered mental status or respiratory depression
- Toradol (ketorolac) 60 mg IM with or without Dilaudid (hydromorphone) 1–2 mg IM (or equipotent narcotic) and Phenergan (promethazine) 25 mg IM or Zofran (ondansetron) 4 mg IM if IV access not readily available
    - Do not use Toradol (ketorolac) if creatinine is elevated
- Do not give increased IV fluids except as needed for dehydration or hypotension

Discharge treatments

- Flomax (tamsulosin) 0.4 mg PO each day for 2-4 weeks if discharged home (can cause passage of larger stones)
- UTI antibiotics if lower urinary tract infection present without pyelonephritis or fever

Discharge symptom treatment options

- Toradol (ketorolac) 10 mg PO QID prn up to 7 days
    - Do not use Toradol (ketorolac) if creatinine is elevated
- Hydrocodone or oxycodone 5–10 mg PO QID prn up to 7 days
- Phenergan (promethazine) 25–50 mg QID PO/PR prn nausea or vomiting

Discharge Criteria

- Pain resolved or tolerable by patient and the patient is agreeable to go home
- No upper tract urinary infection
- No solitary kidney

Discharge instructions

- Kidney stone aftercare instructions
- Follow up within 7–10 days with urologist
- Urine strainer and turn in any stone for analysis

Consult Criteria

- Ureteral stone larger than 6 mm
- Pain and/or vomiting not controlled to clinician or patient's satisfaction
- Uncertain diagnosis
- Concurrent upper tract urinary infection (pyelonephritis)
- Solitary functioning kidney with ureteral calculus
- Pyelonephritis
- Fever

Vital sign and age consult criteria

- Age ≥ 70
- Fever
- Adult heart rate ≥ 110
- Developing hypotension or relative hypotension (SBP < 105 with history of hypertension)

Lab consult criteria

- WBC ≥ 14,000
- Bandemia
- Metabolic acidosis
- Significant electrolyte abnormality
- Glucose ≥ 400 mg/dL in diabetic patient
- Glucose ≥ 300 mg/dL in non-diabetic patient
- Hyperglycemia with metabolic acidosis (decreased serum CO2 or elevated anion gap)
- Hemoglobin decrease > 1 gm
- Creatinine increase > 0.5 from baseline
- Renal insufficiency
- Acute thrombocytosis
- Acute thrombocytopenia

Notes

URINARY TRACT INFECTION PROTOCOL

When using any protocol, always follow the Guidelines of Proper Use (page 16).

Definition

- Bacteriuria with the presence of symptoms

Differential Diagnosis

- Cystitis
- PID
- Ovarian cyst pain
- Gonococcal urethritis
- Nonspecific urethritis (chlamydia or ureaplasma)
- Renal colic
- Bladder outlet obstruction
- Neurogenic bladder
- Pelvic pain disorder
- Endometriosis
- Vaginitis
- Orchitis
- Epididymitis

Considerations

- Female > male incidence until age 50 or in neonates
- 0–3 months of age associated with 30% incidence of sepsis (80% of time the U/A may be normal in neonates with UTI)
- E. coli most common cause
- Sexually active males frequently have prostatitis or urethritis as cause of urinary symptoms (frequently gonorrhea or chlamydia)
- Asymptomatic bacteriuria present in 20% women > 65 years of age
- Elderly often have atypical presentation
    - Altered mental status
    - Confusion

    - Acute incontinence
    - GI symptoms
    - Urinary retention
- Fever and/or vomiting suggest upper tract urinary infection
- Gross hematuria usually present in lower tract infection
- Acute thrombocytosis with upper tract infection (pyelonephritis) may indicate obstruction from ureteral calculus

High risk

- Diabetes
- **Pregnancy**
    - Higher incidence of premature rupture of membranes and fetal demise with UTI (even if asymptomatic)
- Renal failure
- Sickle cell anemia
- Immunocompromise

Complicated UTI

- High risk criteria listed above
- Structural abnormalities
- Mechanical (catheter, stones, stents, instrumentation)
- Functional (reflux or neurogenic bladder)
- Males
- Resistant pathogens

Acute urethral syndrome

- Dysuria without pyuria
- Empiric treatment for STD

Differential of acute urethral syndrome

- Chlamydia
- Gonorrhea
- Herpes
- Vaginitis

Evaluation

- Complete history and physical exam
- Abdominal and costovertebral exam
- Pelvic exam in females and genital exam in males if STD suspected
- U/A – clean catch; catheter specimen if contamination suspected
- CBC if vomiting, fever or tachycardia present
- BMP if diabetic or for dehydration/tachycardia if present
- Prostate and urethral meatus exam in males at risk for STI

Urine culture

- For high risk patient or complicated UTI
- Symptoms after > 2 days of treatment or relapse
- Pyelonephritis

Treatment Options

Asymptomatic bacteriurias do not treat unless

- Pregnant
- Neutropenic
- Abnormal renal functions
- Transplant patient
- Undergoing urologic procedure

Uncomplicated UTI options

- 3 days of one choice below
  - Quinolone
  - Septra (trimethoprim/sulfamethoxazole)
  - Augmentin (amoxicillin/clavulanate)
  - Macrobid (nitrofurantoin) × 7 days
  - 3rd generation cephalosporin
- May use Sanford Guide

Complicated UTI

- Cystitis same as uncomplicated UTI but for 5–7 days of antibiotics

Pyelonephritis

- Antibiotics for 10–14 days
- Consider IM or IV antibiotic first dose if discharged — Rocephin (ceftriaxone) 1–2 gms IV/IM in adults, 50 mg/kg in children – not to exceed adult dose)
- Antibiotics same as for uncomplicated UTI except for parentally dosing

Sexually transmitted diseases

- See Sexually Transmitted Disease Protocol

Pain and nausea medication prn

- Narcotics short course
- OTC medications
- Pyridium 100–200 mg TID (NMT 6 pills)
- Phenergan (promethazine) — may need suppository if actively vomiting)
- Zofran (ondansetron)

Discharge Criteria

- Uncomplicated UTI without toxicity
- Able to hold PO intake and medications down
- Healthy patients with uncomplicated pyelonephritis

Discharge instructions

- UTI aftercare instructions
- Refer to primary care provider or urologist within 7 days as needed

Consult Criteria

- Complicated UTI
- Toxic appearance
- Failed outpatient treatment
- Immunocompromise
- Persistent vomiting
- Unable to hold PO meds down
- Unable to self hydrate
- Pregnancy
- Progressive renal insufficiency

- Poor follow-up
- Male children with first UTI

Vital signs and age consult criteria

- Age ≥ 70
- Age < 24 months
- Adult heart rate ≥ 110
- Hypotension (or relative hypotension: SBP < 105 in patient with hypertension history)
- Pediatric heart rate — see General Patient Criteria Protocol (page 20)

Lab consult criteria

- WBC ≥ 15,000 or < 3,000; neutropenia < 1,000
- Bandemia ≥ 15%
- Acute thrombocytopenia
- Acute thrombocytosis
- Creatinine increase > 0.5 from baseline
- Renal insufficiency
- Increased anion gap
- Significant electrolyte abnormality
- Glucose ≥ 400 mg/dL in diabetic patient
- Glucose ≥ 300 mg/dL in non-diabetic patient
- Hyperglycemia with metabolic acidosis (decreased serum CO_2 or elevated anion gap)

Notes

Chronic Renal Failure Protocol

When using any protocol, always follow the Guidelines of Proper Use (page 16).

Definition

- Decreased kidney glomerular filtration rate (GFR) of less than 60 mL/min

Differential Diagnosis

- Acute renal failure

Considerations

- Normal glomerular filtration rate (GFR) in healthy adult is 120 cc/minute
- Uremia occurs when GFR is 10–20 cc/minute

Main causes

- Diabetes
- Hypertension
- Polycystic kidney disease (inherited)

Signs, Symptoms and Associated Disorders

- Malaise; weakness; fatigue
- Anorexia; nausea; vomiting
- Peptic ulcer disease
- Peripheral neuropathy
- Anemia; thrombocytopenia
- Pruritus
- Volume overload
- CHF
- Hypocalcemia
- Increased infections
- Dialysis catheter infections
- Pericarditis

- Peritonitis in peritoneal dialysis (CAPD) patients

Dialysis disequilibrium syndrome

- Weakness
- Dizziness
- Headache
- Mental status changes in severe cases

Hyperkalemia

- EKG cannot reliably predict K+ level

K+ level

- 5.0–6.5 mEq/L — T wave peaking; shortening QTc interval
- 6.5–8.0 mEq/L — PR interval prolongation; loss of P waves; QRS widening
- Greater than 8.0 mEq/L — IVCD; bundle branch blocks; sine wave complex

Evaluation

- Complete history and physical exam
- Last dialysis noted if currently being treated
- BMP

Testing options

- CBC
- Troponin (frequently elevated due to volume overload and CHF only)
- BNP (commonly very elevated and of questionable utility)
- U/A if producing urine (cath urine sample for fever or lower abdominal pain)
- Chest x-ray if volume overload suspected
- EKG if K+ elevated
- If IV contrast imaging studies desired, discuss with physician

Treatment Options

Emergent hypertension (consult physician promptly)

- Treat with nitroglycerin SL (NTG) up to 3 doses prn
- NTG paste 1–2 inches prn
- Nitroprusside drip IV
- Dialysis if due to volume overload

Asymptomatic hypertension

- Per Hypertension Protocol (usually no treatment needed)

Hyperkalemia > 5.5 mEq/L (consult physician)

- EKG with peaked T waves or widened QRS complex may or may not be seen
- EKG may not reflect degree of hyperkalemia

Calcium gluconate (safer peripheral IV than CaCl) or calcium chloride up to 1 amp IV over 2–3 minutes with patient on monitor

- Calcium chloride 3 three times more potent than calcium gluconate
    - Give 10 ml of calcium gluconate or 5 ml of calcium chloride initially — may repeat as needed per physician
- Duration of action 30–60 minutes
- May be repeated in 5–10 minutes if EKG not improved
- Does not lower serum potassium levels
- Stabilizes cardiac membranes from effects of high potassium
- Controversial whether dangerous or not in Digoxin (digitalis) toxic patients — give Digibind

D50W 1 amp (if patient not hyperglycemic) followed by regular insulin 10 units IV

- Starts to lower K+ by 0.5–1.5 mEq/L in 15 minutes
- Peak effect in 60 minutes

- Effect lasts 4–6 hours
- Recheck blood glucose in 60–75 minutes for hypoglycemia
- If initial blood glucose is ≥ 250, then D50W is not given

Albuterol aerosol inhalation

- 10–20 mg of Albuterol in chamber with a few cc's of NS
- Onset of action within 20–30 minutes
- Peak effect in 90 minutes

Sodium bicarbonate not acutely effective in treating hyperkalemia in renal failure patients

Kayexalate

- 30–60 gms in 20% sorbitol PO
    - Onset of action 1–3 hours
- 60 gms without sorbitol PR
    - Longer onset of action than PO

Dialysis

CHF and volume overload (consult physician prior to treatment)

- BNP usually elevated even in asymptomatic patients

Hypertension treatment options

- NTG SL
- NTG paste 1–2 inches
- NTG drip IV
- Dialysis best treatment

Hypotension

- Rule out sepsis
- IV NS 200 bolus
- Notify physician promptly

Bleeding

- Direct pressure
- DDAVP

CAPD peritonitis

- Consult physician

Discharge Criteria

- Chronic renal failure patient who is stable and at baseline without acute significant electrolyte abnormalities

Discharge instructions

- Chronic renal failure aftercare instructions
- See Hyperkalemia Protocol

Consult Criteria

- Hyperkalemia
- Volume overload
- Heart failure
- Significant electrolyte abnormalities or active comorbidities
- Abnormal vital signs or O2 saturation

Male Genitourinary Protocol

When using any protocol, always follow the Guidelines of Proper Use (page 16).

Urethritis and Epididymoorchitis

Definition

- Infection or inflammation of the urethra, epididymis or testicle

Differential diagnosis for epididymoorchitis

- Testicular torsion
- Mumps
- Trauma
- Hernia
- Tumor — usually painless

Considerations

- Gonorrhea and chlamydia are the main causes and coexist 25–50% of the time
- Urethral discharge
- Tender and swollen epididymis and/or testicle

Gonorrhea

- Dysuria
- Thick purulent discharge from urethra
- Gram negative intracellular diplococci

Chlamydia

- Thinner discharge from urethra
- Little to no discomfort

Evaluation

- Sexual history
- Genital exam
- Smear with intracellular gram negative diplococci can be performed
- Culture

- RPR prn

Treatment options

- Follow CDC guidelines
- May use Sanford Guide
- Analgesics prn
- Rocephin (ceftriaxone) 125 mg IM

  +
- Doxycycline 100 mg PO bid × 7 days to cover chlamydia

Discharge criteria

- Nontoxic patient

Discharge instructions

- Epididymoorchitis aftercare instructions
- Return if worse
- Follow up with PCP or urologist in 3–7 days

Consult criteria

- Systemic toxicity
- Refer to General Patient Criteria Protocol prn (page 20)

Testicular Torsion

Definition

- Torsion of the testicle and spermatic cord with subsequent loss of blood flow to the testicle causing loss of testicular function and eventual testicular death and necrosis

Differential diagnosis

- Torsion of testicular or epididymal appendage (blue dot sign in light skinned patients may be present) — can be discharged home if diagnosed
- Epididymitis
- Epididymoorchitis
- Orchitis
- Hydrocele
- Testicular tumor or carcinoma
- Scrotal edema

- Inguinal hernia
- Fournier gangrene
- Testicular trauma
- Henoch-Schonlein Purpura
- Varicocele
- Appendicitis

Considerations

- True urologic emergency
- Complete torsion occurs with ≥ 360° rotation
- Partial torsion occurs with < 360° rotation
- Testicular salvage rate 90–100% with detorsion within 6 hours of pain onset
- Testicular viability 20–50% after 12 hours
- Peak age is 14 years of age, with second peak in first year of life
- Most torsions rotate inward and toward midline

Signs and symptoms

- Usually rapid onset of unilateral severe testicular pain
- Can occur from activity or trauma
- Can occur during sleep
- High-riding testicle occurs on affected side
- Scrotal swelling
- Nausea and/or vomiting
- Abdominal pain around 20–30%
- Fever not very common
- Cremasteric reflex absent on affected side

Evaluation

- Clinical diagnosis if classic history and findings
- Ultrasound color flow Doppler if unsure of diagnosis
    - 94% sensitive
    - 96% specific

Lab tests not usually very useful (used to evaluate for inflammatory processes with low suspicion of torsion)

- CBC – can be normal or elevated in torsion
- U/A – can have WBC's in 30% of torsions

  - C-reactive protein – not too helpful

Treatment

- Pain control
- Manual rotation of testicles outward like opening a book
  - May need to be repeated 2–3 times to obtain relief
- Emergent surgery if unable to detorse testicle
- Urgent surgery if testicle detorsed
- All testicular torsion patients should have surgery and not be discharged

Consult criteria

- Discuss suspected testicular torsion with physician or urologist immediately

Prostatitis

Definition

- Infection or inflammation of the prostate gland

Differential diagnosis

- Prostate cancer
- Urethritis
- Mechanical back pain
- UTI

Considerations

- Gonorrhea and chlamydia are the main causes in men age < 35 years and coexist 25–50% of the time
- Prostate tender (caution with vigorous palpation if fever or toxicity present)
- Age > 35 years usual cause is bacterial
- Nonbacterial prostatitis is an inflammatory condition without infection
- Chronic prostatitis
  - Increases risk of UTI and BPH

Acute bacterial prostatitis age > 35 years

- Fever

- Chills
- Perineal prostatic pain
- Dysuria
- Obstructive bladder symptoms
- Low back pain
- Low abdominal pain
- Spontaneous urethral discharge

Evaluation options

- U/A
- CBC

Treatment options

Age < 35 years

- Follow CDC guidelines
- May use Sanford Guide
- Analgesics prn
- Rocephin (ceftriaxone) 125 mg IM

  +
- Doxycycline 100 mg PO bid × 10–14 days
- Treatment for sexual partners or refer for treatment for STD

Age > 35 years

- May use Sanford Guide
- Septra DS 1 PO bid × 14–28 days
- Quinolone 14–28 days
- NSAID's and/or narcotics prn

Discharge criteria

- Nontoxic patient
- Refer to General Patient Criteria Protocol prn (page 20)

Discharge instructions

- Prostatitis aftercare instructions
- Return if worse
- Follow up with PCP or urologist in 3–7 days

Consult criteria

- Systemic toxicity

- Urinary retention

Priapism

Definition

- Persistent erection unrelated to sexual desire that is usually painful

Differential considerations

- Penile implant
- Urethral foreign body
- Peyronie disease
- Erection from sexual arousal

Causes

- Idiopathic 35–50% of the time
- Sickle cell anemia
- Leukemia
- Trauma
- Spinal cord injury
- Vasoactive drugs

Low-flow priapism

- Painful
- Ischemia and impotence can occur
- From venous obstruction

High-flow priapism

- From arterial high flow state in penis
- Not usually painful
- Less common than low-flow priapism
- Trauma most frequent cause

Evaluation of priapism

- CBC
- Sickle prep or screen if suspected as a cause
- Color flow ultrasound if not sure if high or low-flow priapism

Treatment options

Low-flow priapism

- Analgesia
- Sickle cell patients may need exchange transfusion
- Terbutaline 0.25 mg SQ may help
- Pseudoephedrine 30–60 mg PO may help
- 1–2 ml of 1% lidocaine with epinephrine 1/100,000 premix injected into proximal corpora cavernosa on lateral penile shaft (one side only) post betadine and alcohol prep – use 27 gauge needle or smaller if possible
    - Aspirate some blood to ensure corpora cavernosa has been entered before injection
    - Caution with coronary artery disease history
    - Hold pressure 30–60 seconds post injection
- Phenylephrine 250–500 mcg can be used instead of 1% lidocaine with epinephrine
- Corpora cavernosa injections usually resolve priapism in 5–15 minutes

High-flow priapism

- Analgesia prn
- Ice packs

Discuss with physician and consult urology immediately

Paraphimosis

Definition

- Entrapment and inability of foreskin to be pulled back over the glans penis in uncircumcised or partially uncircumcised males

Differential diagnosis

- Anasarca
- Balanitis
- Cellulitis
- Insect bite

- Carcinoma
- Penile fracture
- Penile hematoma
- Contact dermatitis
- Hair tourniquet

Considerations
- True emergency
- Can result in penile necrosis

Treatment
- Manual reduction after 5 minutes of ice in exam glove — pushing glans penis under foreskin while holding foreskin in place successful up to 90% of the time
- Dorsal slit of foreskin (consult physician)

Discharge criteria
- Successful reduction of paraphimosis
- No ischemic tissue damage

Discharge instructions
- Referral to urology for circumcision within 7–14 days

Consult criteria
- Inability to reduce the paraphimosis
- Penile tissue ischemic injury

Phimosis

Definition
- Inability to retract foreskin over glans penis

Considerations
- Can lead to venous congestion and eventually tissue damage
- Can lead to paraphimosis

Treatment
- Small hemostat can be passed into foreskin orifice to dilate it and deliver glans penis

Discharge criteria

- Usually can be discharged

Discharge instructions

- Refer to urology

Consult criteria

- Tissue ischemia
- Cellulitis

Hydrocele

Definition

- Collection of serous fluid in scrotum in up to 1% of males

Differential diagnosis

- Orchitis
- Testicular torsion
- Indirect inguinal hernia
- Epididymitis
- Trauma

Considerations

- Usually asymptomatic or subclinical
- Located anterior and superior to testicles
- A light shines through the hydrocele
- Most pediatric cases are congenital
- Can be from trauma, orchitis, or epididymitis

Evaluation options

- History and physical examination only (transillumination)
- CBC
- U/A
- Ultrasound can be used in diagnosis uncertain

Treatment

- Usually no acute treatment needed

Discharge criteria

- Nonpainful, non-inflamed scrotal hydrocele

Discharge instructions

- Hydrocele aftercare instructions
- Refer to urology

Consult criteria

- Painful scrotum
- Scrotal cellulitis
- Fever

Notes

Electrolyte and Acid/Base Disturbances

Section Contents

Hyperkalemia Protocol

Hypokalemia Protocol

Hypernatremia Protocol

Hyponatremia Protocol

Metabolic Acidosis Protocol

When using any protocol, always follow the Guidelines of Proper Use (page 16).

Hyperkalemia Protocol

When using any protocol, always follow the Guidelines of Proper Use (page 16).

Definition

- Elevated serum potassium levels

Differential Diagnosis

- Hypocalcemia

Considerations

- EKG cannot reliably predict K+ level
  - K+ level
    - 5.0–6.5 mEq/L — T wave peaking; shortening QTc interval
    - 6.5–8.0 mEq/L — PR interval prolongation; loss of P waves; QRS widening
    - Greater than 8.0 mEq/L — IVCD; bundle branch blocks; sine wave complex

Causes

- Renal failure
- K+ supplementation
- Hemolysis from blood draw
- Hemolysis
- DIC
- Tissue injury or ischemia

Evaluation

- Complete history and physical exam
- Last dialysis noted if being currently treated
- BMP
- Chest x-ray
- EKG

Testing options

- CBC
- Troponin (frequently elevated due to volume overload and CHF only)

- BNP (commonly very elevated and of questionable utility)
- U/A if producing urine (cath urine sample for fever or lower abdominal pain)
- If IV contrast imaging studies desired, discuss with supervising physician if history of renal disease

Treatment Options

Hyperkalemia > 5.5 mEq/L (consult physician)

- EKG with peaked T waves or widened QRS complex may or may not be seen
- EKG may not reflect the degree of hyperkalemia

Calcium gluconate (safer peripheral IV than CaCl) or calcium chloride (CaCl) up to 1 amp IV over 2–3 minutes with patient on monitor

- Calcium chloride 3 three times more potent than calcium gluconate
    - Give 10 ml of calcium gluconate or 5 ml of calcium chloride initially — may repeat as needed per physician
- Duration of action 30–60 minutes
- May be repeated in 5–10 minutes if EKG not improved
- Does not lower serum potassium levels
- Stabilizes cardiac membranes from effects of high potassium
- Controversial if dangerous in digoxin toxic patients — give Digibind

D50W ½–1 amp (if patient not hyperglycemic) followed by regular insulin 10 units IV

- Starts to lower K+ by 0.5–1.5 mEq/L in 15 minutes
- Peak effect in 60 minutes
- Effect lasts 4–6 hours
- Recheck blood glucose in 60–75 minutes for hypoglycemia
- If initial blood glucose is ≥ 250, then D50W is not given

Albuterol aerosol inhalation

- 10–20 mg of Albuterol in chamber with a few cc's of NS
- Onset of action within 20–30 minutes
- Peak effect in 90 minutes

Sodium bicarbonate not acutely effective in treating hyperkalemia in renal failure patients

Kayexalate

- 30–60 gms in 20% sorbitol PO
  - Onset of action 1–3 hours
- 60 gms without sorbitol PR
  - Longer onset of action than PO

Dialysis

Discharge Criteria

- Mild hyperkalemia < 6.0 mEq/L
- Acceptable treatment response
- Further potassium rises not anticipated

Discharge instructions

- Close follow up
- Hyperkalemia aftercare instructions
- Chronic renal failure aftercare instructions if indicated

Consult Criteria

- Discuss with physician if potassium > 5.5 mEq/L
- End-stage renal disease with abnormal vital signs or O2 saturation
- Significant comorbidities

Notes

HYPOKALEMIA PROTOCOL

When using any protocol, always follow the Guidelines of Proper Use (page 16).

Definition

- Serum potassium level < 3.5 mEq/L

Differential Diagnosis

- Cushing syndrome
- Hypocalcemia
- Hypomagnesemia

Considerations

- Very common
- Increases dysrhythmias
- Increases Digoxin (digitalis) toxicity effects
- Mild 3.0–3.4 mEq/L
- Moderate 2.5–2.9 mEq/L
- Severe < 2.5 mEq/L

Causes

- Diuretics
- Hyperventilation
- Hypomagnesemia
- Poor nutrition
- Diarrhea
- Metabolic alkalosis
- Renal tubular acidosis
- Adrenal conditions
- Hyperaldosteronism
- Gastrointestinal losses (vomiting, diarrhea, NG suction)
- Familial Periodic Hypokalemia Paralysis

Signs and Symptoms

- Severe weakness K+ < 2.5 mEq/L
- Paralysis can occur with rapid development of K+ < 2.0 mEq/L

- Paresthesias
- Muscle weakness
- Muscle cramps
- Constipation
- Cardiac dysrhythmias
- EKG changes
    - Low voltage T waves
    - ST segment depression
    - U waves
    - Small P waves
    - PAC's
    - PVC's

Evaluation

- BMP
- EKG if potassium < 2.5 mEq/L
- Magnesium level not needed usually

Treatment Options

- Oral replacement preferred when indicated
- Oral potassium 40-60 mEq can raise serum potassium 1-1.5 mEq/L; 135-160 mEq PO raises serum potassium 2.5-3.5 mEq/L
- Potassium level < 2.5 mEq/L give IV replacement no faster than 10 mEq per hour
- MgSO4 (magnesium sulfate) replacement can improve potassium replacement
    - 2-4 gms IV over 30 minutes if needed
    - Mg gluconate 200−400 mg PO TID prn if asymptomatic for adults

Discharge Criteria

- Asymptomatic patient
- Able to replenish potassium orally
- Potassium level > 2.5 mEq/L

Discharge instructions

- Hypokalemia aftercare instructions
- Follow up with primary care provider within 5-10 days

Consult Criteria

- Potassium ≤ 2.5 mEq/L
- Symptomatic patient
- EKG changes

Notes

HYPERNATREMIA PROTOCOL

When using any protocol, always follow the Guidelines of Proper Use (page 16).

Definition

- Serum Na+ level > 145 mEq/L

Differential Diagnosis

- Hyperglycemic hyperosmolar state
- Diabetes insipidus
- Salt ingestion
- Hypertonic dehydration

Considerations

Dehydration

- Secondary to volume depletion
- Poor oral intake of fluids
- Commonly seen in nursing home patients
- PEG tube feeding patients
- Bedridden patients
- Stroke patients
- Patients unable to care for self
- Medication induced diuresis
- Accompanied by metabolic acidosis frequently
- High risk condition for mortality in elderly
- Usually in patients with significant comorbidities

Diabetes insipidus

Decreased urine concentration ability of kidneys

- Lithium
- Sickle cell anemia
- Postobstructive diuresis after treatment of bladder outlet obstruction

Decreased secretion of ADH (antidiuretic hormone)

- Brain tumors
- Brain injury
- Cerebral infectious processes

Signs and symptoms

- Altered mental status
- Decreased responsiveness
- Tachycardia
- Hypotension may occur
- Tachypnea
- Poor skin turgor
- Decreased capillary refill
- Dry mucous membranes
- Decreased urine output
- Hard stools

Evaluation Options

- BMP
- CBC
- U/A
- Chest x-ray usually performed to rule out concurrent process
- CT brain if central process suspected
- Urine for spot Na and osmolarity if serum sodium > 170 mEq/L

Treatment Options

- Restore plasma volume first
- Oral rehydration therapy (ORT) preferred over IV in mild to moderate dehydration if appropriate to patient's condition and ability to self-hydrate

Serum Na correction no more than 1 mEq/L per hour

- Too rapid correction may cause cerebral edema

Adult dehydration

Oral Rehydration Therapy (ORT) for mild to moderate dehydration if able to self-hydrate

- Oral rehydration formula (WHO formula, Rehydralyte or Pedialyte) for mild to moderate dehydration or serum CO2 is 14–18 mEq/L or NA+ 146–152 mEq/L

- Zofran (ondansetron) 8 mg chewable tablet if vomiting or 4–8 mg IM
- 15–30 cc every 1–2 minutes for adults (age > 12) for 1–4 hours — start 20 minutes after Zofran (ondansetron) given
- Hold ORT 10 minutes if vomiting occurs then resume
- Reassess for urine production, improved heart rate, and absence of severe vomiting
- Recheck serum CO2 if initially < 17 mEq/L
- Mild dehydration give 50 cc/kg in < 4 hours
- Moderate dehydration give 50–100 cc/kg in 1–4 hours

IV rehydration

- Moderate to severe dehydration (Na+ > 152 mEq/L), give IV NS 150–300 cc/hour over 2–4 hours
- Hypotension or signs of poor organ perfusion (lactic acid > 2), give NS at 500–1000 cc/hour up to 2 liters (consult physician promptly) — caution if CHF history

Pediatric dehydration

Dehydration assessment

Mild ≤ 5%

- Alert
- Mucous membranes variable dry
- Skin turgor normal
- Fontanel flat
- Blood pressure normal
- Heart rate normal
- Capillary refill < 2 seconds
- Urine output decreased

Moderate 6–9%

- Irritable
- Mucous membranes dry

- Skin turgor variably reduced
- Fontanel depressed
- Blood pressure variably orthostatic
- Heart rate tachycardic
- Capillary refill 2–3 seconds
- Urine output decreased — oliguria

Severe ≥ 10%

- Lethargic
- Mucous membranes dry
- Skin turgor reduced
- Fontanel depressed
- Blood pressure orthostatic or hypotensive
- Heart rate markedly tachycardic
- Capillary refill ≥ 4 seconds
- Urine output decreased - oliguria/anuria

Oral Rehydration Therapy (ORT) for mild to moderate dehydration

- Zofran (ondansetron) oral chewable tablet in ED for frequent vomiting
  - 2 mg for 8–15 kg; 4 mg for 15–30 kg; 8 mg for > 30 kg
  - Zofran (ondansetron) 2–4 doses can be prescribed for home if indicated

Oral rehydration formula for mild to moderate dehydration; serum CO2 14–18 mEq/L or serum Na 146–155 mEq/L

- 5 cc every 1–2 minutes for small children by caretaker for < 4 hours — start 20 minutes after Zofran (ondansetron) given
- 5–10 cc every 1–2 minutes for larger children by caretaker for 1–4 hours
- Hold ORT 10 minutes if vomiting occurs then resume
- Reassess for urine production, weight gain, improved HR and alertness, and absence of severe vomiting
- Recheck serum CO2 if initially < 17
- Mild dehydration give 50 cc/kg in < 4 hours

- Moderate dehydration give 50–100 cc/kg over 1–4 hours

Severe dehydration give IV NS bolus 20 cc/kg; may repeat × 2

Exclusion Criteria for Oral Rehydration Therapy

- Age < 6 months of age
- Hematemesis
- Bilious vomiting
- Bloody diarrhea
- VP shunt
- Head trauma
- Focal RLQ tenderness (possible appendicitis)
- Severe dehydration
- Patient vomits 3 or more times after starting ORT

IV therapy criteria and treatment for moderate to severe dehydration

- IV NS hydration for CO2 < 14 mEq/L or Na > 155 mEq/L
- ORT failure
- IV NS 20 cc/kg bolus, may repeat × 2
- Consult physician
- Maintenance IV with D5NS (dextrose decreases return visits)

Discharge Criteria

- Patient responds to rehydration
- Healthy without significant comorbid conditions
- Good social support systems
- Unlikely to acutely become hypernatremic post discharge

Discharge instructions

- Dehydration or hypernatremia aftercare instructions
- Follow up with primary care providers within 1–3 days

Consult Criteria

Discuss with physician

- Patients with significant comorbid conditions or findings
- Serum Na > 150 mEq/L
- Age > 60
- Age < 6 months

Vital signs consult criteria

- Adult heart rate > 100 post treatment
- Hypotension or relative hypotension (SBP < 105 with history of hypertension)
- Orthostatic vital signs
- Pediatric heart rate
    - 0–4 months ≥ 180
    - 5–7 months ≥ 175
    - 6–12 months ≥ 170
    - 1–3 years ≥ 160
    - 4–5 years ≥ 145
    - 6–8 years ≥ 130
    - 7–12 years ≥ 125
    - 12–15 years ≥ 115
    - 16 years or older ≥ 110

Notes

HYPONATREMIA PROTOCOL

When using any protocol, always follow the Guidelines of Proper Use (page 16).

Definition

- Serum sodium level < 135 mEq/L

Differential Diagnosis

- SIADH
- Hepatitis cirrhosis
- Adrenal insufficiency
- Adrenal crisis
- CHF
- Water intoxication
- Gastroenteritis
- Renal failure
- Hypothyroidism
- Nephrotic syndrome

Considerations

- Acute hyponatremia is more symptomatic
- Chronic hyponatremia can be asymptomatic
- Central pontine myelinolysis can occur from too rapid correction of hyponatremia
    - Dysarthria
    - Dysphagia
    - Seizures
    - Altered mental status
    - Quadriplegia
    - Hypotension
- Correction of severe symptomatic hyponatremia should not raise serum sodium level more than 4 mEq/L acutely
- Chronic hyponatremia usually does not need rapid correction (can be dangerous to do so)
- Chronic hyponatremia is much more common than acute hyponatremia

- Serum Na+ is lowered 1.6 mEq/L for every blood glucose level increase of 100 mg% over normal
  - Will correct with correction of hyperglycemia alone
- Children more prone to iatrogenic water intoxication by parents giving excessive water to replace GI fluid losses

Signs and symptoms

- Mild or none in some chronic hyponatremic patients with Na+ > 120 mEq/L

Acute hyponatremia

- Serum sodium > 120 mEq/L
  - Headache
  - Nausea; vomiting
  - Muscle cramps
  - Weakness
  - Anorexia
  - Rhabdomyolysis
- Serum sodium 110–120 mEq/L
  - Hyperventilation
  - Decreased responsiveness
  - Hallucinations
  - Behavior disturbances
  - Incontinence
  - Ataxia
- Serum sodium < 110 mEq/L
  - Posturing
  - Hypertension
  - Bradycardia
  - Impaired temperature regulation
  - Seizures
  - Coma
  - Respiratory arrest

Causes

Hypovolemic

- Excess fluid losses replaced with hypotonic solutions by patient
  - Vomiting
  - Diarrhea

- Third spacing of fluids
- Burns
- Excessive sweating
- Diuretics

Hypervolemic

- Excessive water intake (water intoxication)
- Hepatic cirrhosis
- CHF
- Nephrotic syndrome
- Renal insufficiency

Euvolemic

- Hypothyroidism
- Adrenal insufficiency
- SIADH
- Psychogenic polydipsia

Medications

- Diuretics
- NSAID's
- Oral hypoglycemic agents
- ACE inhibitors
- ARB's
- PPI's

Sodium Requirement (mEq/L)

- Na+ deficit is total body water (Kg × 0.6) times (desired Na – Serum Na)

Hypertonic saline

- 513 mEq/L of NaCl

Normal saline

- 154 mEq/L of NaCl

Lactated ringers

- 130 mEq/L of Na+

Evaluation

- BMP

- Urine spot Na+ level (consider if SIADH suspected)
- Urine osmolarity (if SIADH suspected, which has inappropriately concentrated urine)
- Serum cortisol level if adrenal insufficiency suspected
- TSH and thyroid function tests if hypothyroidism suspected

Treatment Options

Chronic hyponatremia with mild to moderately severe symptoms

(Do not increase serum Na+ by more than 10–12 mEq/L in first 24 hours)

- Hypovolemia: IV NS
- Hypervolemia: restrict free water and sodium
- Euvolemia: restrict free water — may add Lasix (furosemide) short term

Acute hyponatremia — Na+ < 120 mEq/L with severe symptoms (or chronic hyponatremia with severe symptoms such as seizures, coma, severe altered mental status) consult physician

- 3% saline at 100 cc/hr × 2 hours and recheck serum sodium for adults
- Pediatric calculation of TBW (kg × 0.6) × 4 mEq/L = acute Na+ deficit to be replenished over 2 hours
- Do not raise Na+ acutely more than 4 mEq/L

Discharge Criteria

- Asymptomatic serum sodium > 125 mEq/L without comorbid conditions

Discharge instructions

- Follow up within 1–3 days for serum sodium < 130 mEq/L with primary care provider
- Hyponatremia aftercare instructions

Consult Criteria

- Serum sodium ≤ 125

- Comorbid conditions or symptoms
- Refer to General Patient Criteria Protocol prn (page 20)

Notes

METABOLIC ACIDOSIS PROTOCOL

When using any protocol, always follow the Guidelines of Proper Use (page 16).

Definition

- Disease process with an increase in plasma acidity

Differential Diagnosis

- See A CAT MUDPILES below

Considerations

Nonanion gap acidosis

- Diarrhea
- Renal tubular acidosis
- Carbonic anhydrase inhibitors — Diamox (acetazolamide)
- Hypoaldosteronism

Anion gap calculation

- Na+ minus (HCO3 - Chloride)
- Normal range 5–12 ± 3 mEq/L

Respiratory compensation

- Expected pCO2 is 1.5[HCO3] + 8
- If higher, then primary respiratory acidosis exists and there is inadequate respiratory compensation
- Death can result from intubation and ventilation that does not compensate for metabolic acidosis (or maintains sufficient respiratory compensation with hyperventilation if intubated)

Respiratory acidosis

- Acute: HCO3 increased by 1 mEq/L for each 10 mm Hg increase in pCO2
- Chronic: HCO3 increased by 4 mEq/L for each mm Hg increase in pCO2

Anion gap mnemonic — A CAT MUDPILES

A – Alcoholic ketoacidosis
C – Cyanide; carbon monoxide
A – Aspirin; other salicylates
T – Toluene
M – Methanol; metformin
U – Uremia
D – DKA
P – Paraldehyde; phenformin
I – Iron; INH
L – Lactic acidosis (dehydration or tissue ischemia commonly)
E – Ethylene glycol
S – Starvation

Osmolol gap > 10–20 suspect substance ingestion (Normal < 10)

- Gap = Osmolality measured – Osmolality calculated (calculation equation: 2(Na+K) + glucose/18 + BUN/2.8; normal 280–300 mOsm/L)
- Ethanol mg%/4.6 is added to osmolol gap equation if present
- Gap > 50 carries high specificity for toxic alcohol such as methanol, ethylene glycol, or isopropyl alcohol
- Normal gap < 10
- Refer to Toxicology Protocol

Signs and Symptoms

- Tachypnea or Kussmaul respirations
- Tachycardia
- Confusion

Evaluation

- Complete history and physical examination
- CBC
- BMP
- ABG for
    - Severe acidosis
    - Altered mental status

    - Significant tachycardia
- Chest x-ray if indicated
- EKG if indicated

Treatment Options

- Treat underlying process
- pH < 7.0 can consider IV HCO3 (some controversy over degree of acidosis needing this treatment) — consult physician immediately
- See Adult and Pediatric Gastroenteritis Protocols

Discharge Criteria

- Resolving metabolic acidosis with treatable outpatient process
- HCO3 > 17
- Anion gap ≤ 18
- No significant comorbidities

Discharge instructions

- Aftercare instructions relevant to cause of acidosis
- Follow up with primary care provider within 1 day

Consult Criteria

- HCO3 < 18
- Anion gap ≥ 19
- Age ≥ 60
- Condition not likely to improve as outpatient
- Respiratory acidosis
- Hypotension or relative hypotension (SBP < 105 with history of hypertension)
- Toxic appearance
- Adult heart rate ≥ 110
- Pediatric heart rate
    - 0–4 months ≥ 180
    - 5–7 months ≥ 175
    - 6–12 months ≥ 170
    - 1–3 years ≥ 160
    - 4–5 years ≥ 145
    - 6–8 years ≥ 130
    - 7–12 years ≥ 125

- 12–15 years ≥ 115
- 16 years or older ≥ 110

Notes

Head Trauma and Neck Pain

Section Contents

Adult Minor Head Trauma Protocol

Pediatric Minor Head Trauma Protocol

Neck Pain Protocol

When using any protocol, always follow the Guidelines of Proper Use (page 16).

ADULT MINOR HEAD TRAUMA PROTOCOL

When using any protocol, always follow the Guidelines of Proper Use (page 16).

Definition

- Head trauma with Glasgow coma scale ≥ 14 and no focal neurologic deficits or complaints

Differential Diagnosis

- Subarachnoid hemorrhage
- Subdural hematoma
- Epidural hematoma
- Cerebral contusion
- Skull fracture

Considerations

- Loss of consciousness (LOC), amnesia, headache, vomiting and seizures have low sensitivity and specificity for detecting intracranial injury
- Cervical spine exam and evaluation important
- Skull films mainly replaced by CT evaluation of adult head trauma — may consider skull films for laceration > 5 cm or that extends deep to the skull
    - Violent mechanism of injury
- Significant maxillofacial injuries can coexist

Concussion Definitions

Grade 1 concussion

- Transient confusion
- No LOC
- Duration of mental status abnormalities < 15 minutes

Grade 2 concussion

- Transient confusion
- No LOC

- Duration of mental status abnormalities > 15 minutes

Grade 3 concussion

- Loss of consciousness

Postconcussion Syndrome

- Symptoms of headache, dizziness, trouble concentrating days to weeks following a concussion and can persist for months
- Anxiety and depression reported by patients
- Issues of compensation and litigation associated at times with persistent symptoms
- Disequilibrium and vertigo from vestibular concussion
- Reassurance decreases incidence and duration of symptoms
- Avoid narcotics
- Can use mild analgesics
- Can use meclizine or Phenergan (promethazine) for vestibular symptoms
- Rarely seen in young children
- Countries with low litigation have low postconcussion syndrome disability

Evaluation

- CT brain scan for concussion with loss of consciousness
- CT brain scan for patients on Coumadin (warfarin) or Plavix (clopidogrel) with more than trivial injury
- Evaluate for other injuries, especially C-spine
- Retinal exam: hemorrhages present in 65–90% with abuse inflicted head injury
- Detailed neurologic exam
- INR if on Coumadin (warfarin)
- Suspected intracranial injury
- Glasgow coma scale < 15
- Evaluate for other injuries, especially C-spine
- Retinal exam: hemorrhages present in 65–90% with abuse inflicted head injury
- Detailed neurologic exam
- INR if on Coumadin (warfarin)

ENT exam

- Check for hemotympanum
- CSF rhinorrhea
- Battle's sign
- Cranial nerve palsy

New Orleans CT brain criteria (for ordering noncontrast CT brain)

- Normal neurologic exam and one of the following
    - Headache
    - Vomiting
    - Age > 60
    - Persistent anterograde amnesia
    - Drug or alcohol intoxication
    - Visible trauma above the clavicle
    - Seizure

Noncontrast CT brain scan for acute brain injury

(From ACEP/CDC Clinical Policy)

Order noncontrast CT brain scan

- Loss of consciousness
- No loss of consciousness with one of the following:
    - Headache
    - Vomiting
    - Age > 60 years
    - Persistent anterograde amnesia
    - Focal neurologic deficit
    - Coagulopathy
    - Drug or alcohol intoxication
    - Visible trauma above the clavicle
    - Posttraumatic Seizure
    - GCS < 15

Consider noncontrast CT brain scan with no LOC and one of following

- Signs of basilar skull fracture
- Age > 65 years
- Dangerous mechanism of injury (includes)

    - Motor vehicle ejection
    - Pedestrian struck by motor vehicle
    - Fall from > 3 feet or 5 stairs
- Patients on warfarin
    - Minor head trauma patients on warfarin with a normal initial CT brain, it is recommended that 24 hours observation and repeat CT brain scan be perfomed
    - Higher risk with INR > 3.0 for delayed intracranial bleeding

Treatment Options

- Tylenol (no ASA or NSAID's for 36 hours)
- Avoid more potent analgesics so progression of symptoms can be detected
- Head injury instruction sheet
- Return for any neurologic changes
- Follow up with primary care provider or neurologist/neurosurgeon

Discharge Criteria

- Stable condition
- Normal neurologic exam
- No other significant trauma
- No radiologic abnormalities

Discharge instructions

- Head injury aftercare instructions

Consult Criteria

- Age > 65
- Bleeding potential from medications or preexisting disease processes
- Patients on warfarin therapy
- Concussions with loss of consciousness should be discussed with physician
- Dementia
- Persistent vomiting
- Severe persistent headache
- Focal neurologic deficits

- Inadequate home observation

Notes

Reference:

Ann of Emergency Medicine, June 2012 (Vol. 59 | No. 6 | Pages 451-455)

PEDIATRIC MINOR HEAD TRAUMA PROTOCOL

When using any protocol, always follow the Guidelines of Proper Use (page 16).

Definition

- Head trauma with Glasgow coma scale ≥ 14 and no focal neurologic deficits or complaints

Differential Diagnosis

- Subarachnoid hemorrhage
- Subdural hematoma
- Epidural hematoma
- Cerebral contusion
- Skull fracture

Considerations

- Loss of consciousness (LOC), amnesia, headache, vomiting and seizures have low sensitivity and specificity for detecting intracranial injury
- Children < 2 years have a higher risk of skull fracture and intracranial injury after minor mechanisms of injury
    - Skull fracture associated with a 20-fold increase in intracranial injury
    - Most skull fractures are associated with scalp hematomas
- Scalp hematomas indicative of skull fractures is the most sensitive predictor of intracranial injury of the clinical signs of brain injury
- Infant's clinical signs of brain injury less reliable

Postconcussion Syndrome

- Symptoms of headache, dizziness, trouble concentrating days to weeks following a concussion and can persist for months
- Anxiety and depression reported by patients

- Issues of compensation and litigation associated at times with persistent symptoms
- Disequilibrium and vertigo from vestibular concussion
- Reassurance decreases incidence and duration of symptoms
- Avoid narcotics
- Can use mild analgesics
- Can use meclizine or Phenergan (promethazine) for vestibular symptoms
- Rarely seen in young children
- Countries with low litigation have low postconcussion syndrome disability

Evaluation

- Evaluate for other injuries besides head
- Retinal exam: hemorrhages present in 65–90% with abuse inflicted head injury
- ENT exam for:
  - Hemotympanum
  - CSF rhinorrhea
  - Battle's sign
  - Cranial nerve palsy
- Awake, alert and asymptomatic children without LOC usually do not require imaging

CT brain scan

- With loss of consciousness > 30 seconds
- Vomiting
- Severe headache
- Seizure
- Disorientation
- Glasgow coma scale < 15
- Irritability
- Acute focal neurologic deficits
- Slurred speech
- Abnormal gait
- Drowsiness
- Suspected intracranial structural injury
- Have a lower imaging threshold for age < 1–2 years

- Consider CT for asymptomatic infants age < 2–3 months if mechanism more than trivial or a scalp hematoma is present

Treatment Options

- Tylenol (no ASA or NSAID's for 36 hours)
- Avoid more potent analgesics so progression of symptoms can be detected
- Quiet play or activities can be resumed if no significant symptoms
- Head injury instruction sheet
- Return for any neurologic changes
- Follow up with primary care provider or neurologist

Discharge Criteria

- Stable condition
- Normal neurologic exam
- No other significant trauma
- No radiologic abnormalities

Discharge instructions

- Head injury aftercare instructions
- Refer or arrange for follow-up with primary care physician or provider for concussion

Consult Criteria

- Concussion
- Skull fracture
- CT findings of intracranial injury
- Acute neurologic abnormalities
- Intracranial bleeding potential
- Persistent vomiting
- Severe persistent headache
- Focal neurologic deficits
- Inadequate home observation
- Serial visits for head injury symptoms
- Patients on warfarin therapy

Concussion Definitions and Return-to-sports Recommendations

Grade 1 concussion

- Transient confusion
- No loss of consciousness (LOC)
- Duration of mental status abnormalities < 15 minutes
- Return to sports activities same day if all symptoms resolve within 15 minutes
- If second grade 1 concussion occurs then no sports activities until asymptomatic for 1 week

Grade 2 concussion

- Transient confusion
- No LOC
- Duration of mental status abnormalities > 15 minutes
- No sports activities until asymptomatic for 1 week
- If grade 2 concussion occurs same day as a grade 1 concussion then no sports activities until asymptomatic for 2 weeks

Grade 3 concussion

- Loss of consciousness
- No sport activities until asymptomatic for 1 week if LOC was for seconds
- No sports activities until asymptomatic for 2 weeks if LOC minutes or longer

Second grade 3 concussion

- No sport activities until asymptomatic for 1 month
- If intracranial pathology detected on CT, then no sports activities for the remainder of the season and discouraged from any future contact sports ever

NECK PAIN PROTOCOL

When using any protocol, always follow the Guidelines of Proper Use (page 16).

Definition

- Various disorders causing neck pain

Differential Diagnosis

- Muscle strain
- "Whiplash" injury
- Cervical fracture
- HNP
- Soft tissue infection
- Retropharyngeal abscess
- Cervical lymphadenitis
- Spinal stenosis
- Rheumatoid arthritis
- Endocarditis
- Thoracic outlet syndrome

Considerations

- Common neck pain causes
    - Torticollis ("wry neck") from muscle spasm
    - Cervical disc disease
    - Soft tissue disorder
    - Cervical spine injury
    - Muscular and ligament strain
    - Ankylosing spondylitis
        - Can have cranial–cervical disassociation
        - Put in Philadelphia or rigid cervical collar
        - Exercise caution with patient's neck

Torticollis

- Discomfort caused by cervical spine motion
- May be secondary to:
    - C-spine injury
    - Muscle injury

  - Ligamentous injury
- Usually acute in children and of muscular etiology
- Infectious causes
  - URI
  - Cervical adenitis
  - Pharyngitis
  - Retropharyngeal abscess
    - Measurements of retropharyngeal space:
      - At C2: < 7 mm
      - At C6: < 22 mm in adults; < 14 mm in children
  - Epiglottitis
  - Upper lobe pneumonia
  - Meningitis

Evaluation

- Neurologic and neck exam
- If fever present order
  - CBC
  - Soft tissue neck films
  - C-reactive protein if diagnosis not evident
  - CT neck for severe pain and possible deep space infection
- No fever
  - C-spine plain films if injured
  - CT C-spine scan if
    - Significant pain and mechanism of injury
    - Neurologic deficit or complaint

Treatment options

- Benign infectious processes treat per Protocols
- Benign muscular etiology treat with NSAID's and heat or ice
- I&D superficial neck abscess

Discharge criteria

- Benign process
- Chronic stable condition
- Cervical radiculopathy controlled with analgesics

Consult criteria

- Fever
- Meningitis concerns
- Airway concerns
- Severe pain
- Epiglottitis
- Retropharyngeal abscess
- Neurologic deficit

Neck Trauma

Penetrating neck trauma

- Consult physician unless very superficial laceration
- Do not explore Zone 2 penetrating deep neck injuries
    - Angle of mandible to cricoid cartilage
    - Consult physician/surgeon

Cervical spine trauma

- Leave cervical collar on until patient examined and cleared
- Plain C-spine x-ray 3 views

Exclusionary criteria for C-spine films

- No neurologic deficit
- No distracting injuries
- No evidence of intoxication
- Normal mentation
- No posterior midline tenderness

CT C-spine indications

- Moderate to high risk of cervical fracture
- Significant mechanism of injury
- Fracture on plain C-spine films
- Neurologic deficit or complaint
- Inadequate plain C-spine films
- Severe neck pain with normal plain C-spine films
- Patient will not move neck actively (on their own) without external support of patient's hands ("head in hand sign")

- Obtunded patients

Flexion-extension plain films

- Significant pain with negative plain and CT imaging
- Evaluates for ligamentous instability

Treatment options

- If C-spine cleared: analgesics and ice packs prn

Discharge criteria

- Benign neck injury
- No fracture

Discharge instructions

- Neck pain or injury aftercare instructions
- Refer to primary care provider or neurosurgeon within 3 days if not improving
- Avoid discharging with cervical collar if possible

Consult criteria

- Cervical fracture or dislocation/subluxation
- Neurologic deficit or complaint
- Significant pain
- Significant mechanism of injury

Notes

HEENT

Section Contents

Sore Throat Protocol

Otitis Externa Protocol

Eye Protocols

Nosebleed Protocol

ENT Emergency Protocol

Nasal and Facial Fractures Protocol

Dental Injury Protocols

Dental Pain Protocol

When using any protocol, always follow the Guidelines of Proper Use (page 16).

Sore Throat Protocol

When using any protocol, always follow the Guidelines of Proper Use (page 16).

Definition

- Pain located or perceived in the throat or anterior neck region

Differential Diagnosis

- GABHS (Group A beta-hemolytic streptococcus)
- Mononucleosis
- Gonococcal pharyngitis
- Peritonsillar abscess
- Epiglottis
- Retropharyngeal abscess
- Diphtheria (rare)
- Cervical lymphadenitis
- Thyrotoxicosis
- Gastroesophageal reflux

Considerations

- Viral 40%
- Bacterial 30%
- Strep throat - Group A beta-hemolytic Strep (GABHS)
  - 15-30% childhood pharyngitis
  - 5-10% of adult pharyngitis
  - Peak ages 4-11 years
  - Peak months January - May
  - Associated symptoms and findings
    - Sudden onset
    - Odynophagia
    - Fever
    - Headache
    - Abdominal pain
    - Nausea and vomiting;
- Viral pharyngitis
  - Cough
  - Rhinorrhea

- Lack of cervical adenopathy

Viral Pharyngitis

URI

- Treat symptomatically

Mononucleosis

Findings

- Exudative tonsillitis
- Fever
- Posterior cervical chain lymphadenopathy considered diagnostic
- Monospot
  - 90% sensitive age > 5 years
  - 75% sensitive age 2–4 years
  - Less than 30% sensitive age < 2 years
- CBC: 50% lymphocytes, 10% atypical lymphocytes
- Liver function tests elevated in 80–85% of patients up to 3 times normal
- Splenomegaly
- Hepatomegaly
- Encephalitis
- Meningitis

Treatment options

- Treat symptomatically
- No contact sports or gym for 4 weeks after onset of illness
  - Follow up with primary care provider before resuming sports or gym
- Ampicillin or amoxicillin rash can occur if prescribed
- Steroids may decrease symptoms and swelling but may also delay recovery and there is a concern for association with development chronic EBV syndrome
- Steroid dosing if used:
  - Adult or patients heavier than 40 kg: prednisone 40 mg PO daily for 4 days

- Pediatrics: prednisone 1 mg/kg PO daily for 4 days (NMT 40 mg)

Strep throat — GABHS

- Rheumatic fever can be prevented if antibiotic treatment started within 9 days of onset
- Glomerulonephritis cannot be prevented with antibiotic treatment

Evaluation

Centor criteria

- Tonsillar exudates
- Tender anterior cervical lymphadenopathy
- Fever by history
- Absence of cough
  - If 3 present: 40–60% have GABHS
  - If 3 or 4 absent: 80% negative predictive value
  - None or one criterion present: No testing or treatment needed for GABHS

Consider Rapid Strep Tests

- Sensitivity 85–95%
- Specificity 96–99%
- May be positive with carriage state and another cause of acute pharyngitis besides GABHS may exist

Treatment options

- Per Sanford Guide
- Pen VK
- Cephalexin
- Erythromycin or Zithromax (azithromycin) if penicillin allergic (increasing resistance has occurred to macrolides such as azithromycin)
- Steroids one dose
  - Prednisone 40–60 mg PO > 40 kg
  - Prednisone or prednisolone 1 mg/kg PO (NMT 60 mg)

  - Decadron (dexamethasone) 10 mg IM if unable to take PO
  - Decadron (dexamethasone) 0.06 mg/kg IM (NMT 10 mg) if unable to take PO

Epiglottis or suspected epiglottitis

- Now more common in adults than children
- Constitutes an airway emergency — consult anesthesia
- Do not agitate or aggressively exam
  - If patient is in distress
  - Drooling present
  - Tripod position or sniff position present
- Pain on moving thyroid cartilage
- Lateral neck films findings — only obtain in stable patient
  - Thumb sign
  - Vallecula sign — loss of vallecula
  - Review or listen to radiology report
- Notify physician promptly before x-ray if epiglottis suspected or patient in distress

Peritonsillar abscess

- Sore throat 100%
- Fever 26–97%
- Voice change
- Dysphagia
- Drooling
- Headache
- Trismus
- Uvular deviation and peritonsillar bulge
- Neck CT scan may be required to delineate abscess from necrotic lymph node
- Notify physician if diagnosed or suspected

Retropharyngeal abscess

- Usually age 3–5 years

Complications

- Airway compromise
- Aspiration pneumonia

- Internal jugular vein thrombosis
- Carotid artery erosion
- Cranial nerve palsies

History and findings

- Fever
- Dysphagia
- Decreased oral intake
- Stridor or dyspnea
- Neck swelling
- Neck motion pain
- Ill appearing
- Duck-like voice

X-ray findings

- Neck CT scan much more sensitive than lateral neck plain films
- Lateral soft-tissue neck films (neck flexion may cause false positive reading)
- Retropharyngeal space anterior to C2 > 7 mm or > half the width of vertebral body
- Space anterior to C6 > 14 mm in preschool children or > 22 mm in adults

Treatment

- Supplemental oxygen (avoid patient agitation)
- Keep child calm
- Notify physician promptly

Discharge Criteria for Sore throat

- Nontoxic
- No airway obstruction concerns
- Can tolerate oral intake
- Benign diagnosis

Discharge instructions

- Sore throat or pharyngitis aftercare instructions
- Follow up with primary care provider or ENT surgeon within 5 days as needed

Consult Criteria for Sore throat

- Airway compromise
- Toxic
- Dehydration > 5%
- Suspected epiglottitis
- Peritonsillar or retropharyngeal abscess
- Unable to tolerate oral intake
- Immunosuppression

Vital signs consult criteria

- Adult heart rate ≥ 110
- Pediatric heart rate
    - 0–4 months ≥ 180
    - 5–7 months ≥ 175
    - 6–12 months ≥ 170
    - 1–3 years ≥ 160
    - 4–5 years ≥ 145
    - 6–8 years ≥ 130
    - 7–12 years ≥ 125
    - 12–15 years ≥ 120
    - 16 years or older ≥ 115
- Hypotension
- O2 saturation < 95% on room air

Lab consult criteria

- WBC ≥ 18,000 or < 3,000
- Bandemia ≥ 15%
- Acute thrombocytopenia
- Metabolic acidosis

Notes

OTITIS EXTERNA PROTOCOL

When using any protocol, always follow the Guidelines of Proper Use (page 16).

Definition

- Inflammation of the external auditory canal

Differential Diagnosis

- Auditory canal foreign body
- Otitis media
- Chondroma
- Herpes zoster

Considerations

- Caused by breakdown in protective barrier of ear canal
  - Pseudomonas; staph; strep species; fungi
- Pain increased with movement of external ear or touching external ear canal
- Discharge common
- Fever uncommon

Malignant Otitis Externa

- Elderly
- Diabetes
- Immunocompromise (pseudomonas frequent concern)
- Marked swelling
- Headache
- Possible cranial nerve deficit

Evaluation

- Usually none except otoscope and external ear exam
- Serum glucose if diabetic
- Suspected malignant otitis externa
  - CBC
  - C-reactive protein
  - Cultures

CT scan indications

- Neurologic abnormalities
- Toxic appearing patient
- Malignant otitis externa
- Fever

Treatment Options

- Clean ear canal (most important aspect of treatment)
- Irrigate or ear loop curettage (may be difficult due to pain)
  - Use ½ peroxide and ½ water (or water only) – if TM (tympanic membrane) visible and intact (keep liquid near body temperature)
- Can use ear wick if canal markedly swollen – remove in 3 days; replace if canal still very swollen
- NSAID's or narcotics prn

Antibiotic choices

- Acetic acid 2% (Domeboro otic) 4–6 drops q4–6h for 7–10 days or until ear canal normal for 2 days
- Cortisporin otic suspension or solution (has neomycin which can cause allergy) 4 drops qid for 7–10 days or until ear canal normal for 2 days (use suspension if tympanic membrane (TM) perforated)
- Ofloxin 5 drops bid for 7–10 days or until ear canal normal for 2 days (drug of choice for TM perforation)
- Oral antibiotics for facial or neck cellulitis, significant edema of ear canal, or when TM (tympanic membrane) cannot be visualized
- Diabetics may be treated also with ciprofloxacin PO for 10–14 days
- May use Sanford Guide

Discharge Criteria

- Benign otitis externa

Discharge instructions

- Otitis externa aftercare instructions
- Keep ear dry for 3 weeks (no swimming)

- Prophylaxis for future OE after swimming with rubbing alcohol or acetic acid 2% if no TM (tympanic membrane) perforation
- Follow up with primary care provider or ENT surgeon within 7–10 days if needed

Consult Criteria

- Malignant external otitis (needs ENT consultation and IV antibiotics only — no topical antibiotics)
- Fever
- Return visit for same episode
- Glucose ≥ 400 mg/dL in diabetic patient
- Hyperglycemia with metabolic acidosis (decreased serum CO_2 or elevated anion gap)

Notes

EYE PROTOCOLS

When using any protocol, always follow the Guidelines of Proper Use (page 16).

Considerations

- Most conjunctival infections are viral
- Allergic manifestations common
- Contact lens keratitis can be bacterial or from oxygen deficit of cornea

Evaluation

- Visual acuity if complaints of decreased vision
- Examination of
  - Conjunctiva
  - Cornea
  - Pupils
  - Extraocular motion
  - Any discharge
  - For consensual photophobia (light shined in unaffected eye causes pain in affected eye — have affected eye closed during exam)
  - Periorbital tissues
  - Anterior and posterior chambers
  - Visual fields examination as indicated
- See specific conditions below

Conjunctivitis

Allergic

- Itching and redness; watery
- Papillary hypertrophy

Treatment options

- Systemic antihistamine
- Remove offending agent if known
- Choices:
  - Naphcon-A ophthalmic 1–2 drops qid prn
  - Ketorolac ophthalmic 1 drop qid prn

- Low dose steroid eye drops prn — short course
    - Dexamethasone ophthalmic 1–2 drops tid-qid prn or similar ophthalmic steroid
    - Contraindications:
        - Herpes simplex infection (corneal dendrite)
        - Glaucoma
        - Fungal infection

Discharge criteria

- Benign presentation and findings

Consult criteria

- Photophobia
- Visual changes

Viral

- Adenovirus most common
- Watery mucus discharge
- Gritty or foreign body sensation
- HSV: vesicles eyelid margins or periorbital skin; corneal dendrites

Treatment options

- Usually no specific therapy
- Artificial tears prn
- HSV
    - Viroptic ophthalmic drops 1 gtt q2h not to exceed 9 gtts qday
    - Consult physician for herpes infection
    - Ophthalmology referral within 1 day for HSV infection

Bacterial

- Purulent discharge
- Staph most common
- Gonorrhea: profuse purulent discharge
- Chlamydial: mucopurulent discharge; photophobia occasionally
- Contact lens: pseudomonas possible

Treatment options

Common drugs

- Erythromycin eye ointment
- Sulfa eye drops
- Gentamicin eye drops
- All medications given for 7 days

Contact lens complications

- Remove lens until eye normal for 2 days
- Ciloxan 1–2 drops QID × 7 days
- Consult physician

Chlamydia

- Doxycycline 100 BID × 3 weeks
  OR
- Erythromycin 500 mg QID PO × 3 weeks (erythromycin pediatric dose 50 mg/kg PO divided into 4 doses × 14 days — NMT 500 mg per dose)
- Mother of children and other close contacts at risk — treat with doxycycline 100 mg BID × 7 days in age > 8 years, otherwise erythromycin treatment

Gonococcal

- Doxycycline 100 BID × 3 weeks <u>or</u> erythromycin 500 mg QID PO × 3 weeks
- Rocephin (ceftriaxone) 1000 mg IM (can be given daily for 3 days)
- Neonates: Rocephin (ceftriaxone) 50 mg/kg IV daily for 7 days; erythromycin eye ointment QID × 14 days

- May use Sanford Guide

Discharge criteria

- Benign, non-herpetic conjunctivitis

Discharge instructions

- Conjunctivitis aftercare instructions
- Follow up with primary care provider or ophthalmology within 1 day for contact lens

complications, gonococcal or chlamydial infections

- Consult criteria
- Visual change
- Photophobia
- Suspected gonococcal or chlamydial infection
- Significant pain
- Contact lens complications

Infectious Keratitis

Causes

- HSV
- Staph
- Herpes zoster

Evaluation

- Direct visualization
- Fluorescein staining and wood's lamp
- Look for dendritic lesions

Treatment options

HSV

- Viroptic 1 drop q2hr while awake (NMT 9 drops qday)
- Follow up with ophthalmologist within 24 hours

Bacterial (all treatments for 7 days)

- Erythromycin eye ointment
- Sulfa eye drops
- Gentamicin eye drops

Discharge instructions

- Appropriate keratitis aftercare instructions if discharged

Consult criteria

- All infectious keratitis

Blepharitis, Hordeolum (Stye) and Chalazion

Stye

- Painful, swollen, tender and red on eyelid
- Staph 90–95% of the time
- Usually will drain spontaneously

Treatment options

- Warm soaks 3–4 days a day until resolved
- Erythromycin eye ointment or sulfa eye drops or gentamicin eye drops (all for 7–10 days)
- Clean eyelid margins with baby shampoo
- Refer to ophthalmologist in 10–14 days if not resolved

Chalazion

- Treatment similar to Stye

Blepharitis

- Treatment similar to Stye

Discharge instructions

- Appropriate aftercare instructions

Periorbital (Preseptal) Cellulitis

- Usually from S. aureus
- More common in children
- Age < 3 years can progress to bacteremia
- Is anterior to orbital septum

Signs

- Red swollen eyelid
- No vision changes
- Ocular mobility normal
- Conjunctival discharge may be present
- May have minimal pain
    - More severe with orbital cellulitis and helps to differentiate between the two
- Chemosis (conjunctival swelling)

- Fever

Evaluation

- Detailed ocular exam
  - Anterior and posterior chambers
  - Extraocular motion
  - Pupillary examination
  - CT scan may be needed if unable to differentiate from orbital cellulitis
- CBC and blood culture if age < 5 years
- Culture of eye discharge if present

Treatment options

- Augmentin (amoxicillin/clavulanate) 45 mg/kg/day divided bid PO for 10–14 days
- Vancomycin
- Rocephin (ceftriaxone)
- May use Sanford Guide

Discharge instructions

- Periorbital or preseptal cellulitis aftercare instructions
- Follow up in 24 hours with PCP or ophthalmologist

Orbital Cellulitis

- Most commonly from ethmoid sinusitis spread

Findings and symptoms

- May have toxic appearance
- Proptosis
- Limited extraocular motion
- Diplopia
- Significant pain
- Dark red eyelids
- Decreased vision
- Increased intraocular pressure

Complications

- Meningitis
- Cavernous sinus thrombosis
- Vision loss

Evaluation

- Detailed ocular exam
  - Anterior and posterior chambers
  - Extraocular motion
  - Pupillary examination
  - CT scan may be needed if unable to differentiate from orbital cellulitis
- CBC and blood culture if age < 5 years
- Culture of eye discharge if present

Treatment

- Ceftin (cefuroxime) IV and/or per Sanford Guide
- Admission to hospital

Consult criteria

- All suspected or diagnosed orbital cellulitis patients

Corneal Ulcer or Lesions

- Consult physician

Discharge instructions

- Corneal ulcer aftercare instructions

Iritis

- Photophobia — is consensual (light shined into opened normal eye causes pain in closed affected eye due to pupillary reflex)
- Ciliary flush (red injection at edge of cornea circumferentially)
- Cells and flare in anterior chamber; hypopyon more rare
- Miosis
- 50% associated with systemic disease
- Slit lamp exam helpful

Treatment

- Homatropine eye drops 2–5% 1 drop TID
- Steroid eye drops per ophthalmologist
- Consult physician

Discharge instructions

- Iritis aftercare instructions
- Close ophthalmology follow-up

Corneal Abrasion

- Can detect with direct ophthalmoscopy or fluorescein staining
- No consensual photophobia unless iritis present
- Heals in 24–48 hours
- If corneal pain recurs in 2–3 days, it may indicate sloughing of corneal epithelium

Treatment

- No patching
- Can use local anesthetic eye drops at time of exam only (do not prescribe for home pain control since it is mildly cytotoxic and will prevent healing)
- Narcotics PO prn × 2–3 days

Extensive corneal abrasion

- Homatropine 2% sol 1–2 gtt to achieve cycloplegia (pupil dilation) — may repeat q15 min. × 2 prn
- Can prescribe 1–2 gtt QID up to 3 days

Discharge instructions

- Corneal abrasion aftercare instructions
- Follow up in 2–3 days for recheck with primary care provider or ophthalmologist

Ultraviolet Keratitis (Band Keratitis)

- Usually from welding or tanning beds
- Acular (ketorolac) or Voltaren (diclofenic) eye drops 1 gtt QID for several days until eye corneal pain resolved (not longer than 2 weeks)
- Similar evaluation and treatment as corneal abrasion

Discharge instructions

- Ultraviolet (flash burn) keratitis aftercare instructions

Eye Foreign Body

- Usually a foreign body sensation is the chief complaint
- Anesthetic eye drops with proparacaine or tetracaine immediately relieves symptoms for 15 minutes or so
- Patient may or may not be able to localize the foreign body

Examination

- Evert eyelids as needed to locate the foreign body
- If foreign body is not identified, flush under eyelids with eye irrigation fluids to see if symptoms can be resolved
- If foreign body persists after eye flush, use moistened sterile cotton swab to gently swab under eyelids to see if any foreign bodies are found or the patient's symptoms of foreign body sensation resolve
- Check lacrimal duct opening for retained eyelash

Discharge criteria

- Foreign body removed
- No visual changes or significant residual discomfort

Discharge instructions

- Eye foreign body aftercare instructions

Consult criteria

- Retained intraocular foreign body, discuss with physician
- Significant residual pain post foreign body removal
- Acute visual changes or complaints

Corneal Foreign Bodies

- If an iron containing metallic foreign body is present, a rust ring may develop in a few hours
- Examine anterior and posterior ocular chambers — if abnormal discuss with physician or ophthalmologist
- Fluorescein staining can be used as needed to locate foreign bodies and abrasions

- The Provider may opt to not remove small residual rust rings outside of visual axis, and refer to an ophthalmologist for further treatment in 1-3 days

Removal instructions

- After 3-4 drops of eye anesthetic over 1 minute are instilled into the affected eye and the patient has no further complaints of a foreign body sensation or pain, a sterile moistened cotton swab is used to swab across the foreign body to effect removal
- If the cotton swab does not remove the corneal foreign body, an experienced Provider may use a blunt eye spud or eye burr to remove the foreign body
- Consult a physician if not experienced with using a blunt eye spud or eye burr
- If a metallic foreign body has rusted, a residual rust ring will be left after the majority of the central rust area has been removed with the cotton swab
    - A blunt eye spud or eye burr can be used to remove some of the residual rust left, although it is not unusual to not be able to remove it all
- Fresh rust rings are more difficult to remove and after sterile cotton swabbing the residual rust ring can be left to mature in 1-3 days and the patient can then be referred to an ophthalmologist for follow-up

Discharge instructions

- Corneal foreign body aftercare instructions
- Refer to ophthalmology within 3 days
- Return if pain worsens, or photophobia or visual changes develops

Consult criteria

- Discuss with the physician if the residual rust is in the visual axis

Corneal Laceration

- Protective rigid eye shield

- Consult physician and ophthalmologist immediately
- Analgesia and vomiting control IM or IV prn to decrease valsalva

Eyelid Lacerations

Findings to discuss with physician (usually needs referral treatment)

- Tarsal plate involvement
- Eyelid margin
- Tear duct injury
- Orbital septum injury
  - Fat can protrude
- Tissue loss

Globe Injury

- History is important of what patient was doing at time of injury
- Globe injury can be obvious with uveal tissue prolapsing from a wound or pupil, or the eye or papillary shape can be grossly abnormal, or the injury may be subtle
- Small eyelid lacerations can cover or mask perforations of globe
  - Do not close laceration until globe injury is ruled out
- Assess eye motion and visual acuity
  - Visual acuity can be counting fingers at 18 inches or light perception if necessary
  - Critical to avoid pressure on the eye
  - Palpate orbital rims for deformity and crepitus
  - Do not remove any foreign bodies that have penetrated the globe
  - Conjunctival hemorrhage covering 360 degrees of the bulbar conjunctiva can indicate globe rupture
  - Assess pupils for size, shape, afferent defect, direct and indirect pupillary light reflex and the red reflex
  - Examine anterior chamber
  - CT orbital scans are the preferred imaging to evaluate for occult globe injury

Treatment

- Place protective rigid eye shield immediately after assessment

Disposition

- Consult physician and ophthalmologist immediately
- Analgesia and vomiting control IM or IV prn to decrease valsalva and minimize intraocular pressure increases

Chemical Eye Injuries

Alkali burns most serious

- Causes immediate liquefaction necrosis if the pH is very high
- Penetrates the tissue deeply
- Immediate eye lavage with NS for one hour (Morgan lens)
- Exam after lavage
- Notify physician promptly

Acid burns

- Cause coagulation of proteins which can limit depth of injury
- Can use fluorescein to evaluate cornea (exam after lavage if needed)
- Weak acids burns usually managed as outpatient

Evaluation

- Inspection
- After lavage if strong alkali: fluorescein or slit lamp
- Check visual acuity

Treatment

- Significant burns flush with NS using Morgan lens for 30–60 minutes
- Check pH at 5 and 30 minutes of eye lavage to achieve pH 7.3–7.5

- Mild burns with weak acids can be lavaged less (with or without Morgan lens) depending on symptoms
- Use topical eye anesthetic for pain of examination and treatment as needed
- Gentamicin plus erythromycin or bacitracin ophthalmic ointment tid × 5–10 days or until healed for significant chemical burns
- Mild burns without significant damage can be managed with one topical eye antibiotic ointment
- Narcotics or NSAID's PO prn pain

Discharge criteria

- Mild conjunctivitis and keratitis from weak acid chemical burns
- Discuss with physician all chemical eye injuries

Discharge instructions

- Chemical eye injury aftercare instructions
- Refer to ophthalmologist within 1 day if indicated

Consult criteria

- Alkali burns
- Acid burns of moderate or worse severity
- Visual acuity changes

Glaucoma

- Severe pain, ipsilateral visual defects and may see halos around objects
- Nausea and vomiting common with acute closed angle glaucoma
- Steamy and cloudy cornea
- Increase IOP (normal IOP 10–22 mm Hg)
- Mid-dilated pupil and firm globe
- Consult physician promptly

Orbital Blowout Isolated Fracture

- Orbital wall composed of 7 bones
- Occurs usually with larger object than the orbit (baseball; fist)

- Can result in diplopia

Evaluation

- Neurologic exam
- Extraocular motor exam
- Evaluate for associated ocular injuries (present 20–40% of the time)
- Plain facial (water's view best) or CT orbital films
- CT brain scan as per head injury protocols
- Ocular anterior and posterior chamber exam
- TM's (tympanic membrane) exam for hemotympanum
- Grasp upper teeth and palate and pull to assess for Lefort fractures (movement noted)
- Dental exam
- C-spine films prn (see Neck Pain Protocol)

Treatment

- Most patients can be followed as outpatient with plastic surgeon or ophthalmologist in a timeframe determined by the surgeon
- Discuss with physician
- No nose blowing
- Augmentin (amoxicillin/clavulanate) 500 mg TID PO × 10 days or Levaquin (levofloxacin) 750 mg qday PO × 10 days
- Pediatric Augmentin (amoxicillin/clavulanate) dose — 12.5 mg/kg PO bid × 10 days
- Analgesics PO prn
- Ice prn for swelling
- Tetanus if not up to date (see Tetanus Protocol, page 580)

Discharge criteria

- Uncomplicated inferior blowout fracture without extraocular muscle entrapment or other facial fractures or associated conditions

Discharge instructions

- Head injury aftercare instructions
- Orbital blowout fracture aftercare instructions

- Referral to Ophthalmology or plastic surgeon within 7 days

Consult criteria

- Discuss all facial fractures except nasal with physician

Subconjunctival Hemorrhage

- No treatment
- Check PT/INR if on Coumadin (warfarin)
- CBC if constitutional symptoms present

Retinal Detachment

Causes

- Tear in retina

Risk factors

- Near sighted
- Advanced age
- Diabetes
- Sickle cell anemia
- Prior retinal detachment history

Findings and symptoms

- Painless
- Light flashes
- Decreased peripheral vision
- Floaters
- Lowering of curtain over vision in affected eye

Examination includes

- Direct ophthalmoscopy (may need pupils dilated)
- Bedside ultrasound with vascular probe can detect retinal detachment

Treatment

- Elevate head of bed for inferior detachment
- Lay flat for superior detachment

Consult criteria

- Consult physician and ophthalmologist promptly

Central Retinal Artery Occlusion

- True emergency
- Usually from emboli
- 90 minutes to restore vision before irreversible damage
- Evaluate for sickle cell anemia and temporal arteritis

Findings

- Sudden loss of vision in one eye
- Pupil reacts consensually
- Afferent defect to light in affected eye (pupil does not constrict)
- Increased intraocular pressure
- Pale fundus
- Dilated pupil
- Retinal artery may have "box cars" appearance
- Macula has enhanced cherry red appearance (different blood supply)

Treatment

- Gentle massage on globe to attempt dislodging emboli
- Rebreathing bag or mask to increase CO2

IOP treatment

- Timoptic (timolol)
- Diamox (acetazolamide)
- Ophthalmology paracentesis of anterior chamber

Consult criteria

- Notify physician immediately
- Ophthalmologist consult immediately

Central Retinal Vein Occlusion

- Rapid and painless vision loss of one eye
    - Slower onset than retinal artery occlusion
    - From thrombosis of central retinal vein

Findings

- Retinal hemorrhages
- Impressive appearance of fundus with bloody engorgement
    - Optic disc edema

Treatment

- Aspirin

Consult criteria

- All central retinal vein occlusion patients
- All patients with acute vision loss

Hyphema and Hypopyon (Blood or Pus in Anterior Chamber)

- Consult physician

Notes

NOSEBLEED PROTOCOL

When using any protocol, always follow the Guidelines of Proper Use (page 16).

Definition

- Bleeding from nostril, nasal cavity or nasopharynx

Differential Diagnosis

- Nasal foreign body
- Sinusitis
- Barotrauma
- Thrombocytopenia
- Leukemia
- Anticoagulation therapy
- Cocaine abuse
- NSAID use
- ASA use
- Hemophilia
- Von Willebrand's disease
- Trauma

Considerations

- 90% of nosebleeds are anterior
- Most common cause is nose picking
- Hypertension common
- Look for foreign body in young children (suspect if foul smell or discharge present)
- Posterior Epistaxis
    - Less common than anterior Epistaxis
    - Associated with
        - Elderly
        - Hypertension
        - Atherosclerosis

Evaluation

- Attempt visualization of bleeding
- Use nosebleed tray equipment or otoscope
- Have patient clear blood by forcefully blowing nose

- Use suction prn
- Cocaine intranasally can be used for hemostasis and pain control
- If bleeding has stopped and site unknown, take moistened cotton swab and gently stroke suspected area to elicit bleeding
- CBC if suspected significant blood loss or patient is tachycardic or orthostatic
- PT/INR if on Coumadin (warfarin). PTT if on heparin or has Von Willebrand's disease or hemophilia

Treatment Options

- Control anterior nosebleed by pinching all of nose below nasal bone up to 2–4 minutes
- May treat hypertension if > SBP 180 or DBP > 110
    - Repeat BP 10–15 minutes initially, before treatment, to see if BP decreases sufficiently without medication
    - Treat initial SBP > 210 or DBP > 120 if actively bleeding
- IV NS if vital signs or CBC reflect significant bleeding (notify physician promptly)

Silver nitrate

- Silver nitrate stick cautery directly on bleeding site for 5–7 seconds, and then in a circle around bleeding site, holding 5–7 seconds each spot, to form a solid eschar
    - Then hold 2 dry cotton swabs side by side for 60 seconds over cauterized area with enough pressure to stop any bleeding (usually mild pressure is all that is needed)
    - May repeat in places that continue bleeding with more cautery and cotton swabs pressure until bleeding stops

Additional treatments

- Use Rapid Rhino anterior or posterior balloons (or similar intranasal balloons) if silver nitrate cautery not used or ineffective
- Can also use Merocel packing
- Afrin type nasal spray can be used for hemostasis
- Epistaxis thrombin kit for intranasal application

- Septra DS or sinusitis medication Rx per Sanford Guide for 5–7 days if packing or balloon used

Discharge Criteria

- Successful treatment of bleeding
- Anterior nosebleed
- Hemodynamically stable
- No respiratory distress

Discharge instructions

- Nosebleed or epistaxis aftercare instructions
- Packing removal in 2–3 days
- Refer to ENT or primary care provider in 2–3 days
- Antibiotic ointment twice a day for 7–10 days for cautery or after packing removed — gently applied

Consult Criteria

- Unable to stop bleeding
- Posterior nasal bleeding or packing
- Significant blood loss per CBC or vital signs abnormalities
- Tachycardia or orthostatic vital signs
- Coagulopathy secondary to Coumadin (warfarin) or other causes
- Bleeding site not identified or not known whether anterior or posterior

Vital signs and age consult criteria

- Adult HR > 105
- SBP < 90 or relative hypotension (SBP < 105 with history of hypertension)
- Pediatric heart rate
  - 0–4 months ≥ 180
  - 5–7 months ≥ 175
  - 6–12 months ≥ 170
  - 1–3 years ≥ 160
  - 4–5 years ≥ 145
  - 6–8 years ≥ 130
  - 7–12 years ≥ 125
  - 12–15 years ≥ 115

- 16 years or older ≥ 110

Lab consult criteria

- Acute hemoglobin decrease of > 1 gm
- Hemoglobin < 10 gm
- Thrombocytopenia
- INR > 1.2
- PTT > 1.2 times normal

Notes

ENT EMERGENCY PROTOCOL

When using any protocol, always follow the Guidelines of Proper Use (page 16).

Ludwig's Angina

Definition

- Cellulitis (occasionally abscess) involving submandibular and sublingual spaces

Considerations

- Mortality has declined to < 10% since penicillin was introduced
- Can result in elevation of tongue to obstruct airway
- Increased association with diabetes; SLE; neutropenia; alcoholism
- Polymicrobial infection is usual
- Infection of 2nd and 3rd molars most common cause — 80% of cases
- Is a clinical diagnosis
- Assess airway status — may need anesthesia or ENT if difficult intubation likely
- Ability of tongue to be protruded beyond vermillion border excludes sublingual space infection

Signs

- Bilateral submandibular swelling - All
- Elevated or protruding tongue - 19/20
- Fever - 9/10
- Increased WBC - 17/20
- Recent dental extraction or toothache - 8/10
- Neck swelling - 7/10
- Dysphagia - 5/10
- Trismus - 5/10
- Neck pain - 1/3
- Respiratory (stridor; dyspnea; tachypnea) - 7/20
- Dysphonia and dysarthria - 1/5

Evaluation

- Is a clinical diagnosis
- Airway management takes precedence over testing
- CT scanning best modality if needed
- Soft tissue neck and panorex useful when CT not available
- CBC
- BMP

Treatment options

- Antibiotics effective
  - Penicillin + Flagyl (metronidazole)
  - Unasyn
  - Clindamycin
- Surgery
  - Needed 20–65% of time
  - If abscess identified
- Airway management if needed
  - Endotracheal intubation
  - Cricothyroidotomy by physician
  - Notify physician immediately if suspected airway compromise

Complications

- Aspiration
- Mediastinitis
- Pneumonia
- Empyema
- Bacteremia
- Septic emboli
- Pericarditis
- Cavernous sinus thrombosis
- Cerebral abscess

Consult criteria

- All Ludwig's angina cases
- If imminent airway concern, notify physician immediately

Angioedema of Oropharyngeal Area

Considerations

- Affects deeper tissues
- Localized non-pitting edema
- 25% of population experiences urticaria or angioedema during lifetime
- Localized swelling resolves in several days
- Typically involves face and upper lip
- GI tract involvement causes
    - Nausea
    - Vomiting
    - Diarrhea
    - Abdominal pain
    - Esophageal involvement can cause chest pain
- Neurologic involvement rare
- Upper respiratory involvement responsible for mortality

Predictors of need for airway intervention

- Increased age
- Tongue swelling
- Oropharynx swelling
- Odynophagia

Signs

- Respiratory distress
- Stridor
- Voice changes
- Dysphagia

Causes

- Hereditary angioedema (HAE)
- Angiotension converting enzyme inhibitors (ACE) around 70% of patients
    - Increased incidence in African-Americans and women
    - Most occur in first week of therapy
        - But can occur anytime

Treatment options

- Medical management usually suffices
- Stop offending agent if known
- Less responsive to treatment than urticaria
    - Most can be treated with
        - Benadryl (diphenhydramine) 50 mg PO or IM adult; continue for 5–7 days PO
        - Benadryl (diphenhydramine) 1–2 mg/kg PO or IM pediatrics; continue for 5–7 days PO
    - Additional treatment if needed
        - Pepcid (famotidine) 20–40 mg IV/PO for adult
        - Pepcid (famotidine) 0.25 mg/kg IV/PO for pediatric (NMT 40 mg)
    - Consider steroids
        - Prednisone 40–60 mg PO qday for 5–7 days (> 40 kg)
        - Prednisone/prednisolone 1 mg/kg PO qday (children < 40 kg) for 5–7 days
- Airway compromise or significant oropharyngeal swelling (notify physician immediately)
    - Epinephrine
        - Caution if coronary artery disease history present
        - Adult: 0.3 mg SQ; (notify physician promptly)
        - Pediatrics: 0.01 mg/kg SQ – do not exceed adult dose (notify physician promptly)
        - Oxygen prn
    - Responds to fresh frozen plasma (jumbo unit) or C1 esterase inhibitor concentrate
- Consult physician promptly for posterior oropharyngeal angioedema
- Stop ACE inhibitors if currently taking

Discharge criteria

- Observation for 4–6 hours
- Discharge mild lip or non-oropharyngeal angioedema with normal vital signs and no distress

Discharge instructions

- Angioedema aftercare instructions
- Refer to primary care provider within 1 day if not improving, otherwise 3-4 days if improving

Consult criteria

- Discuss all patients with physician

Barotitis Media and Barosinusitis

- Caused by relative negative pressures from descent during flying usually with a coexistent URI or positive pressures from ascent during diving
- Findings that may be seen
  - Loss of TM (tympanic membrane) landmarks, congestion around umbo, hemorrhage into middle ear

Valsalva maneuver

- On airplane descent can be used to prevent occurrence (nostrils pinched and patient blows against a closed mouth forcing air into Eustachian tubes with tympanic membranes feeling the pressure and subsequently moving – do not perform if vertigo present

Treatment options

- For tympanic membrane congestion only
  - Nasal and oral decongestants
- For hemorrhage into middle ear
  - Adult: prednisone 60 mg PO qday for 6 days then taper over 7-10 days
  - Children: prednisone 1 mg/kg PO for 6 days then taper over 7-10 days (do not exceed adult dose)
- Otitis media antibiotics are prescribed if tympanic membrane perforation or discharge noted
  - Keep ear dry
- Narcotics and/or NSAID's prrn for pain

Discharge instructions

- Barotitis or barosinusitis aftercare instructions

- Refer to ENT surgeon if perforation or vertigo present – refer to PCP otherwise
- No altitude traveling till symptoms and findings resolve

Consult criteria

- Discuss with physician immediately any patient with joint pain or swelling, chest pain or dyspnea (order chest x-ray), dizziness, headache, altered mental status or hypotension after diving

Nosebleeds

Considerations

- 90% of nosebleeds are anterior
- Most common cause is nose picking
- Hypertension common
- Look for foreign body in young children (suspect if foul smell or discharge)

Evaluation

- Attempt visualization of bleeding
- Use nosebleed tray equipment or otoscope
- Have patient clear blood by forcefully blowing nose
- Use suction prn to clear blood clots or active bleeding as needed
- If bleeding has stopped and site unknown, take moistened cotton swab and gently stroke suspected area to elicit bleeding
- CBC if suspected significant blood loss or tachycardic or orthostatic
- PT/INR if on Coumadin (warfarin). PTT if on heparin or has Von Willebrand's disease or hemophilia

Treatment options

- Control anterior nosebleed by pinching all of nose below nasal bone up to 2–4 minutes
- May treat hypertension if > SBP 170 or DBP > 110

    - Repeat BP 10–15 minutes initially, before treatment, to see if BP decreases sufficiently without medication
- Treat initial SBP > 210 or DBP > 120 if actively bleeding
- IV NS if vital signs or CBC reflect significant bleeding (notify physician promptly)

Silver nitrate

- Silver nitrate stick cautery directly on bleeding site for 5–7 seconds, and then in a circle around bleeding site, holding 5–7 seconds each spot, to form a solid eschar
    - Then hold 2 dry cotton swabs side by side for 60 seconds over cauterized area with enough pressure to stop any bleeding (usually mild pressure is all that is needed)
    - May repeat in places that continue bleeding with more cautery and cotton swabs pressure until bleeding stops

Additional treatments

- Use Rapid Rhino anterior or posterior balloons (or similar balloons) if silver nitrate cautery not used or ineffective
- Can also use Merocel packing
- Afrin type nasal spray can be used for hemostasis
- Epistaxis thrombin kit for intranasal application
- Septra DS or sinusitis medication Rx per Sanford Guide for 5–7 days if packing or balloon used

Discharge Criteria

- Successful treatment of bleeding
- Anterior nosebleed
- Hemodynamically stable
- No respiratory distress

Discharge instructions

- Nosebleed or epistaxis aftercare instructions
- Packing removal in 2–3 days
- Refer to ENT or primary care provider in 2–3 days

- Antibiotic ointment twice a day for 7–10 days for cautery or after packing removed — gently applied

Consult Criteria

- Unable to stop bleeding
- Posterior nasal bleeding or packing
- Significant blood loss per CBC or vital signs abnormalities
- Tachycardia or orthostatic vital signs
- Coagulopathy secondary to Coumadin (warfarin) or other causes
- Bleeding site not identified or not known whether anterior or posterior

Vital signs and age consult criteria

- Adult HR > 105
- SBP < 90 or relative hypotension (SBP < 105 with history of hypertension)
- Pediatric heart rate
    - 0–4 months ≥ 180
    - 5–7 months ≥ 175
    - 6–12 months ≥ 170
    - 1–3 years ≥ 160
    - 4–5 years ≥ 145
    - 6–8 years ≥ 130
    - 7–12 years ≥ 125
    - 12–15 years ≥ 115
    - 16 years or older ≥ 110

Lab consult criteria

- Acute hemoglobin decrease of > 1 gm
- Hemoglobin < 10 gm
- Thrombocytopenia
- INR > 1.2
- PTT > 1.2 times normal

Notes

Nasal and Facial Fractures Protocol

When using any protocol, always follow the Guidelines of Proper Use (page 16).

Nasal Fractures

- Most common fracture
- X-rays may miss around 50%

Complications

- Septal hematoma
- Associated orbital wall blowout fractures
- Facial fractures with CSF (cerebrospinal fluid) leak – cribriform plate fracture
- Hyphema
- Retinal detachment
- Subconjunctival hemorrhage

CSF rhinorrhea

- Cribriform plate fracture
- Increased by leaning forward
- Increased with jugular compression
- Ring sign (2 rings formed when CSF placed on filter paper)
- Dipstick findings – CSF glucose > 30mg%

Evaluation options

- Physical examination
- Clear nares of blood
- Evaluate for septal hematoma
- CT facial bones if suspected facial fractures
- CT head injury protocols
- C-spine films prn (see Neck Pain Protocol)
- Plain nasal films not usually needed but can be ordered
- CBC if significant blood loss suspected or tachycardia/hypotension
- Tympanic membranes for hemotympanum

- Eye exam of anterior and posterior chambers if suspected eye injury or complaints
- Excessive tearing may indicate nasolacrimal duct injury — if suspected instill fluorescein in eye and exam posterior pharynx (with Wood's light if needed) to see if dye flows into pharynx through intact duct

Treatment options

- Epistaxis controlled with pinching nares together for 2–5 minutes
- Septal hematoma needs immediate drainage
    - Can be drained with 18 gauge needle after cocaine topical anesthesia
    - Rolled cotton swab can help decompress hematoma
    - Packing after drainage for 3–5 days
    - Antibiotics to prevent sinusitis (same as otitis media antibiotics)
- Analgesics prn
- Tetanus if not up to date (see Tetanus Protocol, page 580)

Discharge criteria

- Simple nasal fractures

Discharge instructions

- Nasal fracture aftercare instructions
- Refer to ENT within 7–10 days
- Head injury instructions

Consult criteria

- Septal hematoma
- Associated facial fractures
- Other associated injuries
- Significant blood loss

Orbital Blowout Fractures

- Orbital wall composed of 7 bones
- Occurs usually with larger object than the orbit (baseball; fist)
- Can result in diplopia

Evaluation

- Neurologic exam
- Extraocular motor exam
- Plain facial (water's view best) or CT orbital films
- CT head injury protocols
- Ocular anterior and posterior chamber exam
- TM's (tympanic membrane) for hemotympanum
- Grasp upper teeth and palate and pull to assess for Lefort fractures (movement noted)
- Dental exam
- C-spine films prn (see Neck Pain Protocol)

Treatment

- Antibiotics (same as sinusitis treatment)
- Analgesics prn
- Tetanus if not up to date (see Tetanus Protocol, page 580)

Discharge criteria

- Uncomplicated inferior blowout fracture without extraocular muscle entrapment or other facial fractures or associated conditions
- Head injury instructions should be given to competent alert patient or family member or similar person

Discharge instructions

- Head injury aftercare instructions
- Orbital blowout fracture aftercare instructions
- Referral to Ophthalmology or plastic surgeon within 7 days

Consult criteria

- Discuss all facial fractures except uncomplicated nasal fracture with physician
- Referral to Ophthalmology within 7 days

Mandible Fracture

- Third most common facial fracture
- 20–40% of mandibular fracture patients have associated injuries

- Children age 4–11 years at risk for facial growth disturbance if fracture missed

Findings

- Facial asymmetry
- Malocclusion of teeth
- Paresthesia to lower lip or gums indicate inferior alveolar nerve damage
- Blood in mouth suggests open fracture
- Jaw may deviate to side of fracture

Evaluation

- Airway exam — notify physician immediately if any airway concerns
- Dental exam
- Neurologic exam
- Plain mandible films or panorex
- CT mandible if the plain films not helpful in suspected fracture
- CT head if per head injury protocols or abnormal neurologic exam
- Chest x-ray if missing teeth cannot be located
- C-spine films prn (see Neck Pain Protocol)

Treatment

- Dental antibiotics choices
  - Pen VK 500 mg PO qid × 7–10 days
  - Cleocin (clindamycin) 300 mg PO qid × 7–10 days
  - Erythromycin 250 mg PO qid × 7–10 days
- Tetanus if not up to date (see Tetanus Protocol, page 580)
- See Dental Injury Protocol

Discharge criteria

- Simple nondisplaced mandible fractures
- Soft diet
- Analgesics prn

Discharge instructions

- Mandible fracture aftercare instructions

- Referral to oral surgeon within 1–4 days
- Head injury instructions

Consult criteria

- Discuss all mandible fractures with physician or oral surgeon

Notes

DENTAL INJURY PROTOCOLS

When using any protocol, always follow the Guidelines of Proper Use (page 16).

Considerations

- Injury to primary teeth common in toddlers
- Older children dental injuries commonly from sports
- Assess for other injuries
- Primary tooth eruption from 7 months to 2-3 years of age
- Malocclusion of teeth is a mandible or maxilla fracture until proven otherwise

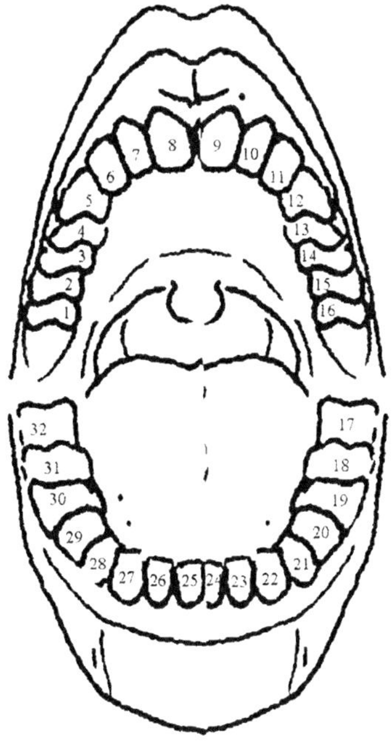

Tooth Fractures

- Ellis class 1: enamel injured only
- Ellis class 2: dentin involved
- Ellis class 3: pulp involved (bloody dental tissue seen)

Dental Avulsions of Permanent Teeth

- 1% loss of successive reimplantation of avulsed per minute that tooth is not replaced in socket
- More than 15 minutes out of socket has poor salvage rate
- After 60 minutes of being out of socket there usually is no salvage rate
- Avulsed teeth should be handled by crown only
- Put in either Hank's solution, milk, or normal saline as a temporizing measure
- Put tooth back immediately after aspirating any clot and irrigating the socket
- Apply a mouth guard (sports mouth guard acceptable)
- Antibiotics: Pen VK 500 mg PO qid for 10 days and see dentist or oral surgeon within one day for further treatment
- It is preferable to discuss with dentist at time of injury

Dental Avulsions of Primary Teeth

- Leave out of mouth

Gingival Lacerations

- Heal well
- Reapproximate with chromic or Vicryl sutures
- Antibiotics of penicillin or erythromycin for 7–10 days or Clindamycin weight or age adjusted tid × 10 days

Lip and Intraoral Lacerations

- Repair from inside out then close skin
- Use absorbable sutures intraorally
- Line up vermillion border if involved
- Antibiotics
  - Pen VK 500 mg PO qid for 7–10 days (weight adjusted for pediatrics)
  - Erythromycin PO tid for 7–10 days if penicillin allergic
  - Clindamycin 300 mg PO tid × 10 days (weight adjusted for pediatrics)
- Refer to Laceration Protocol

Evaluation

- Dental history important to know to determine if teeth worth saving
- Time of injury important
- Palpate and lightly percuss teeth (should be a ping sound normally)
- Remove blood clots
- Check for intraoral lacerations and any through and through involvement
- Check facial bones for looseness (Lefort fractures) but pulling forward on palate or upper maxillary rim
- Plain x-rays for
  - Bony abnormalities
  - Aspirated teeth
  - Foreign bodies (tooth fragments) in lacerations
- Panorex films if available
- Refer to Head Injury Protocols

Treatment

- Enamel fractures do not require immediate treatment
- Class 2 fractures
  - Cover with Dycal (calcium hydroxide paste)
- Class 3 fractures
  - Anesthetize tooth
  - Immediate covering with Dycal
  - Antibiotics
    - Adult
      - Pen VK 500 mg PO qid × 10 days
      - Clindamycin 300 mg PO tid × 10 days
      - Amoxicillin 500 mg PO tid × 10 days
    - Weight adjustment of above antibiotics for pediatrics
- Analgesics prn
- Loose teeth referred to dentist and prescribe a soft diet
- Can use mouth guard to splint very loose teeth
- Move displaced teeth into position post local anesthesia

- Tetanus prophylaxis: (High risk = every 5 years; Low risk = every 10 years)
    - Tetanus IG 250–500 units if high risk and less than 3 tetanus or unknown history of immunizations previously in life — usually with the elderly
- Refer to health department or primary care provider to complete tetanus primary vaccination series if < 2 vaccines given in past
    - See Tetanus Protocol (page 580)

Discharge Criteria

- Ellis class 1 and 2 fractures
- Primary tooth avulsions
- Mildly loose teeth
- Refer to dentist or oral surgeon
    - Ellis class 2 fractures within 24 hours for primary dental avulsions and loose teeth
    - Ellis class 3 fractures dental referral ASAP, no more than next day if possible
- Give avulsed teeth that are not reimplanted to patient to take to dentist

Consult Criteria

- Displaced teeth
- Avulsed permanent teeth
- It is preferable to discuss with dentist at time of injury
- Discuss with physician or dentist Ellis class 2 and 3 fractures

Notes

DENTAL PAIN PROTOCOL

When using any protocol, always follow the Guidelines of Proper Use (page 16).

Differential diagnosis

- Periapical abscess
- Trigeminal neuralgia
- Masticator space infection
- Ludwig's angina
- Retropharyngeal space infection
- Infection after a root canal
- Dental caries

Considerations

- Dental abscess is rare in children
- Abscess can spread more deeply to
  - Bone (osteomyelitis)
  - Cavernous sinus (thrombosis)
  - Maxillary sinus
  - Floor of mouth (Ludwig's angina)
  - Adjacent facial spaces and planes
- Advanced dental disease in children could indicate diabetes mellitus or HIV infection

Evaluation

- Usually history and physical exam only
- Percussion tenderness present
- CBC when patient is toxic appearing
- BMP for tachycardia or history of diabetes or suspicion of undiagnosed diabetes
- Plain films of neck if deeper infections considered
- CT face or neck for suspected deeper infections

Periapical abscess

- Most common dental infection
- Very painful

Treatment options

- I&D with needle if abscess seen
    - Tap water as effective as normal saline for irrigation
- Antibiotics if no pus found or no aspiration performed (choose one below)
    - Pen VK 250 mg PO qid for 7–10 days
    - Clindamycin 150–450 mg PO qid for 7–10 days
    - Metronidazole 500 mg PO bid for 7–10 days
    - Azithromycin 5 day dose pak
    - Erythromycin 250 mg PO qid for 7–10 days
- NSAID's prn
- Hydrocodone prn up to 5 days

Discharge criteria

- Nontoxic patient
- Most dental pain patients

Discharge instructions

- Warm salt water rinses very frequently for 1–5 days. Hold in mouth for several minutes as tolerated
- Warm compresses to painful area several times a day
- Follow up with dentist within 48 hours

Consult criteria

- Deep space infection diagnosed or suspected
- Fever
- Potential for airway compromise

Trauma

Section Contents

Motor Vehicle Accident Protocol

Laceration and Cutaneous Wound Protocol

Bleeding Protocol

Burn Protocol

When using any protocol, always follow the Guidelines of Proper Use (page 16).

MOTOR VEHICLE ACCIDENT PROTOCOL

When using any protocol, always follow the Guidelines of Proper Use (page 16).

Considerations

- Leading cause of death ages 1–37 years
- Complete exam important even when single isolated injury suspected
- Initial assessment critical in determining life threatening processes
- Comorbidities should be addressed
- Liver and spleen most common intra-abdominal injuries followed by small and large intestine in blunt abdominal trauma
- Cervical and lumbar strains common in minor MVA
- Seatbelt marks may indicate deeper injuries

Evaluation

- Patients seen by the practitioner should have minor injuries only
- Alert patients on spine boards can be moved carefully if no suspicion of spine or acute neurologic deficits or significant bony trauma (fractures/dislocations)
- Notify physician immediately for Glasgow scale < 15

Primary survey

- Airway
- Breathing
- Circulation/bleeding
- Disability (neurologic exam)
- Exposure/environment (expose patient and hypothermia evaluation)

- Contact physician immediately if any serious findings found on primary survey
- Significant hemorrhagic vital sign findings, contact physician immediately

- IV NS 500–1000 cc bolus if hypotensive adult (consult physician immediately)
- Pediatrics 20 cc/kg IV NS bolus, may repeat × 2 prn (consult physician immediately)

Secondary survey

- Complete physical exam
- Palpate and inspect all body areas
- Complete neurovascular exam

AMPLE mnemonic for historical key elements

A – Allergies
M – Medications
P – Past history
L – Last meal
E – Events leading to presentation

Estimated Blood and Fluid losses (adults)

	Class I	Class II	Class III	Class IV
Blood loss (cc)	Up to 750	750–1000	1500–2000	> 2000
Blood loss %	Up to 15%	15–30%	30–40%	> 40%
Pulse rate	< 100	> 100	> 120	> 140
Blood pressure	Normal	Normal	SBP < 90	SBP < 70
Capillary refill	Normal	Normal	Delayed	Absent
Pulse pressure	Normal/incr	Decreased	Decreased	Decreased
Respiratory rate	14–20	20–30	30–40	> 35
Urine output (cc/hr)	> 30	20–30	5–15	Negligible
Mental status	Anxious	Anxious	Confused	Lethargic

(Derived from Advanced Trauma Life Support)

Lethal triad for bleeding (each contributes to the others)

- Hypothermia
- Acidosis
- Coagulopathy (frequently too much crystalloid without blood product replacement)

Imaging and Lab Tests (As indicated by exam, history, and mechanism of injury)

- C-spine

- Extremities
- Chest x-ray
  - Deep sulcus sign may indicate pneumothorax when one is not seen in periphery
    - Costophrenic angle deeper than normal
- CT head
- CT abdomen/pelvis; chest if indicated (physician should be involved)

Lab if indicated

- CBC
- BMP
- LFT's
- U/A
- Type and screen or cross

Treatment Options

- Analgesics prn
  - Dilaudid (hydromorphone) 0.5 mg IV or 1–2 mg IM
  - Stadol (butorphanol) 0.5–1 mg IV or 1–2 mg IM
  - Toradol (ketorolac) 30 mg IV or 60 mg IM (if no bleeding possibility present)
    - Do not use Toradol (ketorolac) if creatinine is elevated
- NSAID's or PO narcotics prn (outpatient treatment)
- Tetanus prophylaxis: (High risk = every 5 years; Low risk = every 10 years) Tetanus IG 250–500 units at different site if high risk and less than 3 tetanus or unknown history of immunizations previously in life — usually with the elderly
- Refer to health department or primary care provider to complete tetanus primary vaccination series if < 2 vaccines given in past
  - See Tetanus Protocol (page 580)

Blood/fluid replacement for hemorrhage

- PRBC's/FFP/platelets 2:1:1 ratio
- Avoid > 2 liters of isotonic fluids for acute blood loss before blood products transfusion started
- Avoid hypertension (mean arterial pressure: MAP target of 65) when giving blood or fluids

- Use blood warmer

Head Trauma

Considerations

- Loss of consciousness (LOC), amnesia, headache, vomiting and seizures have low sensitivity and specificity for detecting intracranial injury
- Cervical spine exam and evaluation important
- Skull films mainly replaced by CT evaluation of head trauma
- Evaluate for significant maxillofacial injuries

Concussion definitions

Grade 1 concussion

- Transient confusion
- No LOC
- Duration of mental status abnormalities < 15 minutes

Grade 2 concussion

- Transient confusion
- No LOC
- Duration of mental status abnormalities > 15 minutes

Grade 3 concussion

- Loss of consciousness

Evaluation

- CT per head injury protocols
- Evaluate for other injuries, especially C-spine
- Retinal exam: for hemorrhages
- Detailed neurologic exam

ENT exam

- Check for hemotympanum
- CSF rhinorrhea
- Battle's sign
- Cranial nerve palsy

New Orleans CT criteria (for ordering CT brain)

- Normal neurologic exam and one of the following
    - Headache
    - Vomiting
    - Age > 60
    - Persistent anterograde amnesia
    - Drug-alcohol intoxication
    - Visible trauma above the clavicle
    - Seizure

Discharge criteria

- Stable condition
- Normal neurologic exam
- No other significant trauma
- No radiologic abnormalities

Discharge instructions

- Head injury aftercare instructions
- Tylenol (no ASA or NSAID's for 36 hours)
- Avoid more potent analgesics so progression of symptoms can be detected
- Return for any neurologic changes
- Follow up with primary care provider or neurologist

Consult criteria

- Age ≥ 70 or < 2 years of age
- Bleeding potential
- Concussions
- Dementia
- Persistent vomiting
- Severe persistent headache
- Focal neurologic deficits
- Inadequate home observation

Neck Trauma

Penetrating neck trauma

- Consult physician unless very superficial laceration

- Do not explore Zone 2 penetrating deep injuries
    - Angle of mandible to cricoid cartilage
    - Consult physician

Cervical spine trauma

- Leave cervical collar on until patient examined and cleared
- Plain C-spine x-ray 3 views

Exclusionary criteria for C-spine films

- No neurologic deficit
- No distracting injuries
- No evidence of intoxication
- Normal mentation
- No posterior midline tenderness

CT C-spine indications

- Moderate to high risk of cervical fracture
- Significant mechanism of injury
- Fracture on plain C-spine films
- Neurologic deficit or complaint
- Inadequate plain C-spine films
- Severe neck pain with normal plain C-spine films
- Patient will not move neck actively (on their own) without external support of patient's hands ("head in hand sign")
- Obtunded patients

Flexion-extension plain films

- Significant pain with negative plain and CT imaging
- Evaluation for ligamentous instability

Treatment

- C-spine cleared: analgesics and ice packs

Discharge criteria

- Benign cause of neck pain

Discharge instructions

- Neck injury aftercare instructions

- Refer to primary care provider or neurosurgeon within 3 days if not improving
- Avoid discharging with cervical collar if possible

Consult criteria

- Cervical fracture or dislocation/subluxation
- Neurologic deficit or complaint
- Significant pain
- Significant mechanism of injury

Extremity Trauma

- Refer to specific protocols

Lacerations and Cutaneous Wounds

- Refer to Laceration and Cutaneous Wound Protocol

Discharge Criteria for MVA

- No significant injury that needs admission or acute consultation

Discharge Instructions for MVA

- MVA aftercare instructions
- Refer to appropriate physician specialty within 7–10 days as needed

Consult Criteria for MVA

- As in above sections
- Notify physician immediately for suspected severe trauma
- Significant injuries or mechanism of injury should be seen by physician initially and throughout length of stay
- Severe pain
- Moderate abdominal pain
- Refer to General Patient Criteria Protocol (page 20)
- Hemorrhage from more than minor simple laceration
- Fractures
- Dislocations
- Neurovascular injuries

- Tendon injuries

Notes

LACERATION AND CUTANEOUS WOUND PROTOCOL

When using any protocol, always follow the Guidelines of Proper Use (page 16).

Considerations

- Scalp lacerations with arterial bleeding can cause shock
    - Suture initially instead of pressure dressings with significant arterial bleeding

Anesthetics

- There are two major types of local anesthetics: amides and esters — little cross reactivity
- Maximum safe doses of local anesthetics
    - Lidocaine plain — 4.5 mg/kg
        - Lidocaine with epinephrine — 7 mg/kg
    - Marcaine plain — 2 mg/kg
        - Marcaine with epinephrine — 3 mg/kg

Duration of anesthesia

- Lidocaine without epinephrine lasts 15 minutes locally
    - Regional block lasts longer
- Lidocaine with epinephrine lasts 2–3 hours (avoid in end-circulation areas: fingers, toes, etc.)
- Marcaine lasts 90 minutes to 12 hours

Local anesthetic tips

- If lidocaine mixed with NaHCO3 in 9:1 ratio (90% lidocaine and 10% NaHCO3) it will yield a pH closer to body pH that will not burn with injection
- Warming local anesthetic to body temperature decreases pain of injection
- Topical tetracaine in wound for 20–30 minutes decreases pain of injection

Increased infection risk with

- Foreign body
- Crush injury
- Human or animal bite

Lacerations

Sutures

Nonabsorbable (nylon; polypropylene)

- Retains strength > 60 days; low tissue reactivity
- Use 6'0 on face
- Use 4'0 on rest of body
- May use 3'0 on very high tension areas except on face

Absorbable

- Synthetic is less reactive
- Synthetic has increased strength vs. cat gut
- Wound retains 50% of strength in < 1 week to 2 months
- Plain 5'0–6'0 gut sutures can be used to close the skin margins on children's facial lacerations
    - Avoid using plain gut in high tension areas
    - Vicryl retains strength to 21 days which is too long for external skin closure on facial lacerations
- Plain gut retains strength for 4–5 days

Deep sutures

- Helps relieve skin tension
- Decreases dead space and hematoma formation
- May improve cosmetic outcomes
- Recommend liberal use of deep sutures to approximate skin edges before closure with either skin sutures or tissue adhesives

Staples

- Considered for scalp; trunk; extremity lacerations
- When saving time is essential

Tissue adhesives (Dermabond)

- Reduces the need of suturing in up to 1/3 of lacerations
- Sloughs in 7–10 days
- Not to use if skin margins cannot be manually approximated or held together without a lot of tension
- Use 3–4 coats
- Keep out of laceration
- Caution: too much applied can cause too much heat to be released from the exothermic reaction
- Can be removed with bathing, petroleum or antibiotic gel, or acetone if rapid removal necessary
- May take shower after 24 hours, but avoid bathing or swimming until the adhesive sloughs — usually within 7 days

Evaluation

- Assess for other injuries
- X-ray for foreign bodies or fractures as indicated by history and exam
- Ultrasound may be used to detect foreign bodies depending on level of experience
- Record neurovascular exam prior to anesthesia
- Examine and document any deeper structures involvement
- Tendon involvement or injuries, consult physician
- High pressure injection injuries, consult physician promptly

Treatment Options

Sutures

- On face use 6'0 nylon or equivalent

- Use nylon 4'0 or equivalent on rest of body
- Nylon 3'0 can be used for high tension body lacerations (not on face)
- Vicryl or equivalent absorbable sutures used for deeper layers or intraoral
- Plain 5′0−6′0 gut can be used on children's facial lacerations to avoid later suture removal

Wound preparation

- All foreign material needs to be removed as much as possible
- Flush lacerations deeply with 1% betadine sol. (mix betadine 10% 1:10 with NS) or flush with NS
  - Use 18 gauge IV catheter on syringe after disposing of needle and flush with 20 cc to several hundred cc depending on contamination of laceration
- Superficial lacerations < 0.5 cm deep can be cleaned with betadine (etc.) scrubbing
- Hemostasis by direct pressure
  - Elevation of extremity helpful with point pressure to stop persistent extremity bleeding

Closure techniques

- Keep wound margins flat or everted with the closure
- Avoid wound margin inversion
- Partial muscle injury can be closed by using fascia of muscle
- Lacerations with high risk of infection may need to be left partially or fully open
- Steri–strips or tissue adhesive can be used as indicated

Simple Suture

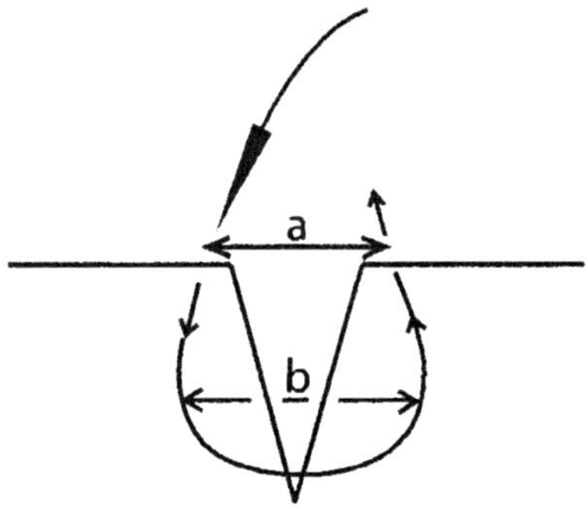

The distance of line (a), the skin entry and exit points, is less than line (b) at the base of the laceration.

- This creates wound eversion which is cosmetically desirable.
- Wound inversion creates a shadow in the laceration site after healing.

Vertical Mattress Suture

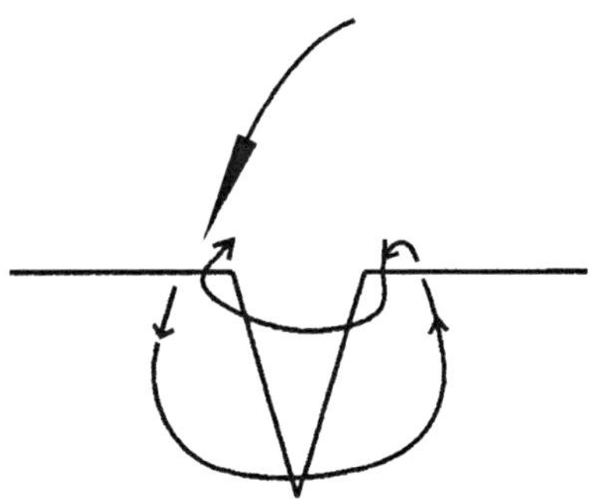

Vertical mattress is used for high tension wounds and when laceration margin eversion is needed.

Antibiotics for

- Tendon or bone involvement
- Septic contamination
- Intraoral lacerations
- Animal/human bites

Aftercare

- Laceration aftercare instructions

- Sutured or stapled lacerations keep clean and gently cleansed after 24–48 hours
- Sutured or stapled lacerations should be protected with nonadherent dressing for 48 hours
- Air dry lacerations after 48 hours of dressing (cover dressing when in contaminated environment)
- Sutured or stapled laceration infection incidence may be reduced with topical antibiotic ointments
- Splint if there is a fracture or tendon injury and prn otherwise
- No antibiotics for clean, simple lacerations that are not animal or human bites

Suture and Staple Removal

- Face 3–5 days
- Neck 4–6 days
- Scalp and trunk 7–10 days
- Upper extremity 10–14 days
- Lower extremity 14–21 days
- Joints 10–21 days

Consult criteria

- Wounds beyond the practitioner's ability to treat
- See General Consult Criteria below

Skin tears

- Common among elderly and long term steroid therapy
- Skin tears can be closed with tissue adhesive if within 8 hours

Class 1 skin tear

- No tissue loss
- Close with surgical tape
- Cover with nonadherent dressing

Class 2 skin tear

- Partial tissue loss

- Manage with absorbent dressings (petroleum based, hydrogels, foams, or hydrocolloids, etc.) for 5–7 days
    - Change daily if needed
    - Use elastic tubular nets to hold in place

Class 3 skin tear

- Complete tissue loss
- Manage same as Class 2 skin tear

Discharge instructions

- Skin tear aftercare instructions
- Follow up with primary care provider or surgeon within 2–5 days as needed

Consult criteria

- Large amount of tissue loss

Plantar puncture wounds

- Rate of cellulitis 2–10%
    - Usually staph or strep
    - Use dicloxicillin or Sanford Guide
- Cleaning alone may be effective
- If foreign body suspected, use plain x-rays if radiopaque, or CT or ultrasound scan otherwise if needed
- Punctures through sweaty moist tennis shoes carries risk of pseudomonas osteomyelitis
    - May prescribe antipseudomonal antibiotic such as Cipro (ciprofloxacin)
- Frequent cleansing and topical antibiotic as treatment at home
- Do not core out puncture wound

Discharge instructions

- Puncture wound aftercare instructions
- Close follow-up within 2–3 days for suspected deep punctures

Consult criteria

- Neurovascular or bone injury

Subungual hematomas

- Treat with nail trephination (burr hole)
- Nail may be removed for disruption of nail or surrounding nail folds

Discharge instructions

- Subungual hematoma aftercare instructions

General Consult Criteria

- Open fracture
- Neurovascular or tendon injuries or deficits
- Muscle bundle totally severed
- Practitioner is uncomfortable repairing laceration
- Human or animal bites

Vital signs and age consult criteria

- Adult heart rate > 100
- SBP < 90 or relative hypotension (SBP < 105 with history of hypertension)
- Pediatric heart rate
    - 0–4 months ≥ 180
    - 5–7 months ≥ 175
    - 6–12 months ≥ 170
    - 1–3 years ≥ 160
    - 4–5 years ≥ 145
    - 6–8 years ≥ 130
    - 7–12 years ≥ 125
    - 12–15 years ≥ 115
    - 16 years or older ≥ 100

Lab consult criteria

- Acute hemoglobin decrease of > 1 gm
- Hemoglobin < 10 gm
- Thrombocytopenia
- INR > 1.5 if checked

Notes

Bleeding Protocol

When using any protocol, always follow the Guidelines of Proper Use (page 16).

Considerations

- Active hemorrhage may be apparent or unsuspected
- Scalp lacerations with arterial bleeding can cause shock
    - Suture initially instead of pressure dressings with significant arterial bleeding
- Medical therapy can precipitate or worsen bleeding

Estimated Blood and Fluid losses (adults)

	Class I	Class II	Class III	Class IV
Blood loss (cc)	Up to 750	750–1000	1500–2000	> 2000
Blood loss %	Up to 15%	15–30%	30–40%	> 40%
Pulse rate	< 100	> 100	> 120	> 140
Blood pressure	Normal	Normal	SBP < 90	SBP < 70
Capillary refill	Normal	Normal	Delayed	Absent
Pulse pressure	Normal/incr	Decreased	Decreased	Decreased
Respiratory rate	14–20	20–30	30–40	> 35
Urine output (cc/hr)	> 30	20–30	5–15	Negligible
Mental status	Anxious	Anxious	Confused	Lethargic

(Derived from Advanced Trauma Life Support)

Lethal triad for bleeding (each contributes to the others)

- Hypothermia
- Acidosis
- Coagulopathy (frequently too much crystalloid without blood product replacement)

Evaluation

- CBC
- PT/INR/PTT if on anticoagulant or have comorbid conditions contributing to bleeding
- Type and screen or cross depending on level of hemorrhage

Treatment

- Direct pressure of bleeding site for 2–5 minutes if actively bleeding when possible
- Exsanguination from extremities where direct pressure ineffective may try tourniquet up to 5 minutes off and on prn (notify physician immediately)

Blood/fluid replacement for hemorrhage

- PRBC's/FFP/platelets 2:1:1 ratio
- Avoid > 2 liters of isotonic fluids for acute blood loss before blood products transfusion started
- Avoid hypertension (mean arterial pressure: MAP target of 65) when giving blood or fluids
- Use blood warmer
- Vitamin K 10 mg IV over 10 minutes (not faster than 1 mg/minute) or IM/SQ/PO prn Coumadin (warfarin) therapy — may take 24–48 hours to affect INR
- FFP can be given to reverse Coumadin (warfarin) effects
- Protamine 1 mg IV for each 100 units of heparin given to reverse anticoagulation prn

Discharge Criteria

- Bleeding without effect on vital signs or hemoglobin level
- Further significant bleeding unlikely
- No coagulopathy

Consult Criteria

- Refer to General Patient Criteria Protocol (page 20)
- Adult tachycardia
- SBP < 90 or relative hypotension (SBP < 110 with history of hypertension)
- Pediatric heart rate
  - 0–4 months ≥ 180
  - 5–7 months ≥ 175
  - 6–12 months ≥ 170
  - 1–3 years ≥ 160
  - 4–5 years ≥ 145
  - 6–8 years ≥ 130

- 7–12 years ≥ 120
- 12–15 years ≥ 115
- 16 years or older ≥ 100

Notes

BURN PROTOCOL

When using any protocol, always follow the Guidelines of Proper Use (page 16).

Considerations

- In children consider child abuse
- Electrical burns may be much worse than suspected
- Evaluate airway and pulmonary system with enclosed building fire or with facial burns
- Consider possible carbon monoxide poisoning in enclosed areas
- Difficult to tell difference between deep second degree burn and third degree burn
- Second degree deep partial thickness burn can become a third degree burn
- Body surface area (BSA) of burn use rule of 9's or the palmer surface of patient is approximately 1% BSA
- Rule of nines for BSA burned is for patients ≥10 years of age
- Depth of burn frequently underestimated
- Size of burn frequently overestimated

Burn depth

First degree

- Epidermis only; no blisters
- Sensation — painful
- Bleeding on pinprick — brisk
- Appearance — light red and dry
- Blanching to pressure — brisk

Second degree superficial partial thickness

- Dermis involved with blisters
- Sensation — painful
- Bleeding on pinprick — brisk
- Appearance — moist and pink
- Blanching to pressure — slow return

Second degree deep partial thickness

- Dermis involved with blisters

- Sensation — dull
- Bleeding on pinprick — delayed
- Appearance — mottled pink or red; waxy white
- Blanching to pressure — none

Third degree full thickness

- Sensation — none
- No bleeding on pinprick
- Appearance — white, charred and dry
- Blanching to pressure — none

Fourth degree

- Involves muscle, fascia or bone

Thermal Burns

Evaluation

Enclosed space fire with smoke

- Airway evaluation
- O2 saturation
- CO (carbon monoxide) level
- CBC
- BMP
- Chest x-ray
- Notify physician promptly

BSA burn < 10%

- Physical exam usually all that is needed if no smoke inhalation history or findings

Treatment options

- Clean with soap and water
- Cool burn with cold tap water
    - Decreases pain
    - Decreases depth and extent of injury
    - Do not use ice or ice water

Blister management

- Leave blisters intact ≤ 3 cm in size
    - Heals faster
- Totally debride any ruptured blisters

- May sterilely aspirate blisters > 3 cm

First degree burns

- Aloe vera and NSAIDs can be used for 1st burns

Superficial 2nd degree burns

- Topical antibiotic or absorptive occlusive dressing
    - Absorptive occlusive dressing is less painful and results in faster healing than antibiotic ointment

Deep 2nd and 3rd degree burns

- Topical antibiotic and refer to surgeon
- Silvadene (silver sulfadiazine) ointment qday for 5-7 days (not on face)
- Aquacel dressing superior to plain Silvadene in healing burns and reducing pain and may be used instead (releases silver sulfadiazine slowly)

Tetanus prophylaxis

- Tetanus toxoid (ADT) 0.5 cc IM if last dose > 5 years
- Tetanus immune globulin 250–500 units IM at different site if < 3 or unknown previous tetanus immunizations
- Refer to health department or primary care provider to complete tetanus primary vaccination series if < 2 vaccines given in past
    - See Tetanus Protocol (page 580)

Discharge criteria

- First degree burns
- Second degree superficial burns < 15% in adults and < 10% in children age 10 or less

Discharge instructions for burns

- Burn aftercare instructions
- Wash burn with soap and water qday and change dressing qday for 5-7 days

- Facial burns use triple antibiotic ointment or polysporin ointment 5-7 days
- Antibiotic PO or IM not usually needed
- Pain treatment with NSAID's and/or narcotics prn (hydrocodone, oxycodone)

Consult criteria

- Second degree superficial burns ≥ 10% in adults and 5% or greater in children
- Deep second degree and third degree burns unless extremely small (<2 cm)
- Burns involving hand; joints; perineum; genitalia; face; eyes; ears
- Comorbid conditions such diabetes, immunosuppression
- Circumferential burns
- Age < 12 months
- All inhalation injuries

Electrical Burns

Considerations

- Household electrical injury can be lethal
- Difficult to estimate degree of injury
- Causes tetany of muscles
- Traumatic injuries common (falls)

Compartment syndrome

- From increased pressure in a muscle or other internal compartment
- Not all signs and symptoms are needed to make diagnosis
- High pressures > 8 hours leads to tissue damage
- Normal tissue pressure is < 10 mm Hg
- Capillary blood flow is compromised at > 20 mm Hg
- Intracompartmental pressures > 30 mm Hg or within 10-30 mm Hg of DBP

Signs and symptoms (not diagnostic)

- Pain

    - Out of proportion to injury
    - On passive stretch of muscles
  - Pallor
  - Paresthesias
  - Paralysis
    - Sensory and motor findings are late signs
  - Poikilothermia — decreased temperature
  - Pulselessness
    - Usually not lost until muscle necrosis has occurred
    - Last sign to develop
  - Tense muscle compartment on palpation

Treatment

  - Consult physician if suspected
  - Keep extremity at level of heart
  - Do not use ice if suspected
  - Remove cast and padding
  - Surgery fasciotomy is usually necessary

Evaluation

- Complete history and physical exam
- Degree of burn and voltage
- Length of time of electrical injury
- Neurologic exam
- EKG and monitor
- CBC
- BMP
- CPK
- U/A for myoglobin if hemoglobin dipstick positive
- Serum myoglobin if U/A positive for hemoglobin

Treatment options

- Treat skin burns same as thermal
- IV NS 200 cc/hr if significant burn injury or suspicion for significant injury for adults and 2 times maintenance rate for pediatrics
- Tetanus toxoid (ADT) 0.5 cc IM if last dose > 5 years

- Tetanus immune globulin 250–500 units IM different site if < 3 or unknown history of previous tetanus immunizations
- Refer to health department or primary care provider to complete tetanus primary vaccination series if < 2 vaccines given in past
    - See Tetanus Protocol (page 580)
- Pain treatment with NSAID's and/or narcotics prn

Discharge criteria

- Low voltage superficial injury
- Normal lab, EKG and vital signs
- Small burn area
- Follow up with primary care provider or plastic surgeon within 2–3 days

Discharge instructions for burns

- Wash burn with soap and water qday and change dressing qday for 5–7 days
- Burn aftercare instructions
- Facial burns use triple antibiotic ointment or polysporin ointment 5–7 days
- Antibiotic PO or IM not usually needed
- Pain treatment with NSAID's and/or narcotics prn (hydrocodone, oxycodone)

Consult criteria

- Loss of consciousness
- Neurologic abnormalities
- High voltage burns
- Abnormal lab, EKG or vital signs
- Large burns or suspected deep tissue injury
- Uncertainty of the extent of injury
- Suspected compartment syndrome

Chemical Burns

Considerations

- Alkali cause deeper injury
- Acids cause more superficial injury usually, depending on pH

Evaluation

- Usually all that is needed is history and physical exam for minor chemical burns

Treatment

- Remove chemical from skin
- Clean with soap and water
- Flush or soak with NS if alkali burn
- Pain treatment with NSAID's and/or narcotics prn

Hydrofluoric acid (HFl) burns

- Intense pain and tissue damage
- Use copious irrigation followed by calcium gluconate gel
- Subcutaneous calcium gluconate may be needed to relieve pain
- TBSA (total body surface area) burn > 5% needs admission to monitor for the development of hypocalcemia
    - If HFI concentration > 50% then 1% TBSA burn needs admission

Tetanus prophylaxis

- Tetanus toxoid (ADT) 0.5 cc IM if last dose > 5 years
- Tetanus immune globulin 250–500 units IM different site if < 3 or unknown history of previous tetanus immunizations
- Refer to health department or primary care provider to complete tetanus primary vaccination series if < 2 vaccines given in past
    - See Tetanus Protocol (page 580)

Discharge criteria

- Minor chemical burns

Discharge instructions for burns

- Wash burn with soap and water qday and change dressing qday for 5–7 days
- Burn aftercare instructions
- Facial burns use triple antibiotic ointment or polysporin ointment 5–7 days

- Antibiotic PO or IM not usually needed
- Pain treatment with NSAID's and/or narcotics prn (hydrocodone, oxycodone)

Consult criteria

- Hydrofluoric acid burns
- Abnormal vital signs
- Diabetes or immunosuppression
- Second degree superficial burns ≥ 10% in adults and 5% or greater in children
- Second degree deep and third degree burns
- Burns involving hand, joints, perineum, genitalia
- Comorbid conditions such diabetes, immunosuppression

Vital sign and age consult criteria for all burn types

- Hypotension or relative hypotension (SBP < 105 with history of hypertension)
- Adult heart rate ≥ 110
- Pediatric heart rate
  - 0–4 months ≥ 180
  - 5–7 months ≥ 175
  - 6–12 months ≥ 170
  - 1–3 years ≥ 160
  - 4–5 years ≥ 145
  - 6–8 years ≥ 130
  - 7–12 years ≥ 125
  - 12–15 years ≥ 115
  - 16 years or older ≥ 110

Notes

Extremity Disorders

Section Contents

Extremity Medical Disorder Protocol

Fracture Protocol

Salter Harris Fracture Protocol

Synovial Fluid Analysis

Shoulder Protocol

Shoulder and Arm Trauma Protocol

Elbow Protocol

Hip Protocol

Knee Soft Tissue Injury Protocol

Knee Disorders Protocol

Ankle Sprain Protocol

Hand, Wrist and Distal Forearm Injury Protocol

Finger Injury Protocol

When using any protocol, always follow the Guidelines of Proper Use (page 16).

EXTREMITY MEDICAL DISORDER PROTOCOL

When using any protocol, always follow the Guidelines of Proper Use (page 16).

Differential Diagnosis

Painful extremity swelling

- Deep venous thrombosis
- Arterial insufficiency
- Tendonitis, bursitis, and arthritis
- Cellulitis
- Abscess
- Septic arthritis
- Gout
- Radiculopathy
- Peripheral neuropathy

Nonpainful extremity swelling

- Congestive heart failure
- Hepatic cirrhosis
- Post-phlebitic syndrome

General Evaluation

- Complete history and physical exam
- Symptom(s) onset and exacerbating factors
- Associated symptoms
- Neurovascular exam
- Document whether Homan's sign and calf tenderness is positive or negative

Deep Venous Thrombosis

Well's DVT criteria

- One point each:
    - Active cancer
    - Paralysis/recent cast immobilization

    - Recently bedridden > 3 days or surgery < 4 weeks
    - Deep vein tenderness
    - Entire leg edema
    - Calf swelling > 3 cm over other leg
    - Pitting edema > other calf
    - Collateral superficial veins
- Two points — alternative diagnosis less likely

High probability: ≥ 3 points

Moderate probability: 1–2 points

Low probability: 0 points

Evaluation

D-dimer (LIA method) — some methods currently in use not reliable

- Useful if negative at cutoff value to rule out DVT or PE
- Negative D-dimer with low to moderate probability Well's DVT score largely excludes venous thromboembolic disease
- Well's criteria high probability: order ultrasound scan regardless of D-dimer result
- Positive — not as useful as negative result which usually rules out VTE disease
    - Frequently positive with hospitalization in past month
    - Chronic bedridden or low activity state
    - Increasingly positive with age without significant acute disease process
    - CHF
    - Chronic disease processes
    - Edematous states

Well's DVT criteria > 1–2 with painful or swollen extremity

- Order D-dimer test (unless patient likely to have positive result regardless of DVT potential)

- Venous Doppler ultrasound of extremity (unless D-dimer negative)
- Coumadin (warfarin) therapy can cause falsely negative D-dimer

Discharge criteria

- Well's DVT criteria low probability
- Negative D-dimer (can be falsely negative with Coumadin (warfarin) therapy)
- Negative ultrasound

Discharge instructions

- Leg pain aftercare instructions
- Follow up with primary care provider in 3–5 days if pain persists
- Return if worse

Consult criteria

- DVT diagnosis
- Suspected DVT diagnosis
- Severe pain

Peripheral Arterial Disease

- Pain worse with activity
- Risk factors same as with coronary disease

Ankle brachial index (ABI)

- Systolic blood pressure at ankle divided by systolic blood pressure in arm
- Normal 0.9–1.1
- Worsening PAD yields decreasing ABI
- Diabetes can interfere with test due to calcinosis

Discharge criteria

- Stable claudication
- Pain resolved
- ASA 81–325 mg PO each day
- Smoking cessation
- Refer to surgeon

Discharge instructions

- PAD aftercare instructions
- Follow up with PCP or general surgeon within 3–5 days

Consult criteria

- Continuous pain
- Severe pain as presenting complaint
- Limb discoloration
- Heart rate > 100
- Hypotension
- Absent pulse
- Decreased temperature to touch

Cellulitis and Abscess

- See Cellulitis and Abscess Protocols

Septic Arthritis

Differential diagnosis

- Cellulitis
- Gout
- Bursitis
- Osteomyelitis
- Rheumatoid arthritis
- Soft tissue injury
- Pseudogout

Considerations

- Rapid onset
- Usually one joint infected
- Joint is very painful; hot; red; fluctuant
- Signs of acute systemic illness may be present
- Fever, chills and sweats frequently present
- See Synovial Fluid Analysis if joint fluid obtained

Evaluation

- History and physical examination
  - Evaluate knee for range of motion as tolerated
- ESR or C-reactive protein

- CBC
- BMP if diabetic
- Knee films
- Ultrasound can be considered
- Joint aspiration if provider experienced
- Joint fluid analysis — see specific protocol

Treatment

- Admission to hospital for drainage and antibiotics

Discharge criteria

- Only with physician consent

Consult criteria

- All septic joint or suspected septic joint patients

Gout

Differential diagnosis

- Cellulitis
- Septic arthritis
- Bursitis
- Osteomyelitis
- Rheumatoid arthritis
- Soft tissue injury
- Pseudogout

Considerations

- Crystal uric acid deposits in joints and tissues
- Most common cause of monoarticular arthritis age > 60
- Increased warmth, redness and joint swelling
- First metatarsophalangeal joint of foot 75% of cases — most common
- Joint fluid: 20,000–100,000 WBC; poor string and mucin clot test; no bacteria (pseudogout similar)
- Risk factors
    - Age > 40
    - Hypertension
    - Diuretics
    - Ethanol intake
    - Obesity

Evaluation

- Clinical evaluation usually all that is needed
- If diagnosis uncertain: CBC, C-reactive protein, x-rays, joint aspiration

Treatment options

- NSAID's high dose 5–10 days
- Narcotics IM or PO prn
- Prednisone 40–60 mg PO qday × 3–7 days

  OR
- Depomedrol (methylprednisolone acetate) 80–120 mg IM
- Allopurinol 50–300 mg PO qday: adjusted for renal function; start after acute episode resolved

Discharge criteria

- Uncomplicated acute gout attack

Discharge instructions

- Gout aftercare instructions
- Follow up with primary care provider within 2–3 days if pain persists

Consult criteria

- Uncertain diagnosis
- Fever history or toxicity
- Tachycardia

Radiculopathy

Lumbar radiculopathy (sciatica)

- Complete history and physical examination
- Check reflexes, SLR (straight leg raise), and neurovascular exam
- Spinal cord compression signs
  - Urinary retention with overflow incontinence or voiding
  - Fecal incontinence and decreased rectal tone and perineal sensation (i.e., cauda equina syndrome — see Back Pain Protocol)
- Healthy non-elderly patients without direct blunt trauma usually need no tests

- Elderly frequently need spine films due to higher incidence of vertebral fractures
- Plain back/pelvic films may be needed in falls, MVC's, direct blunt trauma, depending on severity of injury mechanism
- U/A if renal disease suspected or significant injury mechanism
- D-dimer if aortic dissection considered
- CBC, C-RP (or ESR) for fever with isolated vertebral back pain only without associated symptoms or findings

CT scan of spine

- Compression fracture > 30%
- Burst fracture
- Posterior vertebral involvement
- For back pain out of proportion on exam

- MRI for spinal cord findings or symptoms

Treatment options

- NSAID's prn
- Short narcotic course prn for severe pain — avoid Demerol (meperidine)
- Preferable to minimize bed rest (limit bed rest to no more than 1–2 days if possible, unless a fracture is present)
- Avoid heavy lifting
- Muscle relaxants of questionable usefulness

Discharge Criteria

- Uncomplicated presentation and findings with ability to control pain and ambulate

Discharge instructions

- Back pain aftercare instructions
- Refer to primary care provider
- If HNP suspected: neurosurgery or orthopedic referral
- Orthopedic referral for fractures

Consult Criteria

- Severe pain with inability to ambulate
- Progressive neurologic deficits
- Signs of cauda equina syndrome
- Signs of spinal cord impairment
- Evidence of infectious, vascular, or neoplastic etiologies
- Nontraumatic pediatric back pain
- Fracture
- New onset renal insufficiency or worsening renal insufficiency

Cervical Radiculopathy

Definition

- Compression on cervical spine nerve roots

Considerations

- C7 compression involved 60% of cases
- C6 compression involved 25% of cases
- Younger patients have HNP or injury causing foraminal impingement on nerve root
- Elderly have degenerative changes causing foraminal narrowing and nerve compression

Physical findings

Motor deficits

- C5 — weakness of shoulder abduction
- C6 — weakness of elbow flexion and wrist extension
- C7 — weakness of elbow extension and wrist flexion
- C8 — weakness of thumb extension and wrist ulnar deviation

Sensory dermatomes

- C6 — thumb
- C7 — middle finger
- C8 — little finger
- T1 — inner forearm
- T2 — upper inner arm

Deep tendon reflexes (DTR)

- Biceps DTR tests C5–C6
    - Antecubital fossa
- Brachioradialis reflex test C5–C6
    - Distal radius
- Triceps DTR tests C7–C8
    - Distal triceps tendon posterior and slightly above elbow

Evaluation

- History and physical examination
- Check reflexes, hand grip, shoulder strength and neurovascular exam
- Cervical spine films may be obtained
- Healthy non-elderly patients without direct blunt trauma usually need no tests

Treatment options

- Local ice therapy
- NSAID's
- Hydrocodone or oxycodone prn severe pain
- Semirigid cervical collar for 3-6 weeks
- Physical therapy
- Home exercises

Discharge criteria

- Most patients can be discharged home

Discharge instructions

- Cervical radiculopathy aftercare instructions
- Referral to neurosurgeon or orthopedic spine surgeon within 7-14 days

Consult criteria

- Incapacitating pain
- Central spinal cord compression symptoms
    - Loss of anal sphincter tone
    - Loss of bladder control
    - Weakness of arms and legs
- Central cord syndrome
    - Arms weaker than legs

Peripheral Neuropathy (PN)

Definition

- Disorder of peripheral nerves

Causes

- Usually as a complication of diabetes or alcoholism
- HIV
- Lyme disease
- Guillain–Barre' syndrome
- Cancer (paraneoplastic syndromes)
- Hypothyroidism
- Herpes zoster
- Acute nerve root compression
- Renal failure
- Heavy metal poisoning (lead, etc.)
- Nutritional deficiency

Evaluation

- Complete history and physical exam
- Motor and sensory exam
- Usually no testing on chronic neuropathy
- Acute neuropathy warrants tests directed at possible causes
    - BMP
    - C-reactive protein
    - CBC
    - Lyme titers if indicated
    - TSH if indicated
    - Lead levels if suspected
    - Chest x-ray if sarcoidosis or lung cancer suspected
    - LP if Guillain–Barre' syndrome suspected

Treatment options

- Symptomatic pain treatment
- Treatment directed at underlying cause if possible

Discharge criteria

- Stable chronic peripheral neuropathy

Discharge instructions

- Peripheral neuropathy aftercare instructions
- Follow up with PCP or neurologist as needed for chronic PN
- Follow up for acute neuropathy within 1 day

Consult criteria

- Acute neuropathy from a high comorbidity disease process or from an unknown cause

Nonpainful Extremity Swelling

- Treat underlying condition if feasible
- Elevation
- Compression hose
- Follow up with primary care provider
- Judicious diuretic short term use with caution

General Consult Criteria for Extremity Conditions

- Severe pain
- Acute and progressive arterial insufficiency
- Rapidly spreading rash or cellulitis
- Pain out of proportion to exam
- Crepitus or gas in tissues
- Systemic toxic appearance
- Hypotension or relative hypotension SBP < 105 in patient with hypertension history
- Necrotizing fasciitis or gas gangrene
- Large abscess
- Suspected bony involvement
- Immunocompromise

Vital signs and age consult criteria

- Fever ≥ 102.2°F (39°C)
- Age < 6 months or > 70 years old
- Adult heart rate ≥ 110
- SBP < 90 or relative hypotension (SBP < 105 with history of hypertension)
- O2 Sat ≤ 94% on room air
- Moderate dyspnea

- Pediatric heart rate
  - 0–4 months ≥ 180
  - 5–7 months ≥ 175
  - 6–12 months ≥ 170
  - 1–3 years ≥ 160
  - 4–5 years ≥ 145
  - 6–8 years ≥ 130
  - 7–12 years ≥ 125
  - 12–15 years ≥ 115
  - 16 years or older ≥ 110

Lab consult criteria

- Adult: WBC > 15,000 or < 1,000 neutrophils
- Bandemia ≥ 15%
- Acute thrombocytopenia
- Acute anemia

Notes

FRACTURE PROTOCOL

When using any protocol, always follow the Guidelines of Proper Use (page 16).

Considerations

- Complications
  - Neurovascular injury
  - Open fracture
  - Joint involvement
  - Ligament/tendon injury
  - Displaced and angulated
  - Compartment syndrome
  - Fat emboli — long bones
  - Avascular necrosis
  - Osteomyelitis
- Nondisplaced, closed simple long bone fractures usually can be splinted and discharged with orthopedic follow-up
  - Discuss with physician (except for simple nondisplaced torus fractures)

Compartment syndrome

- From increased pressure in a muscle or other internal compartment
- Not all signs and symptoms are needed to make diagnosis
- High pressures > 8 hours leads to tissue damage
- Normal tissue pressure is < 10 mm Hg
- Capillary blood flow is compromised at > 20 mm Hg
- Intracompartmental pressures > 30 mm Hg or within 10–30 mm Hg of DBP

Signs and symptoms (not diagnostic)

- Pain
  - Out of proportion to injury
  - On passive stretch of muscles
- Pallor
- Paresthesias

- Paralysis
    - Sensory and motor findings are late signs
- Poikilothermia — decreased temperature
- Pulselessness
    - Usually not lost until muscle necrosis has occurred
    - Last sign to develop
- Tense muscle compartment on palpation

Treatment

- Consult physician if suspected
- Keep extremity at level of heart
- Do not use ice if suspected
- Remove cast and padding
- Surgery fasciotomy is usually necessary

Evaluation

- History of injury
- Past history
- Medication history
- Associated symptoms and complete physical exam
- X-rays of affected areas
- Neurovascular/tendon/ligament exam
- Assess for compartment syndrome
- Assess for open fracture or joint

Vertebral Fractures

Considerations

- Compression fractures commonly seen in the elderly secondary to osteoporosis
- Can be pathologic from cancer
- Point tenderness common at fracture site
- May be caused by high impact

Evaluation

- History and physical examination
- Plain films
- CT scan of affected area may be needed for diagnosis

- CT scan for compression fractures ≥ 30% or any posterior element spinal canal involvement
- CT scan of entire spine for acute neurologic complaints or deficits
- Assess for other injuries
- CBC and U/A for significant mechanism of injury

Treatment options

- Pain control with narcotics usually — PO, IM or IV
- Spine immobilization for neurologic complaints or findings
- Elective vertebroplasty
- Early ambulation as tolerated

Discharge criteria

- Uncomplicated vertebral compression fractures < 30% in osteoporosis patients without significant mechanism of injury
- Patient able to ambulate

Discharge instructions

- Vertebral compression aftercare instructions
- Follow up with neurosurgeon or orthopedic surgeon within 7 days

Consult criteria

- Consult physician for compression fractures > 10%
- Acute neurologic deficits or complaints
- Unable to ambulate
- Uncontrollable severe pain
- Posterior element or spinal canal involvement
- Noncompression–type vertebral fractures
- Significant mechanism of injury

Clavicle Fractures

Considerations

- Most common fracture in children
- 80% middle third
- 15% distal third
- 5% proximal third

- May need CT scan for sternoclavicular injuries

Treatment

- Sling for middle and distal end fractures for 4–8 weeks; acromioclavicular sprain and separation
- Proximal sternoclavicular fractures and dislocations, consult physician
- Posterior sternoclavicular dislocation — notify physician promptly if available
  - May have stridor or respiratory distress
  - May have venous congestion of head or neck or affected arm

Posterior sternoclavicular dislocation treatment

- 3–4 inch roll between scapula and spine to extend or open up affected sternoclavicular joint
- Abduct affected shoulder to 90° and extend shoulder to 15° and apply traction with assistant holding trunk still
- If above fails, maintain traction and manually grasp clavicle and pull forward
- Consult orthopedic surgeon for sternoclavicular dislocations

- NSAID's (very effective in children); narcotics prn

Discharge criteria

- Uncomplicated clavicle fracture

Discharge instructions

- Clavicle fracture aftercare instructions
- Referral to orthopedics or PCP within 7–10 days

Consult criteria

- Immediate physician consultation for suspected posterior sternoclavicular joint dislocation
- Neurovascular injury

Scapular Fractures

Considerations

- Can occur with significant trauma to trunk and other injuries
- Evaluate for associated injuries
- Type 1: body of scapula
- Type 2: coracoid and acromion
- Type 3: neck and glenoid
- Shoulder x-rays needed
- CT may be needed if going to surgery for repair

Treatment options

Type 1

- Sling
- Analgesics
- Consult physician

Type 2 and 3

- Per physician and orthopedic consultation

Discharge criteria

- Uncomplicated Type 1 scapular fracture

Discharge instructions

- Scapular fracture aftercare instructions
- Follow up with trauma or thoracic surgeon within 5–10 days

Consult criteria

- Type 2 and 3 scapular fractures
- For any significant associated injuries
- Discuss all scapular fractures with physician prior to discharge

Humerus Fractures

Considerations

- Fall on outstretched hand frequent cause
- Usually elderly
- Younger patients with epiphyseal injuries of growth plate

- Shoulder tense and swollen
- Obtain AP and lateral shoulder x-rays
- Evaluate for neurovascular injury
- Proximal humerus – Axillary nerve
- Humeral shaft – Radial nerve

Treatment

- Sling
- Physical therapy
- Narcotics prn
- Children can take Tylenol prn

Discharge criteria

- Uncomplicated and minimally displaced proximal closed humerus fracture

Discharge instructions

- Humerus fracture aftercare instructions
- Orthopedic referral within 7 days

Consult criteria

- Orthopedic consultation for severely angulated or comminuted fracture
- Orthopedic consult for pediatric humerus fractures
- Discuss with physician all humerus fractures prior to discharge

Shoulder, Hip, Knee, Wrist, Elbow, and Ankle Dislocations

- Analgesics
- Evaluate for associated injuries
- Consult physician

Rib Fractures – Isolated

Considerations

- First and second rib fractures associated with high impact and significant mechanism of injury

Evaluation

- Complete history and physical examination

- Chest x-ray
- Rib films
- Chest CT scan may be needed for high mechanism of injury and abnormal vital signs or hypoxia
- Ultrasound can detect subtle rib fractures
- U/A to check for kidney injury in low posterior rib fractures
- Evaluate for associated injuries

Treatment options

- Narcotics prn
- NSAID's prn
- Rib belt not recommended due to causing atelectasis and pneumonia

Discharge criteria

- Simple 1 or 2 rib fractures
- No pulmonary abnormality (pulmonary contusion or pneumothorax)

Discharge instructions

- Rib fracture aftercare instructions
- Follow up with PCP or trauma surgeon within 7–10 days

Consult criteria

- If more than 2 ribs fractured
- Pulmonary abnormality on chest imaging
- Hypoxia or respiratory distress

Forearm Fractures

Torus fractures of distal forearm

- Splint and sling
- Analgesics
- Torus fracture aftercare instructions
- Orthopedic referral within 10 days

Colles, Smith and Barton's fractures

- Consult physician
- Respective fracture aftercare instructions

- OCL sugar tong splint and sling for Colles fracture if discharged
- Analgesics

Radius and ulnar midshaft fractures

- Consult physician

Elbow Fractures

Considerations

- X-ray may or may not show radial head fractures
- Anterior or posterior fat pad sign on x-ray is from blood from fracture or sprain pushing on the fat pad
- Posterior fat pad associated more frequently with fracture

Evaluation

- Elbow x-ray
- Neurovascular examination
- Assess for associated injuries

Treatment options

- Sling
- OCL posterior splint may be needed
- Analgesics prn

Discharge criteria

- Nondisplaced simple proximal radius fracture
- X-ray reveals fat pad sign without obvious fracture

Discharge instructions

- Elbow fracture aftercare instructions
- Inform patient and family that the x-ray shows a fat pad sign that may indicate a fracture present, even if no fracture seen at that time
- Follow up with orthopedic surgeon within 10 days

Consult criteria

- Proximal ulnar fracture
- Distal humerus fracture
- Supracondylar fracture
- Neurovascular deficits
- Neurologic complaints

Metacarpal Fractures

Nondisplaced, nonangulated transverse fracture

Evaluation

- X-ray
- Neurovascular exam

Treatment

- Dorsal splint for 3–4 weeks
- Sling
- Analgesics prn

Discharge criteria

- Simple closed fracture

Discharge instructions

- Metacarpal fracture aftercare instructions
- Follow up with orthopedic or hand surgeon within 7–10 days

Consult criteria

- Open fracture
- Neurovascular deficit or complaint

Transverse, angulated and displaced fracture

- Consult physician

Spiral or oblique fracture

- Consult physician

Hip and Femur Fractures

- Consult physician
- Pain control

Patella

Fracture

Nondisplaced with extensor function intact

Evaluation

- Knee x-ray with sunrise view
- Assess neurovascular status

Treatment

- Knee immobilizer
- Analgesics
- Crutches

Discharge criteria

- Closed simple patella fracture with intact extensor function

Discharge instructions

- Patella fracture aftercare instructions
- Orthopedic referral

Consult criteria

- Displaced > 3 mm or extensor function loss

Dislocation

Evaluation

- Same as patella fracture

Treatment

- Reduce dislocation
- Knee immobilizer
- Analgesics

Discharge criteria

- Closed simple reduced patella fracture

Discharge instructions

- Patella dislocation aftercare instructions
- Orthopedic follow-up within 10 days

Consult criteria

- Nonreducible patellar dislocation

Tibial Plateau and Midshaft Fractures

Considerations

- Tibial plateau fractures may be difficult to see on plain x-ray
- CT scan of knee frequently reveals a more extensive fracture than plain film

Evaluation

- Knee or tibial/fibula x-ray
- CT scan of knee may be needed or requested for tibial plateau fractures
- Neurovascular examination
- Assess for associated injuries

Treatment

- Pain control IM or IV
- Splint knee in extension for tibial plateau fracture
- Splint lower leg if needed prior to physician exam

Consult criteria

- Discuss with physician all tibial fractures

Fibula Proximal, Midshaft and Displaced Distal Fractures

Evaluation

- X-ray
- Neurovascular examination
- Assess for associated injuries

Treatment

- Pain control IM or IV
- Splint as needed

Consult criteria

- Discuss these fractures with a physician

Nondisplaced Distal Fibula Fracture

Evaluation

- X-ray
- Neurovascular examination
- Assess for associated injuries
- Ligament examination as tolerated

Treatment

- Walking boot
- Crutches
- Analgesics

Discharge criteria

- Simple closed nondisplaced fibular fracture
- Normal neurovascular examination

Discharge instructions

- Ankle sprain and distal fibular fracture aftercare instructions
- Follow up with orthopedic surgeon within 7–10 days

Consult criteria

- Neurovascular injury
- Open fracture

Knee Strain

- See Knee Soft Tissue Injury Protocol

Foot Fractures and Dislocations

Tarsal or midfoot

- Consult physician
- Analgesics

Metatarsal fractures

Nondisplaced

- Boot
- Crutches
- Analgesics

- Orthopedic referral

Displaced

- Consult physician

Calcaneus fractures

- Posterior splint
- Analgesics prn
- Consult physician

Consult Criteria

- Acute neurovascular deficits or injury
- Suspected compartment syndrome
- Nonreducible dislocations
- Open fractures, joints or dislocations

Notes

SALTER HARRIS FRACTURE PROTOCOL

When using any protocol, always follow the Guidelines of Proper Use (page 16).

Definition

- Disruption of the cartilaginous plates of the physeal area or growth plate that may or may not involve a fracture of the adjacent bone in children

Salter Pneumonic

- Salter 1 — **S**lip of growth plate
- Salter 2 — **A**bove (fracture extends above growth plate)
- Salter 3 — **L**ow (fracture extends below growth plate)
- Salter 4 — **T**hrough (fracture above and below plate)
- Salter 5 — **E**ntire (crush fracture of growth plate area)
- Salter 6 — **R**ing (injury to the perichondral ring or periosteum)

Considerations

- The cartilage growth plate can be weaker than ligaments in children
- Sprains in children can actually be Salter 1 fractures that are not evident on initial x-ray
- Plain x-rays may depict widening of growth plate as only sign of a fracture
- Comparison x-rays of uninjured opposite extremity can be helpful with Salter 1 fractures
- CT scans may be necessary to delineate degree of injury in severely comminuted Salter fractures
- Growth acceleration (uncommon) or growth arrest can occur with Salter fractures
- Long term follow-up at 6 and 12 months important
- Salter 1 fracture of the great toe with subungual hematoma represents an open fracture

Growth plate (physeal) fractures at increased risk of growth arrest are

- Distal femur
- Distal tibia
- Distal radius and ulna
- Proximal tibia
- Triradiate cartilage — acetabulum in children

Evaluation

- History of injury
- Examination for neurovascular and tendon injuries
- Examination for remote undisclosed injuries
- X-ray of injured area
- Comparison x-rays if needed of opposite uninjured extremity

Treatment

- Most Salter 1 and 2 fractures can be treated, if mildly displaced, with reduction if needed and splinting and follow-up in 7–10 days
- Salter 3 and 4 usually require open reduction and fixation
- Salter 5 fractures are rarely diagnosed acutely and treatment is usually delayed because of the delay in diagnosis
- Antibiotics for great toe Salter fractures with subungual hematoma that are discharged — Augmentin (amoxicillin/clavulanate) or cephalosporin
    - Considered an open fracture (preferable to discuss with physician)
- Pain medications as needed

Discharge Criteria

- Nondisplaced Salter 1 and 2 fractures
- Reduced Salter 1 and 2 fractures

Discharge instructions

- Salter Harris fracture aftercare instructions
- Follow up in 7–10 days preferably with orthopedic surgeon

- Instructions in various pediatric "sprains" that could be a nondisplaced Salter 1 fracture

Consult Criteria

- Displaced Salter fractures
- Open Salter fractures
- Neurovascular deficits
- Tendon deficits
- Salter 3–6 fractures

Notes

SYNOVIAL FLUID ANALYSIS

When using any protocol, always follow the Guidelines of Proper Use (page 16).

Normal

- Transparent clarity
- Clear color
- WBC < 200/ml
- PMN's < 25%
- Culture negative
- No crystals
- Mucin clot firm
- Glucose approximates blood levels

Noninflammatory

- Transparent clarity
- Yellow color
- WBC 200–2000/ml
- PMN's < 25%
- Culture negative
- No crystals
- Mucin clot firm
- Glucose approximates blood levels
- Associated conditions: rheumatic fever, trauma, osteoarthritis

Inflammatory

- Cloudy clarity
- Yellow color
- WBC 200–50,000/ml
- PMN's > 50%
- Culture negative
- Crystals can be present if gout or pseudogout are etiology
- Mucin clot friable
- Glucose decreased
- Associated conditions: SLE, Lyme disease, gout, pseudogout, spondyloarthropathies

Septic

- Cloudy clarity
- Yellow color
- WBC 25,000/ml to often > 100,000/ml
- PMS's > 50%
- Culture often positive
- No crystals
- Mucin clot friable
- Glucose very decreased
- Fever
- C-reactive protein elevated

Notes

SHOULDER PROTOCOL

When using any protocol, always follow the Guidelines of Proper Use (page 16).

Shoulder conditions

Impingement syndrome encompasses

- Supraspinatus tendonitis
- Bicipital tendonitis
- Subacromial bursitis

Supraspinatus tendonitis

- Middle aged
- Subacute or chronic pain in shoulder
- Top of shoulder tender distal to acromion
- Abduction beyond 80–120 degrees limited from pain
- X-rays may be normal or show erosions and calcifications in tendon

Bicipital tendonitis

- Pain in anterior shoulder
- Tenderness along long head of biceps and bicipital groove
- Flexion painful with elbow extended
- Rotation restricted by pain
- Flexion against resistant causes pain

Subacromial bursitis

- Least common of shoulder musculotendinous cuff disorders
- Most painful and acute of the 3 impingement disorders
- Any movement of shoulder causes pain
- Shoulder diffusely tender
- May have fever and elevated ESR

Treatment Options

- Severe pain — rest in sling short-term
- Ice packs with severe pain
- NSAID's prn

- Gravity-assisted range of motion pendulum exercises started in hours to days
- Physical therapy
- 1 cc of Depomedrol (methylprednisolone acetate) 40–80 mg/cc or Kenalog (triamcinolone) 10–20 mg/cc mixed with 1 cc of 1–2% plain lidocaine, injected through normal skin if Provider is experienced performing injections

Discharge Criteria

- Uncomplicated case

Discharge instructions

- Shoulder tendonitis and bursitis aftercare instructions
- Referral to primary care provider or orthopedics if pain persists in 7–10 days

Consult Criteria

- Suspected septic shoulder joint

Thoracic outlet syndrome

- Compression of the neurovascular bundle as it passes out of the thoracic outlet above first rib and behind the clavicle
- May be associated with a cervical rib

3 types of thoracic outlet syndrome

Neurologic (most common)

- C8 and T1 roots most commonly affected
- Pain is in medial arm, forearm, and ring and fifth fingers
- Nocturnal paresthesias
- Weakness
- Cold intolerance
- Neck pain (trapezius)
- Occipital headache
- Anterior chest wall pain
- Raynaud's phenomenon

Venous

- Extremity
  - Swelling
  - Cyanosis
  - Paresthesias

Arterial (most serious and least common)

- Pain
- Coldness
- Numbness
- Pallor
- Seen in young patients with vigorous activity history
- Seen with emboli

Examination

- Provocative tests not reliable

Elevated arm stress test (EAST)

- Most reliable for all three types
- Arms at 90° to body and elbow flexed 90°
  - Hands opened and closed for 3 minutes
- Symptom reproduction is a positive test

Adson's test

- Palpate both radial arteries while patient turns head side to side
- Loss of pulse positive for arterial type

Testing options

- Chest x-ray for cervical rib and pulmonary disease
- Cervical spine
- Duplex scan of arm

Treatment options

- NSAID's
- Narcotics prn

Discharge criteria

- Benign presentation

Discharge instructions

- Thoracic outlet aftercare instructions
- Refer to thoracic surgeon

Consult criteria

- Arterial insufficiency
- Severe pain
- Severe neurologic deficit
- Suspected spinal cord etiology

Rotator Cuff Tear (RCT)

Considerations

- 90% with minimal or no injury
- Tenderness of middle third of shoulder
- Unable to abduct shoulder in massive tears
- Weak abduction and pain with minor tears
- Palpable crepitus with movements
- Painless or tolerable passive abduction
- Atrophy with long standing RCT

Treatment options

- Severe pain — rest in sling short term
- Ice packs with severe pain
- NSAID's prn; narcotics prn
- Gravity-assisted range of motion pendulum exercises started in hours to days
- Physical therapy
- Local lidocaine injection 2 cc prn through normal skin (if Provider has experience with injections)
- No steroid injections

Discharge criteria

- Uncomplicated injury

Discharge instructions

- Rotator cuff tear aftercare instructions
- Referral to orthopedics for major RCT tear within 7 days

Consult criteria

- Discuss major tears with physician

Acromioclavicular (AC) Injuries

Acromioclavicular sprain

- Partial tear of capsule of AC joint
- Usually in young or middle aged with injury to AC joint
- AC joint tender and may be slightly swollen
- Attempted abduction > 60 degrees causes pain
- X-rays show normal AC joint

Treatment

- Sling initially
- Early motion encouraged
- Avoid hyperabduction for 3 weeks
- Avoid heavy lifting for 6 weeks
- Ice packs
- NSAID's prn; narcotics prn

Discharge criteria

- Uncomplicated injury

Discharge instructions

- AC sprain aftercare instructions
- Primary care provider or orthopedic follow up within 10–14 days

Acromioclavicular subluxation

- Complete tear of AC joint capsule
- AC joint markedly swollen
- Outer end of clavicle may protrude slightly upward
- Attempted abduction > 60 degrees causes pain
- X-rays without weights may be normal
- X-rays with 10-lb weights show widened AC joint

Treatment

- Sling initially

- Early motion encouraged
- Avoid hyperabduction > 90 degrees for 3–4 weeks
- Avoid heavy lifting for 2 months
- Ice packs
- NSAID's prn; narcotics prn

Discharge criteria

- Uncomplicated injury

Discharge instructions

- AC injury aftercare instructions
- Primary care provider or orthopedic follow up within 10–14 days

Consult criteria

- Complicated injury
- Neurovascular injury or complaints

Notes

Shoulder and Arm Trauma Protocol

When using any protocol, always follow the Guidelines of Proper Use (page 16).

General Evaluation

- History of injury; past history; medication history
- Associated symptoms and complete physical exam
- X-rays
- Neurovascular/tendon/ligament exam
- Assess for compartment syndrome
- Assess for open fracture or joint

Acromioclavicular (AC) Injuries

Acromioclavicular sprain

- Partial tear of capsule of AC joint
- Usually in young or middle aged with injury to AC joint
- AC joint tender and may be slightly swollen
- Attempted abduction > 60 degrees causes pain
- X-rays show normal AC joint

Treatment

- Sling initially
- Early motion encouraged
- Avoid hyperabduction for 3 weeks
- Avoid heavy lifting for 6 weeks
- Ice packs
- NSAID's prn; narcotics prn

Discharge criteria

- Uncomplicated injury

Discharge instructions

- AC sprain aftercare instructions
- Primary care provider or orthopedic follow-up within 10–14 days

Acromioclavicular subluxation

- Complete tear of AC joint capsule
- AC joint markedly swollen
- Outer end of clavicle may protrude slightly upward
- Attempted abduction > 60 degrees causes pain
- X-rays without weights may be normal
- X-rays with 10-lb weights show widened AC joint

Treatment

- Sling initially
- Early motion encouraged
- Avoid hyperabduction > 90 degrees for 3–4 weeks
- Avoid heavy lifting for 2 months
- Ice packs
- NSAID's prn; narcotics prn

Discharge criteria

- Uncomplicated injury

Discharge instructions

- AC injury aftercare instructions
- Primary care provider or orthopedic follow-up within 10–14 days

Consult criteria

- Complicated injury
- Neurovascular injury or complaints

Clavicle Fractures

Considerations

- Most common fracture in children
- 80% middle third
- 15% distal third
- 5% proximal third
- May need CT scan for sternoclavicular injuries

Treatment

- Sling
    - Middle and distal end fractures for 4–8 weeks

    - Acromioclavicular sprain and separation
- Proximal sternoclavicular fractures and dislocations — consult physician
- Posterior sternoclavicular dislocation — notify physician promptly if available
    - Needs immediate reduction to prevent life threatening complications
    - May have stridor or respiratory distress
    - May have venous congestion of head or neck or affected arm

Posterior sternoclavicular dislocation treatment

- 3-4 inch roll between scapula and spine to extend or open up affected sternoclavicular joint
- Abduct affected shoulder to 90° and extend shoulder to 15° and apply traction with assistant holding trunk still
- If above fails, maintain traction and manually grasp clavicle and pull forward
- Consult orthopedic surgeon for sternoclavicular dislocations

- NSAID's (very effective in children); narcotics prn

Discharge criteria

- Uncomplicated clavicle fracture

Discharge instructions

- Clavicle fracture aftercare instructions
- Follow up with PCP or orthopedic surgeon within 10 days

Consult criteria

- Immediate physician consultation for suspected posterior sternoclavicular joint dislocation

Scapular Fractures

Considerations

- Can occur with significant trauma to trunk and other injuries
- Evaluate for associated injuries

- Type 1: body of scapula
- Type 2: coracoid and acromion
- Type 3: neck and glenoid

Evaluation

- Shoulder x-rays
- Chest x-ray
- CT may be needed if going to surgery for repair

Treatment

Type 1

- Sling
- Analgesics
- Consult physician

Type 2 and 3

- Physician and orthopedic consultation

Discharge criteria

- Uncomplicated Type 1 scapular fracture

Discharge instructions

- Scapular fracture aftercare instructions
- Follow up with trauma or thoracic surgeon within 5–10 days

Consult criteria

- Type 2 and 3 scapular fractures
- For any significant associated injuries
- Discuss all scapular fractures with physician prior to discharge

Humerus Fractures

Considerations

- Fall on outstretched hand
- Usually elderly
- Younger patients with epiphyseal injuries of growth plate
- Shoulder tense and swollen
- Obtain AP and lateral shoulder x-rays
- Evaluate for neurovascular injury

- Proximal humerus: axillary nerve (test deltoid sensation)
- Humeral shaft: radial nerve (test for wrist drop and 1st web space sensation loss)

Treatment

- Sling
- Physical therapy
- Narcotics prn
- Children may take   prn
- Orthopedic referral within 7 days

Discharge criteria

- Uncomplicated and minimally displaced proximal closed humerus fracture

Discharge instructions

- Humerus fracture aftercare instructions
- Orthopedic referral within 7 days

Consult criteria

- Orthopedic consultation for severely angulated or comminuted fracture
- Orthopedic consult for pediatric humerus fractures
- Discuss with physician all humerus fractures prior to discharge

Shoulder (Glenohumeral) Dislocation

Considerations

Anterior dislocation

- Most common: 95–97%
- Axillary nerve most common neurovascular injury
  - Assess with pinprick over lateral shoulder
- Median and ulnar injuries rare
  - Median nerve
    - Decreased sensation to thumb
    - Index and middle finger sensation impaired
    - Thumb opposition weak

    - Ulnar nerve
        - Decreased sensation and weakness of 4th and 5th fingers
        - Abduction and adduction of 4th and 5th fingers very weak or impossible to perform
        - Flexion of the 4th and 5th metacarpophalangeal joints with interphalangeal joints extended is weak or impossible to perform
- Patient holds arm adjacent to body
- Any motion causes severe pain
- Rounded shoulder contour is lost
- Hill-Sachs humeral head deformity present in 50%: no treatment
- Bankart fracture — glenoid rim fracture

Posterior dislocation

- 2–4% of dislocations
- Occurs with seizures, direct anterior shoulder trauma and falls on outstretched hand
- Arm held across chest
- External rotation blocked
- X-ray can be deceptive — less overlap of humeral head and glenoid on AP view

Luxatio Erecta (inferior dislocation)

- 0.5% of glenohumeral dislocations
- Arm held over head
- High complication rate
- 60% neurological injury — most commonly axillary nerve
- Rotator cuff tear > 50%

Evaluation

- Neurovascular exam
- Shoulder x-ray AP and lateral (or Y-view)

Treatment options

- Conscious sedation frequently needed (consult physician)
- Sling for 3–6 weeks in younger patients

- Sling for 1–2 weeks in age > 40 years
- Faster healing if arm in 15 degrees external rotation (may be hard to accomplish)

Anterior dislocations

External Rotation method

- Patient supine
- Adduct arm and flex 90° at elbow
- Slowly rotate arm externally
- Reduce shoulder before reaching coronal plane

Scapular rotation

- Patient prone
- 5–15 pounds of hanging weights
- Rotate inferior scapula medially and superior scapula laterally

  OR
- Patient sitting
- Assistant provides traction on wrist with other hand pushing against chest
- Rotate inferior scapula medially and superior scapula laterally

Traction-counter traction (Modified Hippocratic Technique)

- Sheet over flexed forearm and tied around Provider's waist with countertraction with sheet around axilla by assistant
- Be careful of injuring brachial plexus
- Gentle internal and external rotation with traction by Provider

Stimson technique

- Patient in prone position and secured from falling off table
- Arm hanging off table with axilla and brachial plexus protected
- 20 lb. weights taped or attached to forearm or wrist/hand
- Wait 20 minutes

- Shoulder will usually reduce or will need minimal traction at the 20 minute timeframe
- Can be done without sedation or pain treatment occasionally

Posterior dislocations

- Traction along long axis of arm with anterior pressure on posterior shoulder

Luxatio Erecta (inferior dislocation)

- Overhead traction in upward and outward direction on arm with countertraction towards feet with sheet on injured shoulder

Discharge criteria

- Uncomplicated dislocation

Discharge instructions

- Shoulder dislocation aftercare instructions
- Refer to orthopedic surgeon within 7–10 days

Consult criteria

- Discuss all shoulder dislocations with physician
- Neurovascular injury
- Compartment syndrome
- Orthopedic consult if irreducible dislocation
- Orthopedic consult if associated fracture excluding Hill-Sachs deformity

Notes

ELBOW PROTOCOL

When using any protocol, always follow the Guidelines of Proper Use (page 16).

Considerations

- Tendonitis is usually from overuse
- "Tennis elbow" is most common elbow complaint orthopedists see

Lateral Epicondylitis ("Tennis Elbow")

- Chronic overuse syndrome
- Occupations that require a rotary motion at the elbow
- Increased with grasping motions (handshake) or twisting motions
- Point tenderness over lateral epicondyle
- X-rays usually normal
- Ice or heat — whichever provides the greatest relief

Treatment options

- Elimination of offending activity
- Rest
- NSAID's prn
- Splinting or "tennis elbow bands"

Discharge criteria

- All uncomplicated cases

Discharge instructions

- Elbow tendonitis aftercare instructions
- Follow with PCP or orthopedic surgeon as needed

Consult criteria

- Orthopedic referral for refractory cases

Medial Epicondylitis

- Less common than lateral epicondylitis
- Tenderness over medial epicondyle

- May be associated ulnar neuritis with loss of sensation over palmar 5th finger and lateral palmar surface of 4th finger

Treatment options

- Similar to lateral epicondylitis
- Oral steroids for 1 week in nondiabetics can be used for ulnar neuritis

Discharge criteria

- All uncomplicated cases

Discharge instructions

- Elbow tendonitis aftercare instructions
- Follow with PCP or orthopedic surgeon as needed

Consult criteria

- Orthopedic referral for refractory cases

Olecranon Bursitis

- Usually a painless cystic swelling
- Can be painful from trauma, infection or cryptogenic cause
- Transudate fluid if aspirated is from chronic inflammation

Treatment options

Nonpainful bursitis

- Sterile lateral bursal aspiration if experienced (avoid bone and joint)
- 1 cc of 1–2% plain lidocaine mixed with 1 cc Depomedrol (methylprednisolone acetate) 40–80 mg/cc or Kenalog (triamcinolone) 10–20 mg/cc prn if Provider experienced with injections (do not introduce needle into bursa through cellulitis)
- Elbow ace wrapping

Painful bursitis

- Fluid needs evaluation (culture and gram stain)

- Heat if infectious etiology
- Heat or ice if cryptogenic etiology — whichever provides the greatest relief

Traumatic bursitis

- Ice × 2 days
- Elbow ace wrapping
- NSAID's prn; narcotics prn

Discharge criteria

- Nonpainful or minimal painful bursitis
- Not infected

Discharge instructions

- Olecranon bursitis aftercare instructions

Consult criteria

- Infected olecranon bursitis

Nursemaid Elbow

- Peak age 1–4 years
- Toddler pulled up by arm or similar type traction on arm
- Cries for a few minutes and stops usually
- Arm appears normal
- No other history; occasionally no helpful history
- Usually does not need x-ray if history and exam consistent with nursemaid elbow
- X-ray if performed is negative for acute process
- Perform x-ray if unsure of diagnosis

Treatment

- Elbow flexed 90 degrees
- Fully pronate elbow and then supinate
- If performed correctly will feel or hear click
- Patient cries transiently
- Provider leaves room and returns in 5–10 minutes
- Hold an object for toddler to grasp with affected arm to demonstrate resolution

Discharge criteria

- All patients without other concerns (abuse) or other injuries

Discharge instructions

- Nursemaid elbow aftercare instructions

Consult criteria

- If child abuse suspected

Notes

HIP PROTOCOL

When using any protocol, always follow the Guidelines of Proper Use (page 16).

Septic Hip

Considerations

- Most common cause of painful hip in infants
- Rapid onset of pain
- Fever
- Elevated ESR and C-reactive protein
- Hip flexed
- All motion of hip resisted
- X-rays show externally rotated hip soft tissue outline

Evaluation

- Neurovascular exam
- Hip and pelvis x-rays
- Hip joint aspiration by specialist if indicated
- Synovial fluid analysis (see Synovial Fluid Analysis as needed)

Treatment

- Orthopedic admission for hip lavage and antibiotics

Consult criteria

- Suspected septic hip joint

Transient Synovitis

Considerations

- Self-limited disease of children age 3–10 years
- Etiology unknown (viral infection etiology postulated)
- Males twice as likely as females to have
- Crying at night in very young
- Antalgic gait or limp
- Usually afebrile; may have low-grade fever

- Hip held in flexion and slight abduction with external rotation
- 1/3 has no decreased hip motion
- Hip may be tender to palpation and painful to passive motion

Evaluation options

- Neurovascular exam
- CBC
- ESR
- Aspiration of hip by specialist if fever > 99.5; ESR > 20; or there is severe pain with movement
- Hip and pelvis x-rays
- Ultrasound as needed

Treatment

- Local heat and massage
- Bed rest for 7–10 days
- No weight bearing
- Close follow-up

Discharge criteria

- Discuss all pediatric hip pain with physician
- Diagnosis firm
- Provide transient hip synovitis aftercare instructions

Consult criteria

- Uncertain diagnosis
- Septic hip suspected

Legg-Calve-Perthes' Disease (Avascular Necrosis of Femoral Head)

Considerations

- Caused by loss of blood supply to hip
- Insidious onset
- Limp often presenting complaint
- Aching in groin and thigh
- Tender over anterior hip joint

- Age 4–10 years most common; range 2–18 years of age
- Male > female prevalence
- 20% bilateral
- Leg externally rotated

Evaluation

- Neurovascular exam
- CBC
- ESR
- Hip and pelvis x-rays
- Ultrasound helpful
- Bone scan diagnostic

Treatment

- NSAID's prn; Tylenol prn
- Non-weight bearing
- Physical therapy
- Crutches

Discharge criteria

- Most patients
- Adequate pain control is achievable

Discharge instructions

- Legg-Calve-Perthes' Disease aftercare instructions

Consult criteria

- Discuss with physician
- Severe pain not controlled by medications
- Poor social situation not allowing non-weight bearing

Slipped Capital Femoral Epiphysis (SCFE)

Considerations

- Most patients obese
- Male peak age 13–15 years
- Female peak age 11–13 years
- More common in males

- Bilateral hips in 1/3 of cases
- Present with limp
- Pain referred to knee, thigh, groin or hip
- Commonly with leg externally rotated
- Flexion is restricted
- Do not ambulate if SCFE suspected

Evaluation

- Neurovascular exam
- CBC
- ESR
- C-reactive protein
- AP and frog leg lateral of both hips
- Klein line is a line drawn parallel to lateral femoral neck that does not transect epiphysis; normally it does transect epiphysis in healthy hips

Treatment

- Immobilization
- Non-weight bearing

Consult criteria

- Immediate orthopedic consult

Hip Fracture

Considerations

- Elderly fall most common reason
- Affected leg externally rotated

Evaluation

- Hip and pelvis x-rays
- CT scan if plain hip x-ray without definite fracture but there is high suspicion of hip fracture
- Neurovascular exam
- Assess for other injuries
- Evaluate for acute medical condition if the cause of injury

Treatment

- Pain control

Consult criteria

- All hip fracture patients
- All suspected hip fracture patients

Hip Dislocation

Considerations

- Posterior dislocation most common
- Frequently seen with total hip replacement

Evaluation

- Hip and pelvis x-rays
- Neurovascular exam
- Assess for other injuries or conditions

Treatment

- Pain control

Consult criteria

- Consult physician

KNEE SOFT TISSUE INJURY PROTOCOL

When using any protocol, always follow the Guidelines of Proper Use (page 16).

Differential Diagnosis

- Knee strain
- Anterior cruciate ligament tear or strain
- Posterior cruciate ligament tear or strain
- Medial meniscus tear
- Lateral meniscus tear
- Medial collateral tear or strain
- Lateral collateral tear of stain
- Patellar dislocation

Considerations

- Effusions occurring within 6 hours suggest ligament or cartilage injury
- Grade 1: microscopic ligament injury
- Grade 2: severe stretch with partial tear
- Grade 3: complete ligament disruption

Ottawa Knee Rule for obtaining x-rays (any of the following) for injuries < 24 hours and age > 18

- Inability to bear weight (walk 4 steps) immediately and presently
- Patellar tenderness
- Fibular head tenderness
- Age > 55 years
- Unable to flex knee > 90 degrees

Examination

- Palpate for areas of tenderness
- Check for knee effusion

Lachman's test

- Knee held in 15–30 degree flexion and move tibia forward
- Positive if motion visible; motion more than in uninjured knee
- Suggests anterior cruciate ligament (ACL) tear

McMurray's test

- Flex knee fully
- Rotate externally or internally and extend the knee
- Painful click on extension suggests meniscus injury
    - Internal rotation: lateral meniscus
    - External rotation: medial meniscus

Apley's test

- Patient in prone position
- Knee flexed
- Compression of foot into knee while rotated — suggests meniscus injury
- Distraction of foot from knee while rotated — suggests ligament injury

- Neurovascular exam
- Knee x-ray if indicated
    - Evaluate for fracture, dislocation and effusion

Treatment Options

- Ice
- Elevation
- Knee immobilizer prn
- Crutches prn
- Analgesics: NSAID's, narcotics prn

Discharge Criteria

- Uncomplicated injury

Discharge instructions

- Knee injury aftercare instructions

- Referral to orthopedic surgeon for grade 2–3 ligament injury or suspected meniscus injury suspected within 7–10 days
- Primary care provider follow-up for grade 1–2 sprains and contusions within 7–10 days

Consult Criteria

- Neurovascular injury
- Open joint injury
- Grossly unstable joint

Notes

KNEE DISORDERS PROTOCOL

When using any protocol, always follow the Guidelines of Proper Use (page 16).

Considerations

- Most nontraumatic knee conditions are degenerative or inflammatory
- Blood cultures may be positive in septic arthritis
- Consult physician for acute neurovascular deficits

Synovial fluid analysis

Normal

- Transparent clarity
- Clear color
- WBC < 200/mL
- PMN's < 25%
- Culture negative
- No crystals
- Mucin clot firm
- Glucose approximates blood levels

Noninflammatory

- Transparent clarity
- Yellow color
- WBC 200–2000/mL
- PMN's < 25%
- Culture negative
- No crystals
- Mucin clot firm
- Glucose approximates blood levels
- Associated conditions: rheumatic fever, trauma, osteoarthritis

Inflammatory

- Cloudy clarity
- Yellow color
- WBC 200–50,000/mL
- PMN's > 50%
- Culture negative

- Crystals can be present if gout or pseudogout or none
- Mucin clot friable
- Glucose decreased
- Associated conditions: SLE, Lyme disease, gout, pseudogout, spondyloarthropathies

Septic

- Cloudy clarity
- Yellow color
- WBC 25,000/mL to often > 100,000/mL
- PMS's > 50%
- Culture often positive
- No crystals
- Mucin clot friable
- Glucose very decreased
- Fever
- C-reactive protein elevated

Osgood-Schlatter's Disease

Considerations

- Childhood disorder
- Males 10–15 years of age
- Aseptic necrosis within tibial tuberosity
- Pain, swelling and erythema over anterior tibial tuberosity
- Pain during resisted extension
- Pain on kneeling
- Slow onset
- Lateral knee x-ray may or may not show fragmentation of the tibial tubercle
- Clinical diagnosis

Treatment options

- Avoid climbing, running, kicking until pain has resolved

Discharge criteria

- All patients usually

Discharge instructions

- Osgood–Schlatter's disease aftercare instructions

Consult criteria

- Orthopedic referral if condition persistent

Prepatellar and Superficial Infrapatellar Bursitis

Considerations

- "Housemaid knee"
- Swelling of involved area

Treatment options

- Avoid kneeling
- Aspirate fluid if experienced with procedure
- May inject 1 cc of triamcinolone 40/cc with 1 cc lidocaine if experienced (do not inject if cellulitis present)
- Ace wrap

Discharge criteria

- Noninfected bursitis

Discharge instructions

- Patellar bursitis aftercare instructions

Consult criteria

- Infected bursitis suspected

Deep Infrapatellar and Anserine Bursitis

Considerations

- Excessive weight bearing
- Pain at rest
- Increased pain with resisted extension
- Pain is felt in knee and may refer to hip, thigh or lower leg
- Swelling may occur
- Tenderness deep to patellar tendon

Treatment options

- Minimize weight bearing
- Avoid climbing, jumping, running, squatting
- Ice packs
- Quadriceps exercise when pain allows
- Range of motion exercises
- Corticosteroid injection prn (if Provider is experienced)
- NSAID's prn; narcotics prn

Discharge criteria

- Noninfected bursitis

Discharge instructions

- Knee bursitis aftercare instructions

Consult criteria

- Infected bursitis
- Orthopedic referral if not resolving

Baker's Cyst

Considerations

- Effusion of semimembranosus bursa
- Predisposes to chronic knee effusion
- Mass behind knee up to 5 × 5 cm
- X-rays may or may not show DJD

Treatment options

- May aspirate if experienced
- Ace wrap prn
- NSAID's prn

Discharge criteria

- Nonseptic joint
- Orthopedic referral

Discharge instructions

- Baker's cyst aftercare instructions

Consult criteria

- Uncertain diagnosis

Chondromalacia Patella

Considerations

- Degeneration of the patellar cartilage
- Any age
- Usually no injury
- Positive Patellar Grind Test — pushing on patella while moving knee into extension causes pain

Treatment options

- Avoid climbing, jumping, running, squatting

Discharge criteria

- Usually most patients

Discharge instructions

- Chondromalacia patella aftercare instructions

Consult criteria

- Orthopedic or primary care provider referral if not resolving

Osteoarthritis (DJD)

Considerations

- Related to increasing age
- Can result from previous injuries or knee surgery
- Knee effusion may be present
- Knee feels like it "gives way" occasionally
- Range of motion limited

Treatment options

- Minimize wear and tear activities
- NSAID's prn; narcotics prn for severe pain — short course
- Oral steroids for 7 days prn if not diabetic
- Knee immobilizer prn
- Crutches or walker prn

Discharge criteria

- Nonseptic knee joint

Discharge instructions

- Knee osteoarthritis aftercare instructions

Consult criteria

- Orthopedic referral for severe knee pain

Gout

Differential diagnosis

- Cellulitis
- Septic arthritis
- Bursitis
- Osteomyelitis
- Rheumatoid arthritis
- Soft tissue injury
- Pseudogout

Considerations

- Crystal uric acid deposits in joints and tissues
- Most common cause of monoarticular arthritis age > 60
- Increased warmth, redness and joint swelling
- First metatarsophalangeal joint of foot involved 75% of the time — most common involved joint
- Joint fluid: 20,000–100,000 WBC; poor string and mucin clot; no bacteria (pseudogout similar)
- Risk factors
    - Age > 40
    - Hypertension
    - Diuretics
    - Ethanol intake
    - Obesity

Evaluation

- Clinical evaluation usually all that is needed
- If diagnosis uncertain may order
    - CBC
    - C-reactive protein
    - X-rays

- Joint aspiration if experienced Provider

Treatment options

- NSAID's high dose 5–10 days
- Narcotics IM or PO short course prn
- Steroids prn
  - Prednisone 40–60 mg PO qday × 3–7 days

    OR
  - Depomedrol (methylprednisolone acetate) 80–120 mg IM
- Allopurinol 50–300 mg PO qday — adjusted for renal function; start after acute episode resolved
- Follow up with primary care provider within 2–3 days if pain persists

Discharge instructions

- Gout aftercare instructions

Consult criteria

- Uncertain diagnosis
- Fever or toxicity
- HR ≥ 110

Septic Arthritis

Differential diagnosis

- Cellulitis
- Gout
- Bursitis
- Osteomyelitis
- Rheumatoid arthritis
- Soft tissue injury
- Pseudogout

Considerations

- Onset is rapid
- Usually one joint infected
- Joint is very painful; hot; red; fluctuant
- Signs of acute systemic illness may be present
- Fever, chills and sweats frequently
- C-reactive protein elevated
- See Synovial Fluid Analysis

Treatment
- Admission to hospital for drainage and antibiotics

Discharge criteria
- Only with physician consent

Consult criteria
- All septic joint patients

Notes

Ankle Sprain Protocol

When using any protocol, always follow the Guidelines of Proper Use (page 16).

Definition

- Stretching or tearing of the ankle's ligaments

Differential Diagnosis

- Ankle fracture
- Ankle dislocation

Considerations

- 85–90% involves lateral ligaments
- Age < 10 years with traumatic ankle pain and no fracture on x-ray likely have Salter type 1 fracture
- Stress testing acutely often limited by pain
- Nonweight bearing for several days has been shown to improve long-term outcomes for all sprains
- Ankle sprain grades
    - Grade 1: Ligament stretching without tearing or instability on exam
    - Grade 2: Some ligament tearing without instability, but more swelling and ecchymosis than grade 1
    - Grade 3: Complete tearing of ligaments with gross instability, marked swelling and ecchymosis and pain

Ottawa Rule for ordering ankle x-rays. Can defer x-ray if no criteria present below

- Bony tenderness distal 6 cm of posterior edge or tip of tibia or fibula, or either malleolus
- Bony tenderness base of 5th metatarsal or navicular bone
- Inability to take 4 unassisted steps at time of injury and when being evaluated

Evaluation

- Assess ankle for instability

- Drawer test — anterior
- Assess inversion and eversion for instability
- Neurovascular exam
- Examine for associated ipsilateral leg injuries
- Examine for other remote injuries
- Evaluate as needed for the cause of injury

Treatment Options

- Ice and elevation
- Mild to moderate sprains can be treated with elastic wrap, air splint or plastic boot.
    - Can be weight bearing or nonweight bearing per Provider's discretion
- Severe sprains (ligament laxity) or severe pain — plastic boot or OCL posterior splint and crutches
- Consider nonweight bearing for 5–10 days to improve long-term outcome
- Nondisplaced distal fibula fractures can be treated with OCL posterior splint or plastic boots and crutches
- NSAID's, Tylenol, or narcotics prn — avoid Demerol (meperidine)

Discharge Criteria

- Sprains with intact ankle mortise, closed, with no acute neurovascular deficits
- Potential Salter 1 fractures

Discharge instructions

- Ankle sprain aftercare instructions
- Refer to grade 1 and 2 sprains to primary care provider
    - Permissible to refer to orthopedics
- Refer grade 3 or severe sprains to orthopedics within 7–10 days
- Nonweight bearing for 3 weeks improves outcomes
- Refer potential Salter 1 fractures to PCP or orthopedic surgeon for recheck in 10 days

Consult Criteria

- Grossly unstable ankle joint or disrupted ankle mortise

- Potential open ankle joint
- Acute neurovascular deficits
- Fractures (excluding nondisplaced distal fibula fractures)

Notes

Hand, Wrist, and Distal Forearm Injury Protocol

When using any protocol, always follow the Guidelines of Proper Use (page 16).

General Recommendations

Evaluation

- X-ray all orthopedic hand and wrist injuries with mechanism of injury that could cause fractures or dislocations
- Assess neurovascular status and for tendon/ligament deficits

Treatment

- Reduce dislocations if experienced
- NSAID's or narcotics prn for pain
- Tetanus prophylaxis prn (see Tetanus Guidelines, page 580)

Discharge criteria

- Simple, nondisplaced, nonrotated closed long bone fractures can be splinted and discharged with orthopedic follow-up usually
  - Discuss with physician (except simple nondisplaced torus fractures)
- Simple dislocations that have been reduced

Consult criteria

- Wrist or proximal metacarpal dislocations
- Open injuries
- Acute neurovascular deficits
- Tendon/ligament injuries

Considerations

Complications

- Neurovascular injury
- Open fracture

  - Joint involvement
  - Ligament/tendon injury
  - Displaced and angulated
  - Compartment syndrome
  - Fat emboli — long bones
  - Avascular necrosis
  - Osteomyelitis
- Nondisplaced, closed simple long bone fractures can be splinted and discharged with orthopedic follow-up usually
  - Discuss with physician (except simple nondisplaced torus fractures)

Compartment syndrome

- From increased pressure in a muscle or other internal compartment
- Not all signs and symptoms are needed to make diagnosis
- High pressures > 8 hours leads to tissue damage
- Normal tissue pressure is < 10 mm Hg
- Capillary blood flow is compromised at > 20 mm Hg
- Intracompartmental pressures > 30 mm Hg or within 10–30 mm Hg of DBP

Signs and symptoms (not diagnostic)

- Pain
  - Out of proportion to injury
  - On passive stretch of muscles
- Pallor
- Paresthesias
- Paralysis
  - Sensory and motor findings are late signs
- Poikilothermia — decreased temperature
- Pulselessness
  - Usually not lost until muscle necrosis has occurred
  - Last sign to develop
- Tense muscle compartment on palpation

Treatment

- Consult physician if suspected
- Keep extremity at level of heart
- Do not use ice if suspected
- Remove cast and padding
- Surgery fasciotomy is usually necessary

Human Bite or Clenched Fist Injury

- Augmentin (amoxicillin/clavulanate) preferred antibiotic x 10–14 days
- Need operative irrigation and surgical exploration emergently unless very superficial
- Usually presents late
- Do not perform primary repair of laceration
- Consult physician
- See Human and Animal Bite Protocol

Boxer's Fracture (4th and/or 5th Metacarpal Shaft)

Considerations

- Usually from punching with a closed fist

Evaluation

- X-ray
- Assess for neurovascular and tendon injury
- Assess for human teeth injury

Treatment

- Treat with OCL ulnar gutter or boxer's splint
- Sling
- Analgesics

Discharge criteria

- Simple closed fracture with < 40 degrees angulation

Discharge instructions

- Boxer's fracture aftercare instructions
- Refer to orthopedic or hand surgeon within 7 days

Consult criteria

- 40 degrees or more of angulation needs reduction (consult physician)
- Salter fractures consult physician
- Open fracture
- Human bite

High Pressure Injection Injuries

- Consult physician promptly

Dislocations of the MP Joint

Evaluation

- X-ray
- Assess for neurovascular and tendon injury
- Assess for human teeth injury

Treatment

- May reduce if seen right after injury without x-ray if there is no doubt to diagnosis
- Metacarpal block may not be needed if seen immediately after injury
- Push your thumb on dorsal surface of hand and distally on proximal phalanx to reduce
- Splinting may not be necessary

Discharge criteria

- Closed simple MP joint dislocations that are reduced

Discharge instructions

- MP joint aftercare instructions
- Refer to orthopedic or hand surgeon within 7–10 days

Consult criteria

- Unable to reduce
- Open joint
- No associated fracture

Scaphoid Fracture or Suspected Fracture

Considerations

- Most common carpal fracture
- Snuffbox tenderness
- Complication of avascular necrosis may occur
- High malpractice fracture when missed

Evaluation

- X-ray — may need special views
- Assess for neurovascular and tendon injury

Treatment

- Thumb spica splint and sling if fracture diagnosed or suspected
  - Cast for 12 weeks placed by outpatient referral provider

Discharge criteria

- Closed simple scaphoid fracture
- See Shoulder and Arm Trauma Protocol

Discharge instructions

- Scaphoid fracture aftercare instructions
- Orthopedic or hand surgeon referral within 7–10 days if diagnosed or suspected

Consult criteria

- Open fracture
- Neurovascular, tendon or ligament deficit

Carpal Bone Fractures or Dislocations

- Consult physician (see Scaphoid Fracture above)

Colles and Smith Fractures

Considerations

- Involves distal forearm
- Colles is a dorsal angulation and Smith fracture volar angulation of fracture
- Angulation ≤ 10 degrees can be treated without reduction anatomically

- Intra-articular step-off > 1–2 mm needs orthopedic consultation
- Ulna is usually within 2 mm of radius at wrist
- Treatment varies depending on age and activity level

Evaluation

- X-ray (lateral, AP and oblique)
- Neurovascular examination
- Ligament and tendon examination

Treatment

- Sugar tong splint
- Sling
- Reduction of significant angulation
- Surgery needed commonly

Discharge criteria

- Consult criteria not met
- Simple closed fracture

Discharge instructions

- Colles or Smith fracture aftercare instructions
- Follow up with orthopedic surgeon within 7 days

Consult physician

- Intra-articular step-off > 1–2 mm
- Dorsal tilt 10%
- Volar tilt > 20%
- Radial shortening > 3 mm
- Loss of radial angle
- Neurovascular injury
- Open fracture
- Ligament disruption
- Lunate and perilunate wrist dislocations

Notes

FINGER INJURY PROTOCOL

When using any protocol, always follow the Guidelines of Proper Use (page 16).

General Evaluation and Considerations

- X-ray all finger injuries with mechanism of injury with potential to cause fractures or dislocations
- Assess neurovascular status and for tendon/ligament deficits
- Consult on all open injuries or with acute neurovascular deficits
- Consult on tendon/ligament injuries except as discussed below
- NSAID's or narcotics prn for pain
- Consult for proximal and middle phalanx fractures
- Nondisplaced distal phalange fractures may be splinted in extension and referred to orthopedic or hand surgery

Mallet Finger

- Avulsion of the DIP extensor tendon
- Distal 1 inch volar foam aluminum splint with 110 degrees extension for 6 weeks
- Can splint up to 6 weeks post injury
- Surgery only option if injury 2 months old (Refer to orthopedic or hand surgeon)
- Refer to primary care provider, orthopedic or hand surgeon for recent injury

Avulsion of the Flexor Profundus Tendon DIP Joint

- Jamming injury (usually children)
- Palmar middle phalanx and dorsal DIP joint swollen and tender
- Unable to actively flex distal phalanx
- Splint in position of function (normal resting position of an uninjured finger)
- Orthopedic referral for surgery

PIP Joint Dislocation

- Usually from hyperextension injury
- May reduce if seen right after injury without x-ray if there is no doubt to diagnosis
- Local digital anesthesia may not be needed if seen immediately after injury
- Push distal phalanx back into alignment and x-ray
- Splint in full extension for 3 weeks
- Refer to orthopedic or hand surgeon

Avulsion of the Central Extensor Slip

- Difficult to diagnose at time of injury because of swelling
- Boutonniere deformity of the PIP joint is frequently a late finding
- Due to forceful PIP joint flexion
- Splint in full extension for 3 weeks if suspected or diagnosed
- Refer to orthopedic or hand surgeon within 7–10 days

Avulsion of the Volar Carpal Plate PIP Joint

- Hyperextension injury or a recently reduced PIP joint dislocation
- Joint movements very painful and limited
- Palmar surface very tender
- Abnormal extension of joint possible on exam
- Splint in full extension for 3 weeks if suspected or diagnosed
- Refer to orthopedic or hand surgeon within 3–7 days

Tear or Avulsion of the Collateral Ligament

- Instability of lateral PIP joint in either direction
- Splint in 15-20 degrees at PIP joint and 70 degrees at MP joint for 3 weeks
- Refer to orthopedic or hand surgeon

Gamekeeper Thumb

- Tenderness over first metacarpal phalangeal joint of thumb
- Rupture of ulnar collateral ligament

- Joint opens up with radial stress > than other thumb
- Associated avulsion fracture is common
- Thumb spica
- Refer to orthopedic or hand surgeon within 3–7 days

Notes

Pediatrics

Section Contents

Pediatric Fever Protocol

Benign Febrile Seizure Protocol

Crying Infant Protocol

URI and Sinusitis Protocol

Otitis Media Protocol

Pediatric Asthma Protocol

Bronchiolitis Protocol

Croup Protocol

Pediatric Dehydration and Gastroenteritis Protocol

Pediatric Diarrhea Protocol

When using any protocol, always follow the Guidelines of Proper Use (page 16).

PEDIATRIC FEVER PROTOCOL

When using any protocol, always follow the Guidelines of Proper Use (page 16).

Definition

- Rectal temperature > 100.4°F (38°C)

Differential Diagnosis

- Viral infections
- Localized bacterial infections
- Bacteremia
- Sepsis
- Urinary tract infection
- Heat illness

Considerations

- Risk of occult bacteremia has declined markedly with pneumococcal and HIB vaccines
- Males < 6 months without a source of fever have a UTI 7% of the time
- Females < 12 months without a source of fever have UTI 8% of the time
- 0–8 weeks of age at higher risk of bacterial infection — especially 0–4 weeks of age
- Serious bacterial infection (SBI) can occur without fever
- Hypothermia during infection portends a higher risk
- Fever is not dangerous in of itself unless ≥ 105°F (40.6°C)
- Viruses are the most common cause of fever
- Treating fever has no effect on decreasing febrile seizures
- Otitis media by itself does not cause fever usually
- Pneumonia frequently has a normal pulmonary auscultatory exam

Evaluation

Children 3–36 months of age

- Complete history of fever, any prior treatments and associated symptoms
- Baseline dehydration assessment, see Pediatric Dehydration Protocol
- Assess interaction, feeding and alertness
- Nontoxic patients with viral source of fever may need no further evaluation
- CXR
    - O2 saturation < 95% on room air
    - Tachypnea or respiratory distress
    - WBC ≥ 15,000 with cough
- Fever ≥ 102°F (38.9°C) without source
    - CBC; Consider CXR
    - U/A in males < 6 months; uncircumcised male < 12 months; females < 24 months
    - Blood culture × 1 can be considered if WBC ≥ 15,000 or neutrophil count > 10,000
- Dehydration > 5% order BMP (See Pediatric Diarrhea Protocol for baseline dehydration assessment and treatment)
- Urinary complaints order U/A
- Decreased alertness or distress
    - CBC, chest x-ray, blood culture × 1, U/A, urine culture – discuss performance of a lumbar puncture with physician

Treatment Options

- Fever may be treated; if patient not uncomfortable, it may not need to be treated unless ≥ 104°F (40°C) Alternating Tylenol with ibuprofen not officially recommended and does not control fever any better than single antipyretic medication alone
- Fever ≥ 102°F (38.9°C) without a source and patient is nontoxic and feeding normally
    - Can be treated with Rocephin (ceftriaxone) 50 mg/kg IM
    - Can have no treatment, but needs close follow up within 12–24 hours

- Fever with a source in patient without toxicity or distress
  - Viral: treat symptoms
  - Suspected bacteria infection: appropriate antibiotic
  - May use Sanford Guide
- Fever with or without a source and patient toxic or in distress
  - Consult physician promptly

Discharge Criteria

- Healthy prior to fever onset
- No significant risk factors (prematurity or comorbid conditions)
- Nontoxic and healthy appearance
- Less than 5% dehydration (serum $CO_2 \geq 18$ if checked)
- Feeding well
- Reliable caregivers and access to follow-up
- WBC < 15,000 and patient appears well

Discharge instructions

- Pediatric fever aftercare instructions
- Return if patient becomes less active or appears worse
- Follow up with primary care provider in 2–3 days if fever persists

Consult Criteria

- Appears toxic, has poor alertness, decreased interaction or in distress
- Fever ≥ 104.5°F (40.3°C)
- Greater than 5% dehydration
- Poor feeding
- No source of fever
- Immunosuppression
- Splenectomy
- Seizure

Vital signs and age consult criteria

- Fever ≥ 104.5°F (40.3°C)

- Age < 90 days
- O_2 saturation < 95% on room air
- Pediatric heart rate
    - 0–4 months ≥ 180
    - 5–7 months ≥ 175
    - 6–12 months ≥ 170
    - 1–3 years ≥ 160
    - 4–5 years ≥ 145
    - 6–8 years ≥ 130
    - 7–12 years ≥ 125
    - 12–15 years ≥ 120
    - 16 years or older ≥ 115
    - Hypotension

Lab and x-ray consult criteria

- WBC ≥ 15,000 or < 3,000; absolute neutrophils < 1,000
- Bandemia ≥ 15%
- Acute thrombocytopenia
- New onset anemia
- Serum CO_2 < 18 mEq/L
- Metabolic acidosis
- Glucose ≥ 200 mg/dL
- Significant pneumonia
- Pleural effusion

Notes

BENIGN FEBRILE SEIZURE PROTOCOL

When using any protocol, always follow the Guidelines of Proper Use (page 16).

Definition

- A seizure event in infancy or childhood usually occurring between three months and five years of age, associated with fever, but without evidence of intracranial infection or other defined cause

Differential Diagnosis

- Meningitis
- Encephalitis
- Subdural and epidural infections
- Bacteremia and sepsis
- Epilepsy

Considerations

- Affects 2–4% of all children < 5 years of age
- Occurs in early childhood
- Usually occurs in children with systemic viral infection
- Majority last < several minutes
- Rate of serious infections are equivalent to febrile patients without seizures
- Increased rate of febrile seizures on day of DTP vaccination and 8–14 days after MMR vaccination
- Patients with febrile seizure have slightly higher rate of developing epilepsy
- No evidence that treatment with seizure medications decreases future febrile seizures
- No evidence of future cognitive differences in patients with febrile seizures
- Fever treatment does not alter developing febrile seizures
- Mild postictal phase usual
- Occurs in families to some extent

Types

Simple febrile seizure

- Lasts < 15 minutes
- Generalized
- Occurs only once in 24 hours

Complex febrile seizure

- Lasts > 15 minutes
- Focal features at any time
- Recurs within 24 hours

Evaluation

- Complete history and physical exam
- Serum glucose
- Routine labs usually not indicated
- Lab and x-rays if significant comorbid disease suspected (bacterial infection suspected)
- CT head for focal findings
- Lumbar puncture considered for age < 18 months for any of the following
    - History of irritability, decrease feeding, or lethargy
    - Abnormal appearance or mental status after postictal period
    - Signs of meningitis; severe headache
    - Complex febrile seizure
    - Slow postictal clearing of mentation
    - Pretreatment with antibiotics

Treatment Options

- No specific treatment for simple febrile seizure
- Reassure parents
- Treat any serious underlying cause of fever (see Pediatric Fever Protocol or other appropriate protocols)

Complex febrile seizures

- Intubation if airway not secure
- IV NS KVO
- Oxygen
- Lorazepam 0.05–0.1 mg/kg IV prn; may repeat q10–15 minutes prn (NMT 6 mg)

- Diastat (diazepam rectal gel) if no IV available
    - Age up to 5 years: 0.5 mg/kg
    - Age 6–11 years: 0.3 mg/kg
    - Age > 12 years: 0.2 mg/kg
    - Round up to available dose: 2.5, 5, 7.5, 10, 12.5, 15, 17.5, 20 mg/dose
- Midazolam IV/IM/PR/ET/intranasal 0.1–0.2 mg/kg/dose; not to exceed a cumulative dose of 10 mg)

Status epilepticus (beware of "too slow and too low" treatment)

- Lorazepam 0.1 mg/kg IV (NMT 10 mg total dose)
- Cerebyx (fosphenytoin) 15–20 mg/kg IV at 100 mg/minute if no response in 5 minutes to lorazepam or midazolam (Versed)
- Keppra (Levetiracetam) 20 mg/kg IV

Drugs that can be used if lorazepam, midazolam or Cerebyx (fosphenytoin) fail per physician

- Pentobarbital 1 mg/kg boluses IV to maximum 5 mg/kg per physician
- Valproic acid 15 mg/kg over 1–5 minutes (NMT 40 mg/kg)
    - 5 mg/kg/hr drip
- Phenobarbital 20 mg/kg IV at 100 mg/hr per physician

Management of refractory status epilepticus (consult physician immediately)

- Referral to an intensive care unit
- Anesthetic agents such as midazolam, propofol or barbiturates (thiopental, pentobarbital) for generalized convulsive status epilepticus
- Non-anesthetic anticonvulsants such as phenobarbital or valproic acid for nonconvulsive status epilepticus

Discharge Criteria

- Normal neurologic exam
- Simple febrile seizure

- Source of fever can be treated as an outpatient
- All seizures are to be discussed with physician prior to discharge
- Contact primary care physician or provider to alert of visit and arrange follow-up

Discharge instructions

- Benign febrile seizure aftercare instructions
- Return if seizure recurs
- Return if patient appears worse
- Close follow-up within 1 day preferable

Consult Criteria

- Discuss all seizures with physician
- Complex febrile seizure
- Suspected or diagnosed serious underlying infection
- Neurologic abnormality
- History of irritability
- Poor feeding
- Lethargy
- Abnormal appearance or mental status after postictal period
- Signs of meningitis
- Severe headache
- Slow postictal clearing of mentation
- Very recent or concurrent treatment with antibiotics
- Appears toxic, has poor alertness, decreased interaction or distress
- Greater than 5% dehydration
- No source of fever
- UTI — follow UTI Protocol

Vital signs and age consult criteria

- Age < 6 months
- Pediatric heart rate
    - 0–4 months ≥ 180
    - 5–7 months ≥ 175
    - 6–12 months ≥ 170
    - 1–3 years ≥ 160
    - 4–5 years ≥ 145

- Fever ≥ 104.5°F (40.3°C)
- Hypotension

Lab and x-ray consult criteria

- WBC ≥ 15,000 or < 3,000; absolute neutrophils < 1,000
- Bandemia ≥ 15%
- Thrombocytopenia
- New onset anemia
- Metabolic acidosis
- Glucose ≥ 200 mg/dL
- Hyperglycemia with metabolic acidosis (decreased serum CO_2 or elevated anion gap)
- Significant pneumonia
- Pleural effusion

Notes

CRYING INFANT PROTOCOL

When using any protocol, always follow the Guidelines of Proper Use (page 16).

Definition

- Crying child that presents without discernible cause of distress

Differential Diagnosis

- Otitis media is most common cause
- Infant colic
- Viral illness with anorexia
- Dehydration
- UTI
- Corneal abrasion
- Ocular foreign body
- Oropharynx foreign body
- Hair tourniquet syndrome (hair wrapped around toe or penis)
- Brown recluse spider bite
- Clavicle or tibial fracture
- Gastrointestinal prodrome
- GERD
- Intussusception
- DTP reaction
- PSVT
- Intracranial abnormality or infection
- Congenital cardiac disease (check for decreased femoral pulses)
- Child abuse (nonaccidental trauma)

Considerations

- Crying stimulated by
  - Unmet need: hunger; thirst; desire for attention
  - Distress: anger; discomfort; pain
- Healthy infants: crying levels increase from birth and peak at 6–8 weeks of life

- Crying follows circadian rhythm — clusters late afternoon or early evening
- Infants that won't stop crying in the exam area is more predictive of serious illness

Colic — recurrent paroxysmal attacks of crying lasting several hours

- Drawing up legs
- Abdomen may appear distended
- Bowel sounds increased
- Flatus may be passed

Colic rules of 3

- Lasting 3 or more hours
- Occurring 3 or more days per week
- Lasting minimum of 3 weeks
- No specific cause identified

Treatment options

- Short trial of hypoallergenic formula
- Stop cow's milk
- Treatments that are not effective
    - Simethicone
    - Lactase enzymes
    - Soy based formula
    - Fiber enriched foods
    - Carrying infant more
    - Care ride stimulators
    - Chiropractic manipulation

Evaluation

- History and physical exam reveals the majority of causes (71%)
- Consider rectal and genital exam if cause not evident
- Consider U/A
- Tests are aimed at suspected causes of excessive crying
- Evaluate for child abuse and order tests as indicated by exam and history

Treatment Options

- Observe for 1–2 hours to see if crying ceases
- Aimed at cause of crying

Discharge Criteria

- Patient stops crying in exam area
- Normal vital signs
- O2 saturation > 95%
- No serious illness detected
- Cause of crying determined to be benign and can be treated as outpatient
- Contact primary care physician or provider to alert of visit and arrange follow-up

Consult Criteria

- Patient will not stop crying
- O2 saturation ≤ 94%
    - Toxic appearance; poor interaction and activity
    - Greater than 5% dehydration — post rehydration
    - Poor response to treatment
    - Worrisome abdominal tenderness
    - Petechial rash
    - Altered mental status
    - Significant disease causation of crying

Vital signs consult criteria

- Pediatric heart rate
    - 0–4 months ≥ 180
    - 5–7 months ≥ 175
    - 6–12 months ≥ 170
    - 1–3 years ≥ 160
    - 4–5 years ≥ 145
- Hypotension

Lab consult criteria

- WBC ≥ 15,000 or < 3,000
- Bandemia ≥ 15%
- Thrombocytopenia
- Serum CO2 < 18 mEq/L post rehydration

- Initial serum CO_2 < 17 mEq/L

Notes

URI AND SINUSITIS PROTOCOL

When using any protocol, always follow the Guidelines of Proper Use (page 16).

Definition

- Infection of the nasopharynx, larynx, or sinuses

Differential Diagnosis

- Rhinitis
- Sinusitis
- Laryngitis
- Bronchitis
- Bronchiolitis
- Pneumonia
- Gastroesophageal reflux
- Candidiasis

Considerations

- Sinusitis (rhinosinusitis) is usually viral
- Viral sinusitis difficult to differentiate from bacterial sinusitis early in the course
- Children are 20–100 times more likely to have viral rhinosinusitis then bacterial sinusitis
- Viral rhinosinusitis
    - Congestion
    - Cough
    - Nasal discharge up to 14 days
- Acute bacterial sinusitis is associated with prolonged symptoms lasting more than 10–14 days
- Diagnosis of acute bacterial sinusitis should be made on clinical grounds
- CT scan may help in unclear cases. Plain films are rarely helpful
- Antibiotics should not be used to treat nonspecific URI symptoms in previously healthy patients
- Acute bacterial sinusitis does not require antibiotic treatment, especially if symptoms are mild or moderate

- Up to 75% of sinusitis resolves in 1 month without antibiotic treatment
- Severe or persistent moderate symptoms of bacterial sinusitis should receive antibiotic treatment
- Fever not common
- Acute invasive fungal rhinosinusitis
  - Can be caused by Candida, Aspergillus and Phycomycetes species — found in patients with:
    - Diabetes (especially with very high serum glucose levels)
    - Cancer
    - Hepatic disease
    - Renal failure
    - Other immunosuppressive conditions or diseases
- Sinusitis has same pathogens as otitis media

Signs of sinusitis

- Mucopurulent rhinorrhea
- Nasal congestion
- Facial pain, pressure or fullness
- Decreased sense of smell
- Severe headache, malaise, fever
- Pain exacerbation with head movement
- Retro-orbital pain (ethmoid sinus)
- Dental pain (maxillary sinus)
- Ear fullness

Evaluation

- Nasal exam
- Percussion of sinuses for tenderness
- Transillumination for frontal and maxillary sinus opacification
- CBC: severe sinusitis

CT scan indications

- Facial swelling
- Orbital or periorbital swelling
- Visual or mental status changes
- Consider for severe headache

Treatment Options

- Nasal saline for young children
- Antipyretic treatment prn
- Warm compresses to face prn
- Nasal steroids up to 15 days can be considered
- Mucolytics (guaifenesin) can be used to thin secretions — efficacy unknown

Antihistamines

- Without benefit
- Can worsen congestion and sinus pain by thickening of mucus and decreasing drainage
- Can use for allergic rhinosinusitis without bacterial infection

Antibiotics — for persistent moderate symptoms or severe symptoms and are the same as for otitis media

- Amoxicillin drug of choice
- Augmentin (amoxicillin/clavulanate)
- Omnicef (cefdinir)
- Macrolides
- May use Sanford guide

Discharge Criteria

- Uncomplicated rhinosinusitis
- Nontoxic

Discharge instructions

- URI and/or sinusitis aftercare instructions
- Follow up with primary care provider within 10–14 days if symptoms persist

Consult Criteria

- Toxic patients
- Abnormal vision
- Severe headache
- Altered mental status
- Facial swelling
- Vomiting

- Sphenoid sinusitis

Vital signs and age consult criteria

- Fever ≥ 103°F (39.4°C) if felt to be solely from sinusitis
- Age ≥ 80 or < 3 months
- Adult heart rate ≥ 110
- Pediatric heart rate
    - 0–4 months ≥ 180
    - 5–7 months ≥ 175
    - 6–12 months ≥ 170
    - 1–3 years ≥ 160
    - 4–5 years ≥ 145
    - 6–8 years ≥ 130
    - 7–12 years ≥ 125
    - 12–15 years ≥ 120
    - 16 years or older ≥ 115
- Hypotension
- O2 saturation < 95% on room air

Lab consult criteria

- WBC ≥ 15,000 or < 3,000
- Bandemia ≥ 15%
- Acute thrombocytopenia

Notes

OTITIS MEDIA PROTOCOL

When using any protocol, always follow the Guidelines of Proper Use (page 16).

Definition

- Infection of the middle ear with acute onset, presence of middle ear effusion, and signs of middle ear inflammation

Differential Diagnosis

- Bell's palsy
- Dental pain
- TMJ pain
- URI
- Mastoiditis
- Ear canal foreign body
- Barotitis media
- Herpes zoster
- Pharyngitis
- Sinusitis
- Serous otitis media

Considerations

- Viruses 35%; S. pneumoniae 25%; H. influenzea 23%; M. catarrhalis 15%; mixed bacteria 10%
- Most commonly occurs 6–36 months of age
- One-half of patients have fever
- Otitis media by itself should not be considered as the source of fever
- Usually associated with URI
- History can include: earache, irritability, rhinitis, GI symptoms, poor feeding, fever, pulling at ear
- Mild cases resolve without antibiotics 80% of the time within 1 week
- Fever is defined as rectal temperature > 38 °C or 100.4°F; Axillary temperature is unreliable

Treatment considerations

- Antibiotics increases resolution by another 13%

- 50% of patients will have residual middle ear fluid 1 month after antibiotic treatment so rechecking ears in 10–14 days may be unwarranted unless symptoms continue
- Antihistamines, decongestants, and steroids have no proven effectiveness
- High dose amoxicillin overcomes drug resistance
- Red TM's (tympanic membrane) can also be from fever and crying
- Pneumatic otoscopy most accurate method in diagnosing otitis media
- Otitis media with bulging TM's warrant immediate antibiotic treatment
- Otitis media without bulging TM's will likely clear spontaneously — can delay antibiotics 48–72 hours to see if spontaneous resolution of symptoms occurs
- Antibiotic treatment warranted for age < 6 months or older children > 36 months
- Mastoiditis is the same antibiotic treatment PO as otitis media

Evaluation

- Rectal temperature for age < 3 years unless patient cooperates with oral measurement to nurse's satisfaction
- Feeding, irritability, urine output and fever history
- CBC, chest x-ray, and U/A for fever ≥ 101°F (38.3°C) without a source (no URI symptoms for example)
- BMP for > 5% dehydration
- WBC ≥ 15,000 without a source for fever — get chest x-ray and one blood culture
- Obtain history of recent antibiotics treatment
- Evaluate for TM (tympanic membrane) perforation
- Complete H&P, including nuchal exam

Treatment Options

- Wait and see for 48–72 hours for symptom resolution for red TM's without bulging is acceptable for ages 6 months to 36 months
- Auralgan for otalgia in nonperforated TM (tympanic membrane) prn

Antibiotic options

- Amoxicillin 80 mg/kg divided TID for 7–10 days — preferred first line drug
- Augmentin (amoxicillin/clavulanate) 80 mg/kg divided TID for 7–10 days
- Zithromax (azithromycin) 10 mg/kg day 1, then 5 mg/kg qday for following 4 days
- Rocephin (ceftriaxone) 50 mg/kg IM × 1 dose (NMT 1,000 mg)
- Septra (trimethoprim/sulfamethoxazole) 0.4 mg/kg BID PO or 0.5 cc/LB BID PO for 7–10 days
- Cefuroxime 30 mg/kg BID for 7–10 days
- May use Sanford Guide

Discharge Criteria

- Uncomplicated otitis media

Discharge instructions

- Otitis media aftercare instructions
- Follow up with primary care provider in 7–10 days if symptoms persist

Consult Criteria

- Toxic patient
- Dehydration > 5 % who have not responded to ORT (see Pediatric Dehydration Protocol)
- Pneumonia
- Age < 3 months
- Fever of unknown etiology

Vital signs consult criteria

- Hypothermia < 95°F (35°C)
- Fever ≥ 104.5°F (40.3°C)
- Pediatric heart rate
  - 0–4 months ≥ 180
  - 5–7 months ≥ 175
  - 6–12 months ≥ 170
  - 1–3 years ≥ 160
  - 4–5 years ≥ 145
  - 6–8 years ≥ 130

- 7–12 years ≥ 125
- 12–15 years ≥ 120
- 16 years or older ≥ 110
- O2 saturation < 95% on room air

Lab consult criteria

- WBC ≥ 15,000 or < 3,000
- Bandemia ≥ 15%
- Acute thrombocytopenia

Notes

PEDIATRIC ASTHMA PROTOCOL

When using any protocol, always follow the Guidelines of Proper Use (page 16).

Definition

- Reversible acute bronchospasm and airway resistance secondary to infectious, allergic, environmental or internal stimuli

Differential Diagnosis

- Panic disorder
- Pneumonia
- Bronchitis
- Bronchiolitis
- Aspiration
- CHF
- COPD
- Anaphylaxis
- URI
- Vocal cord dysfunction
- Laryngospasm
- Epiglottitis
- Croup
- Retropharyngeal abscess

Considerations

- Cough is commonly the first symptom
- Viral URI or allergens or environmental stimuli most common causes of asthma
- Severe episode may have decreased breath sounds without wheezing
- Steroids very useful

Peak flow % of predicted (age > 5 yrs old)

- Mild asthma ≥ 70
- Moderate 40–69%
- Severe < 40%

Principles of Asthma Management

- Recognizing severity of exacerbation
- Using correct therapy
- Identify and treat any precipitants
- Make correct disposition

Evaluation

- Complete history and physical exam
- Assess respiratory effort
- Assess hydration status
- CBC and/or BMP for significant tachycardia and fever
- O2 saturation measurement
- Consider peak flows before and after aerosols for age 5 years or higher
- Check radiology interpretations if completed prior to discharge if chest x-ray performed

Chest x-ray if

- Pneumonia suspected
- Significant respiratory distress
- Respiratory distress not responsive to aerosols

Treatment Options

- Supplemental oxygen for O2 Sat < 95% on room air or significant respiratory distress
- Albuterol (with or without atrovent) aerosols up to 3 treatments total every 15–20 minutes prn

Additional treatment options if needed for severe exacerbations (notify physician promptly)

- Continuous Albuterol with or without atrovent and notify physician promptly
- Terbutaline 0.25 mg SQ prn q15–20 minutes up to 3 as needed for age ≥ 12 years
- Terbutaline 0.005–0.01 mg/kg SQ q15–20 minutes up to 3 — age < 12 years (NMT 0.4 mg per dose)
- Epinephrine 0.01 mg/kg in children not to exceed adult dose

- MgSO4 (magnesium sulfate) 25–50 mg/kg IV over 10–20 minutes per physician (NMT 2 gm) for children

Steroid treatment options useful for moderate to severe exacerbations (caution with diabetes)

Effectiveness starts around 6 hours after dosing

- Prednisolone 1 mg/kg PO

  OR

- Decadron (dexamethasone) 0.6 mg/kg IV or IM (NMT 10 mg)

Discharge treatment options

- Albuterol MDI with spacer prn at home
- Albuterol syrup per weight for patients unable to use MDI
- Antibiotics not needed usually
- If bacteria infection suspected, use Sanford Guide

Discharge systemic steroid treatment (caution if diabetic)

- Prednisolone or prednisone 1 mg/kg PO × 5 days (NMT 60 mg/dose)
- May give Decadron (dexamethasone) 0.6 mg/kg IM (NMT 10 mg) if PO route not usable

Discharge inhaled steroids

- Consider inhaled steroid Rx only after acute exacerbation has resolved
  - Prescribe double dose if already on single strength dose

    OR

  - Advair diskus bid – age > 3 years (combination of long acting beta-agonist and steroid) to be used only after acute exacerbation has resolved
    - Use 100/50 strength dose bid for age 4–11 years
    - Use adult strength for age ≥ 12 years

Discharge Criteria

- Good response to therapy
- Peak flow ≥ 70% predicted if checked (age 5 years or higher)
- O2 saturation ≥ 94% on room air
- < 5% dehydrated post ORT (oral rehydration therapy) if needed
- Good follow-up and compliance

Discharge instructions

- Follow up with primary care provider in 1–5 days depending on severity of illness and response to treatments
- Provide pediatric asthma aftercare instructions

Consult Criteria

- Insufficient response to treatment
- Work of breathing moderate to severe post Rx
- Wheezing not resolving adequately
- Patient or family of child feels patient is too dyspneic to go home
- Peak flow < 70% predicted if checked
- Moderate respiratory distress
- Age < 6 months
- > 5% dehydration post rehydration
- Poor feeding
- Unable to self-hydrate
- O2 saturation < 94% on room air post treatment
- Significant comorbid conditions
    - Pediatric heart rate
        - 0–4 months ≥ 180
        - 5–7 months ≥ 175
        - 6–12 months ≥ 170
        - 1–3 years ≥ 160
        - 4–5 years ≥ 145
        - 6–8 years ≥ 130
        - 7–12 years ≥ 125
        - 12–15 years ≥ 120
        - 16 years or older ≥ 110

Notes

BRONCHIOLITIS PROTOCOL

When using any protocol, always follow the Guidelines of Proper Use (page 16).

Definition

- Bronchiolitis is an acute infectious disease process of the lower respiratory tract that occurs primarily in young infants, most often in those aged 2–24 months, that may result in obstruction of small airways

Differential Diagnosis

- Asthma
- Pneumonia
- Bronchitis
- Congenital heart disease
- Aspiration
- Foreign body obstruction
- Congestive heart failure
- Bronchopulmonary dysplasia (prematurity history)

Considerations

- Age < 2 years usually
- Fall and spring peaks
- RSV usual cause
- Wheezing and tachypnea usually present
- Hypoxia not uncommon
- Variable response to bronchodilators
- Steroids not effective
- Dehydration and poor feeding not uncommon
- Fever usually low grade
- Rhinorrhea and cough
- Apnea more commonly seen in infants < 2 months of age or premature infants
- Hydration treatment helpful

Higher risk

- Prematurity
- Bronchopulmonary dysplasia history

- Cardiac history

Evaluation

- Complete history and physical
- O2 saturation measurement
- Work of breathing assessment
- Dehydration assessed
- Chest x-ray
- CBC and BMP if moderate to severe respiratory distress or > 5% dehydration
- RSV testing usually not needed
- RSV testing if admitted, history of prematurity or cardiopulmonary disease history

Treatment Options

- Supplemental O2 if O2 saturation < 93%
- Trial with Albuterol aerosol with or without atrovent – may repeat × 2 as needed
- Oral or IV hydration for dehydration. Refer to Pediatric Diarrhea Protocol
- No steroids unless history of asthma

Discharge Criteria

- Feeding well
- Absence of significant respiratory distress
- O2 saturation ≥ 94% on room air
- < 5% dehydrated post ORT (oral rehydration therapy) if given
- Good follow-up and compliance
- Contact primary care physician or provider to alert of ER visit and arrange follow-up

Discharge instructions

- Bronchiolitis aftercare instructions
- Follow up with primary care provider within 1–2 days
- Return if symptoms worsen
- Return if activity or feeding decreases

Consult Criteria

- Age < 6 months — discuss with physician
- Significant respiratory distress post treatment or respiratory rate > 60/minute
- O2 saturation < 94% on room air post treatment
- Family feels patient is too dyspneic to go home
- > 5% dehydration after any rehydration treatment
- Poor feeding
- Unable to self-hydrate
- Persistent vomiting
- History of apnea
- Significant comorbid conditions
- Toxic appearance
- Respiratory fatigue
- Hypotension
- Heart rate
  - 0–4 months ≥ 180
  - 5–7 months ≥ 175
  - 6–12 months ≥ 170
  - 1–3 years ≥ 160

Notes

CROUP PROTOCOL

When using any protocol, always follow the Guidelines of Proper Use (page 16).

Definition

- Infection of the upper respiratory tract (trachea) that is usually of a viral etiology and causes varying degrees of obstruction and is usually self-limited

Differential Diagnosis

- Epiglottitis
- Retropharyngeal abscess
- Foreign body in trachea
- Foreign body in esophagus
- Peritonsillar abscess
- Subglottic stenosis
- Tracheomalacia
- Vocal cord paralysis

Considerations

- Most common in 6 months to 6 years of age
- Peak is 2 years of age
- Parainfluenza virus most common, followed by RSV and Influenza
- Seal-like barking cough
- Stridor at rest indicates increased risk
- Can be life threatening
- Drooling may indicate epiglottis
- Lab tests usually not needed unless patient appears dehydrated or in significant distress; Defer blood tests when respiratory distress is present
- Imaging not required in mild cases that respond to treatment
- Neck AP & lateral for stridor at rest or significant respiratory distress
    - Consult physician before obtaining films if in significant distress
- Chest x-ray findings
    - Steeple sign indicative of croup on neck film

- Thumb or vallecula sign (loss of vallecula) indicative for epiglottitis
- Retropharyngeal swelling for abscess

Severity assessment

Mild severity

- Occasional barking cough
- No audible stridor at rest
- Either no or mild suprasternal or intercostal retractions

Moderate severity

- Frequent barking cough
- Easily audible stridor at rest
- Suprasternal and sternal retractions at rest, with little or no agitation

Severe severity

- Frequent barking cough
- Prominent inspiratory and occasionally expiratory stridor
- Marked sternal retractions
- Agitation and distress

Impending respiratory failure

- Barking cough (often not prominent)
- Audible rest stridor
- Sternal retractions may not be marked (fatigue)
- Lethargy or decreased mentation
- Often dusky appearance if no supplemental oxygen given

Evaluation

- Complete history and physical exam
- Patients can sit on parent's lap for exam
- O2 saturation measurement
- Assess respiratory effort and for respiratory distress
- Assess for dehydration
- BMP if > 5% dehydrated clinically

- CBC if toxic — hold blood draw if severe respiratory distress
- If drooling or in sniff position consult physician immediately
- Avoid actions that agitate patient

Imaging studies

- Not required in mild cases that respond to treatment
- Chest x-ray and soft tissue neck films in cases without adequate response to treatment or moderate or greater severity if clinical situation safely permits

Treatment Options

- Humidified oxygen if O2 saturation < 95%
- Racemic epinephrine if stridor at rest — observe for 2 hours for recurrence of stridor at rest
- Decadron (dexamethasone) 0.6 mg/kg IM (do not exceed 10 mg)

  OR
- Decadron (dexamethasone) 0.15–0.6 mg/kg PO (NMT 10 mg) or prednisolone 1–2 mg/kg PO (NMT 60 mg); Single dosing effective for mild to moderate croup
- Consider prednisolone 1–2 mg/kg PO × 5 days
- Avoid steroids in varicella (chickenpox)
- Cool mist vaporizer (or night air) may help
- Antibiotics rarely needed
- Follow up with primary care provider within 24 hours
- Check radiology interpretations prior to discharge if completed

Discharge Criteria

- Mild croup
- Moderate or severe croup with good response to therapy (discuss with physician)

Discharge instructions

- Croup aftercare instructions
- Refer to primary care provider or notify of visit and arrange follow-up

- Return if symptoms worsen

Consult Criteria

- Stridor at rest unresponsive to treatment
- Moderate to severe croup post treatment
- Notify physician promptly if severe severity assessment or impending respiratory failure
- Dehydration > 5% unresponsive to oral hydration
- Epiglottitis
- Pharyngeal area abscess
- Suspected foreign body
- O2 saturation ≤ 95% on room air after treatments
- Moderate to severe respiratory distress
- Depressed sensorium
- Poor oral intake
- Poor home situation

Vital signs consult criteria

- Pediatric heart rate
  - 0–4 months ≥ 180
  - 5–7 months ≥ 175
  - 6–12 months ≥ 170
  - 1–3 years ≥ 160
  - 4–5 years ≥ 145
  - 6–8 years ≥ 130
- Hypotension
- Age > 5 years

Lab consult criteria

- WBC ≥ 15,000 or < 3,000
- Acute thrombocytopenia
- Bandemia ≥ 15%
- Metabolic acidosis

Notes

PEDIATRIC DEHYDRATION AND GASTROENTERITIS PROTOCOL

When using any protocol, always follow the Guidelines of Proper Use (page 16).

Definition

- Acute inflammatory or infectious process of the stomach and intestines

Differential Diagnosis

- Colitis
- Appendicitis
- Cholecystitis
- Pancreatitis
- Peptic ulcer disease
- GERD
- Biliary colic
- Renal colic
- Bowel obstruction
- Inflammatory bowel disease
- Pyloric stenosis in infants
- Volvulus in infants
- Diabetic ketoacidosis

Considerations

- Degree (%) of acute weight loss indicates degree of dehydration
- Decreased serum CO2 and increased anion gap early indicators of dehydration
    - BUN and creatinine rise later
- Vomiting may occur in early gastroenteritis prior to diarrhea
- Vomiting by itself may indicate mechanical obstruction if without fever or diarrhea
- Vomiting with fever only may be from a UTI
- Viral infections are the usual etiology
- Antibiotics not usually indicated

  - Use Sanford guide prn
- Oral rehydration therapy (ORT) preferred over IV in mild to moderate dehydration

Dehydration assessment

Mild < 5%

- Alert
- Mucous membranes variable dry
- Skin turgor normal
- Fontanel flat
- Blood pressure normal
- Heart rate normal
- Capillary refill < 2 seconds
- Urine output decreased

Moderate 6–9%

- Irritable
- Mucous membranes dry
- Skin turgor variably reduced
- Fontanel depressed
- Blood pressure variably orthostatic
- Heart rate tachycardic
- Capillary refill 2–3 seconds
- Urine output decreased — oliguria

Severe ≥ 10%

- Lethargic
- Mucous membranes dry
- Skin turgor reduced
- Fontanel depressed
- Blood pressure orthostatic or hypotensive
- Heart rate markedly tachycardic
- Capillary refill ≥ 4 seconds
- Urine output decreased — oliguria/anuria

Evaluation

- Detailed history and PE
- Assess patient activity and interactions
- Perform baseline dehydration assessment
- BMP if appears moderate to severely dehydrated

- CBC if patient appears less active

  OR

  Pediatric heart rate
  - 0–4 months ≥ 180
  - 5–7 months ≥ 175
  - 6–12 months ≥ 170
  - 1–3 years ≥ 160
  - 4–5 years ≥ 145
  - 6–8 years ≥ 130
  - 7–12 years ≥ 125
  - 12–15 years ≥ 120
  - 16 years or older ≥ 115
- Check U/A if vomiting and fever only symptoms
- Consider imaging if obstruction suspected
- Stool studies prn

Treatment Options

- < 5% dehydration by weight (or serum CO2 > 18 mEq/L) small frequent feedings with pedialyte/rehydrate, etc. up to 24 hours
- Zofran (ondansetron) oral chewable tablet in ED for frequent vomiting
  - 2 mg for 8–15 kg; 4 mg for 14–30 kg; 8 mg for > 30 kg
  - Zofran (ondansetron) 2–4 doses can be prescribed for home if indicated

Oral Rehydration Therapy (ORT) for mild to moderate dehydration

- Oral rehydration formula (WHO formula, Rehydralyte or Pedialyte) for above vital signs; mild to moderate dehydration or serum CO2 14–18 mEq/L
  - 5 cc every 1–2 minutes for small children by caretaker for < 4 hours — start 20 minutes after Zofran (ondansetron) given
  - 5–10 cc every 1–2 minutes for larger children by caretaker for 1–4 hours
  - Hold ORT 10 minutes if vomiting occurs then resume

  - Reassess for urine production, weight gain, improved heart rate and alertness, and absence of severe vomiting
  - Recheck serum CO2 if initially < 17 mEq/L
  - Mild dehydration give 50 cc/kg in < 4 hours
  - Moderate dehydration give 50–100 cc/kg within 1–4 hours
- Severe dehydration give IV NS bolus 20 cc/kg; may repeat x 2

Exclusion criteria for Oral Rehydration Therapy

- Age < 6 months of age
- Hematemesis
- Bilious vomiting
- Bloody diarrhea
- VP shunt
- Head trauma
- Focal RLQ tenderness (possible appendicitis)
- Severe dehydration
- Patient vomits 3 or more times after starting ORT

IV therapy criteria and treatment for moderate to severe dehydration

- IV NS hydration for CO2 < 14 mEq/L
- ORT failure
- IV NS 20 cc/kg bolus, may repeat × 2
- Consult physician
- Up to 2 times maintenance IV with D5NS after any vigorous NS rehydration therapy is completed if patient is to be further observed (dextrose clears ketosis faster and decreases return visits)

Discharge Criteria

- Nontoxic patients with mild dehydration
- Patients responding to rehydration with significantly improved vital signs, normal alertness and interaction
- CO2 ≥ 18 mEq/L if rechecked
- Improved urine output in mild to moderate dehydration

Discharge instructions

- Pediatric dehydration, gastroenteritis, vomiting or diarrhea aftercare instructions
- Frequent small feedings of 10 cc of pedialyte or rehydrate every 10 minutes at home as needed for continued symptoms
- Resume regular diet (except milk initially) as soon as symptoms start resolving
    - May need to change to soy formula in infants
- Follow up with primary care provider within 1–2 days if symptoms not improving sufficiently at home

Consult Criteria

- Toxic appearance
- Greater than 5% dehydration post rehydration
- Poor response to treatment
- Worrisome abdominal tenderness
- Petechial rash
- Seizure

Vital signs consult criteria

- **Pediatric heart rate —** post rehydration therapy
    - 0–4 months ≥ 180
    - 5–7 months ≥ 175
    - 6–12 months ≥ 170
    - 1–3 years ≥ 160
    - 4–5 years ≥ 145
    - 6–8 years ≥ 130
    - 7–12 years ≥ 125
    - 12–15 years ≥ 120
    - 16 years or older ≥ 115
- Hypotension develops or orthostatic vital signs

Lab consult criteria

- Serum CO2 < 18 mEq/L post rehydration
- Initial serum CO2 < 17 mEq/L
- WBC ≥ 15,000 or < 3,000
- Bandemia ≥ 15%
- Acute thrombocytopenia

Notes

PEDIATRIC DIARRHEA PROTOCOL

When using any protocol, always follow the Guidelines of Proper Use (page 16).

Definition

- Increased fluid content of stool and frequency of bowel movements usually secondary to viral or bacterial infection

Differential Diagnosis

- Inflammatory bowel disease
- Irritable bowel syndrome
- Malabsorption syndromes

Considerations

- Degree (%) of acute weight loss indicates degree of dehydration
- Serum CO2 and increased anion gap early indicators of dehydration
- BUN and creatinine rise later
- Viruses 70–80% — Bacteria 10–20% — Parasites 5% — Use Sanford guide prn
- Can be from allergy, food intolerance, malabsorption or inflammatory causes.
- Oral rehydration therapy (ORT) preferred over IV in mild to moderate dehydration.

Dehydration assessment

Mild < 5%

- Alert
- Mucous membranes variable dry
- Skin turgor normal
- Fontanel flat
- Blood pressure normal
- Heart rate normal
- Capillary refill < 2 seconds
- Urine output decreased

Moderate 6–9%

- Irritable
- Mucous membranes dry
- Skin turgor variably reduced
- Fontanel depressed
- Blood pressure variably orthostatic
- Heart rate tachycardic
- Capillary refill 2–3 seconds
- Urine output — oliguria

Severe ≥ 10%

- Lethargic
- Mucous membranes dry
- Skin turgor reduced
- Fontanel depressed
- Blood pressure orthostatic or hypotensive
- Heart rate markedly tachycardic
- Capillary refill ≥ 4 seconds
- Urine output decreased — oliguria/anuria

Evaluation

- Detailed history and PE
- Assess patient activity/interaction
- Perform baseline dehydration assessment
- BMP for moderate to severe dehydration
- CBC and patient appears less active

    OR

    Pediatric heart rate is

    - 0–4 months ≥ 180
    - 5–7 months ≥ 175
    - 6–12 months ≥ 170
    - 1–3 years ≥ 160
    - 4–5 years ≥ 145
    - 6–8 years ≥ 130
    - 7–12 years ≥ 125
    - 12–15 years ≥ 120
    - 16 years or older ≥ 115
- Check U/A if vomiting and fever only symptoms
- Consider imaging if obstruction suspected
- Stool studies prn (consider rotavirus antigen)

Oral Rehydration Therapy (ORT) for Mild to Moderate Dehydration

- Oral rehydration formula (WHO formula, Rehydralyte or Pedialyte) for above vital signs; mild to moderate dehydration or serum CO2 14–18 mEq/L
  - 5 cc every 1–2 minutes for small children by caretaker for < 4 hours
  - 5–10 cc every 1–2 minutes for larger children by caretaker for 1–4 hours
  - Hold ORT 10 minutes if vomiting occurs then resume
  - Reassess for urine production, weight gain, improved heart rate and alertness, and absence of severe vomiting
  - Recheck serum CO2 if initially < 17 mEq/L
  - Mild dehydration give 50 cc/kg in < 4 hours
  - Moderate dehydration give 50–100 cc/kg within 1–4 hours

Severe dehydration give IV NS bolus 20 cc/kg; may repeat × 2 prn

Exclusion criteria for Oral Rehydration Therapy

- Age < 6 months of age
- Hematemesis
- Bilious vomiting
- Bloody diarrhea
- VP shunt
- Head trauma
- Focal RLQ tenderness (possible appendicitis)
- Severe dehydration
- Patient vomits 3 or more times after starting ORT

IV Therapy Criteria and Treatment for Moderate to Severe Dehydration

- IV NS hydration for CO2 < 14 mEq/L
- ORT failure
- IV NS 20 cc/kg bolus, may repeat × 2 prn
- Consult physician

- Maintenance IV with D5NS (Dextrose decreases return visits)

Discharge Criteria

- Nontoxic patients with mild dehydration.
- Patients responding to rehydration with significantly improved vital signs, normal alertness and interaction
- CO2 ≥ 18 mEq/L, with weight gain and improved urine output in mild to moderate dehydration

Discharge instructions

- Pediatric dehydration or diarrhea aftercare instructions
- Frequent small feedings of 10 cc of pedialyte or rehydrate every 10 minutes at home as needed for continued symptoms
- Resume regular diet (except milk initially) as soon as symptoms start resolving
    - May need to change to soy formula in infants
- Follow up with primary care provider within 1–2 days if symptoms not improving sufficiently at home

Consult Criteria

- Toxic appearance
- Greater than 5% dehydration post rehydration
- Poor response to treatment
- Worrisome abdominal tenderness
- Petechial rash
- More than 1 visit for same episode of diarrhea

Vital signs consult criteria

- **Pediatric heart rate** — post rehydration therapy
    - 0–4 months ≥ 180
    - 5–7 months ≥ 175
    - 6–12 months ≥ 170
    - 1–3 years ≥ 160
    - 4–5 years ≥ 145
    - 6–8 years ≥ 130
    - 7–12 years ≥ 125
    - 12–15 years ≥ 120

    - 16 years or older ≥ 115
- Hypotension develops or orthostatic vital signs

Lab consult criteria

- Serum CO_2 < 18 mEq/L post rehydration
- Initial serum CO_2 < 17 mEq/L
- WBC ≥ 15,000 or < 3,000
- Bandemia ≥ 15%
- Acute thrombocytopenia

Notes

Geriatrics

Section Contents — one protocol

Geriatrics Protocol

When using any protocol, always follow the Guidelines of Proper Use (page 16).

GERIATRICS PROTOCOL

When using any protocol, always follow the Guidelines of Proper Use (page 16).

Basic Ethical Principles

- Beneficence – act in the patient's best interest
- Autonomy – treatment guided by patient's wishes
- Family responsibility – plays a central role in care of the geriatric patient
- Advance directives – follow wishes of patient and family in care

General Considerations of Elderly

- Live in high density environments
- May have poor nutritional status
- May have altered immune function
- Have multiple medical problems
- Take multiple medications
- May delay seeking medical consultation
- Subtle alterations in appearance or behavior may be only indication of serious infections

Pharmacology in the Elderly

Risk factors for adverse drug reactions

- Advanced age and living alone
- Female gender
- Chronic use of medications
- Polypharmacy
- Institutionalization
- Multiple medical problems (especially hepatic or renal insufficiency)

Adverse drug presentations

Confusion

- Anticholinergics
- Antihistamines
- Antidepressants
- Antihypertensives

- Antipsychotics
- Narcotics
- Sedatives
- Digoxin (digitalis)
- Steroids
- NSAID's
- Diuretics

Dementia

- Antihistamines
- Phenothiazines
- Tricyclic antidepressants

Depression

- Sedatives
- Beta–blockers
- Steroids
- Oral diabetic medications
- Ethanol
- NSAID's
- Narcotics

General weakness

- Digoxin (digitalis)
- Diuretics

Nausea

- Digoxin (digitalis)
- Theophylline
- Macrolide antibiotics (erythromycin)
- Iron
- Narcotics
- Steroids
- L-dopa
- ASA

Postural hypotension

- Angina medications
- Hypertension drugs
- Antidepressants
- Antihistamines

- Sedatives
- Beta–blockers

Renal insufficiency
- Digoxin (digitalis)
- Diuretics

Syncope/presyncope
- Cardiac drugs
- Hypertension drugs

Urinary incontinence
- Antipsychotics
- Diuretics
- Beta–blockers
- Medications causing fecal impaction
- Sedatives

Urinary retention
- Anticholinergics
- Antihistamines (especially in elderly men with BPH)

Hallucinations
- Anticholinergics

Drugs causing falls
- Antidepressants
- Antihistamines
- Antipsychotics
- Sedatives
- Nitroglycerin

Principles of safe medication usage
- Consider medications as a potential cause for presentation for medical care
- Educate patient about potential adverse reactions
- Obtain drug levels or monitoring tests of medications where appropriate
- Determine compliance and noncompliance of drug use

- Exercise care in prescribing medications that may have an adverse reaction to drugs the patient is currently taking
- Keep refills and number of pills small if appropriate
- Start low and go slow with dosing

Common Lab Findings in Elderly

- Frequently normal
- Fasting blood glucose: 135–150 mg/dL
- Normal creatinine with evidence of decreased creatinine clearance
- Higher ESR – up to 40 mm/hr
- Hemoglobin – women 11 gm/dl; men 11.5 gm/dl
- BUN – up to 28–35 mg/dL

Delirium in the Elderly

- Acute organic brain syndrome manifested by impaired thinking, confusion, deficits in attention, fluctuating course, impaired speech and other symptoms and signs of impaired cognition

Causes of delirium

Medications and substances

- Ethanol
- Anticholinergics
- Antihistamines
- Sedatives
- Narcotics
- Antidepressants
- Lithium
- Neuroleptics
- Tagamet (cimetidine)

Withdrawal

- Ethanol
- Benzodiazepines
- Narcotics

Metabolic

- Electrolyte abnormalities (Na and Ca)

- Hypoglycemia and hyperglycemia
- Acid-base disturbance
- Dehydration
- Hypoxia
- End organ insufficiency – liver, kidney and lungs
- Vitamin deficiency — thiamine, folate
- Fever or hypothermia

Infectious

- Urinary tract infection
- Encephalitis or meningitis
- Pneumonia
- Sepsis
- Influenza

Neurologic

- Brain tumor
- Subdural hematoma
- Intracerebral hemorrhage
- Seizure disorder
- CVA

Endocrine

- Hyperthyroidism
- Hypothyroidism
- Parathyroid — hyper and hypoparathyroidism

Cardiovascular

- Congestive heart failure
- Arrhythmia
- Acute myocardial infarction

Conditions that mimic delirium

- Dementia
- Depression
- Schizophrenia
- Mania
- Wernicke's aphasia

Evaluation of delirium

- CBC
- BMP
- LFT's
- U/A
- Chest x-ray
- EKG

Ordered as indicated

- Drug levels
- Thyroid studies
- Urine drug screen
- Blood alcohol
- Blood cultures
- CT brain scan
- Lumbar puncture for CSF analysis
- Urine culture

Treatment of delirium

- Treat underlying illness
- Restore any fluid or electrolyte imbalances
- Discontinue unnecessary medication that is contributing to delirium (discuss with physician)

Consult criteria for delirium

- Discuss all cases with physician
- Physician should examine all delirium or acute altered mental status patients

Temporal Arteritis

- True emergency of the elderly
    - Age of onset 50–70 years of age
    - Six times more common in females than in males
- Headache localized over eye or to scalp
- Fever, malaise and weight loss are associated symptoms
- Jaw claudication is important associated symptom
- Frequently associated with polymyalgia rheumatica (joint and muscles aches)
- ESR 50–100

- C-reactive protein elevated usually
- Vision loss can occur early in course of disease

Treatment

- Prednisone 40–80 mg PO qday or divided bid for several months to one year

Disposition

- Minimal symptoms can be treated as outpatient
- Severe symptoms or question of eye involvement should be admitted with IV high dose steroid treatment and ophthalmology consultation obtained

Discharge instructions

- Temporal arteritis aftercare instructions
- Follow up with PCP within 1 day
- Return for visual changes

Consult criteria

- Discuss all temporal arteritis cases with physician

Falls in Elderly

Causes

- Environmental or accidental: 30–50% of patients
- Gait, balance, weakness or deconditioning: 10–25% of patients
- Sensation of dizziness: 5–20% of patients
- Syncope: 2–10% of patients
- Orthostatic hypotension: 2–15% of patients
- Drop attacks: 1–10% of patients
- Other: 1–10% of patients

Physical examination

- Orthostatic blood pressures
    - Postural blood pressure changes can occur after standing for 10 minutes and so blood pressure should be checked again at 10–15 minutes if low orthostatic blood pressure is suspected as cause of the fall

- Core body temperature
- Skin for evidence of trauma, pallor
- HEENT for vision loss, hearing deficits, cranial nerve deficits, nystagmus
- Neck for carotid bruit, meningeal signs
- Chest auscultation for rales
- Heart for aortic stenosis murmur, arrhythmias
- Extremities for fractures, motion limitations, DJD findings
- Neurologic for altered mental status, focal neurologic deficits, loss of position sense

Lab and x-ray evaluation options as indicated

- CBC
- BMP
- Chest x-ray
- X-ray of injured areas
- U/A
- UDS and blood alcohol
- EKG
- Medication levels
- CT brain scan

Discharge criteria

- Cause of fall benign and no serious injury
- Good social and home support systems if needed

Consult criteria

- Cause of fall requires admission
- New medical condition causing fall
- Significant abnormal lab or imaging study
- Fracture
- See General Patient Criteria Protocol (page 20)

Notes

Gynecology

Section Contents

Vaginal Bleeding Protocol

Pelvic Pain Protocol

Pregnancy Complications Protocol

When using any protocol, always follow the Guidelines of Proper Use (page 16).

VAGINAL BLEEDING PROTOCOL

When using any protocol, always follow the Guidelines of Proper Use (page 16).

Definition

- Abnormal vaginal bleeding

Differential Diagnosis

- Dysfunctional uterine bleeding (anovulatory bleeding)
- Spontaneous abortion
- Threatened abortion
- Uterine fibroids
- Cervical and endometrial polyps
- Pelvic tumors
- Atrophic endometrium (postmenopausal)
- Systemic disorders
- Hypothyroidism

Considerations

- See Pregnancy Complications Protocol if pregnant
- Usually from a benign etiology
- Rule out pregnancy — negative menstrual and sexual histories do not rule out pregnancy
- Causes besides pregnancy need evaluation
- Average tampon holds 5–15cc of blood; average pad holds 15–30 cc of blood
- Postmenopausal vaginal bleeding needs to be evaluated for cancer

Evaluation Options

- Gestational history
- Last normal menstrual period noted
- Current medications (anticoagulants, hormones)
- Pelvic exam (delay for pregnancy > 20 weeks)
- CBC if tachycardia or hypotension present, or worrisome history for significant hemorrhage
- UCG
- Serum quantitative HCG if known to be pregnant

- Rh type if pregnant
- Type and screen if tachycardic
- PT/PTT/INR if indicated
- Type and cross match if hypotensive and notify physician promptly

Estimated Blood and Fluid losses (adults)

	Class I	Class II	Class III	Class IV
Blood loss (cc)	Up to 750	750–1000	1500–2000	> 2000
Blood loss %	Up to 15%	15–30%	30–40%	> 40%
Pulse rate	< 100	> 100	> 120	> 140
Blood pressure	Normal	Normal	SBP < 90	SBP < 70
Capillary refill	Normal	Normal	Delayed	Absent
Pulse pressure	Normal/incr	Decreased	Decreased	Decreased
Respiratory rate	14–20	20–30	30–40	> 35
Urine output (cc/hr)	> 30	20–30	5–15	Negligible
Mental status	Anxious	Anxious	Confused	Lethargic

(Derived from Advanced Trauma Life Support)

Treatment Options

Dysfunctional uterine bleeding (DUB) with stable vital signs

- Estrogen 2.5 mg PO QID: add provera 10 mg qday for 7-10 days when bleeding subsides
- Combination oral contraceptives
    - Nortrel 1/35 one PO bid × 7 days until bleeding stops, then 1 PO qday × 2 weeks
- Provera 10 mg PO qday × 10 days
    - Bleeding will resume when hormone therapy is finished
- NSAID's can be used to decrease bleeding and pain

IV NS 500cc bolus

- If heart rate ≥ 120
- If SBP < 90
- If SBP < 105 and heart rate ≥ 110 with history of hypertension
- Notify physician promptly

Discharge Criteria

- Pregnancy — see Pregnancy Complications Protocol
- Benign vaginal bleeding such as DUB or irregular menses with heart rate ≤ 100, SBP > 90, and SBP ≥ 105 in patients with hypertension history

Discharge instructions

- Vaginal bleeding aftercare instructions
- Referral to OB/GYN within 1–10 days depending on severity of symptoms

Consult Criteria

- Pregnancy — see Pregnancy Complications Protocol
- Ectopic pregnancy or possible ectopic pregnancy
- Fever
- Severe abdominal or pelvic pain
- Purulent vaginal discharge
- Continued heavy vaginal bleeding
- Return visit for same vaginal bleeding episode
- Postmenopausal vaginal bleeding

Vital signs and age consult criteria

- Age ≥ 55
- SBP < 90 or relative hypotension (SBP < 105 with history of hypertension)
- Adult heart rate > 100
- Orthostatic vital signs

Lab consult criteria

- Hemoglobin decrease > 1 gm
- Hemoglobin < 10 gms
- WBC ≥ 15,000
- Bandemia ≥ 15%
- Increased anion gap or metabolic acidosis
- Thrombocytopenia
- Elevated coagulation studies
- Creatinine increase > 0.5 from baseline
- Elevated LFT's

Notes

PELVIC PAIN PROTOCOL

When using any protocol, always follow the Guidelines of Proper Use (page 16).

Definition

- Female pelvic pain

Differential Diagnosis

- Pelvic inflammatory disease (PID)
- Ectopic pregnancy
- Normal pregnancy
- Ovarian cyst
- Endometriosis
- Ovarian torsion
- Uterine fibroids
- Chronic pelvic pain syndrome
- UTI
- Renal colic

Considerations

- Must be differentiated from GI or urologic causes of pain
- Bilateral tubal ligation does not always prevent pregnancies — order UCG on all BTL patients that would be fertile otherwise

Evaluation

- Pelvic and abdominal exam
- UCG on fertile females
- U/A
- CBC for
    - Fever
    - Tachycardia
    - Hypotension
    - Moderate to severe pain
- BMP for
    - Dehydration
    - Tachycardia

    - Hypotension
    - Diabetes
- C-reactive protein may be helpful for inflammatory disease or PID

Pelvic ultrasound when
- Pregnant
- Suspected ovarian torsion
- Suspected ruptured ovarian cyst with tachycardia
- Suspected tubo-ovarian abscess (TOA)

Pelvic Inflammatory Disease (PID)

Definition
- Spectrum of the female genital tract infection to include uterus, tubes, ovaries and peritoneum

Differential diagnosis
- Ectopic pregnancy
- Normal pregnancy
- Ovarian cyst
- Endometriosis
- Ovarian torsion
- Uterine fibroids
- Chronic pelvic pain syndrome
- UTI
- Renal colic

Considerations
- Common in females of reproductive age
- Gonorrhea and chlamydia are most common causes
- Important to treat sexual partners
- Can lead to tubo-ovarian abscess

Symptoms and findings
- Can cause peritonitis
- Usually bilateral pelvic pain and tenderness
- Associated with vaginal discharge frequently
- Dyspareunia
- Cervical motion tenderness usually bilateral

- Fever and chills
- Nausea and vomiting

Evaluation

- Pelvic and abdominal exam
- CBC
- UCG (unless hysterectomy history)
- U/A
- Consider RPR
- Consider C-reactive protein
- LFT's if right upper quadrant tenderness for Fitz-Hugh-Curtis syndrome
- Cultures for gonorrhea and chlamydia; wet prep
- Consider pelvic ultrasound if TOA suspected
- CT abdominal/pelvis scan if appendicitis suspected

Treatment options

Outpatient

- Rocephin (ceftriaxone) 250 mg IM

  +

- Doxycycline 100 mg PO BID × 14 days

  +

- Flagyl (metronidazole) 500 mg PO BID × 14 days (avoid ethanol)
- Treatment for sexual partners or refer for treatment for STD
- NSAID's and/or narcotics prn
- Phenergan (promethazine) prn
- May use Sanford Guide
- Follow CDC recommendations

Inpatient

- Cefotetan 2 gms IV

  +

- Doxycycline 100 mg IV
- Consult physician

Discharge criteria

- Mild to moderate pain
- Does not meet consult criteria

Discharge instructions

- PID aftercare instructions
- Follow up in 3 days to monitor treatment effectiveness
- Return if pain or fever worsens

Consult criteria

- Uncertain diagnosis or toxic appearance
- Suspected pelvic abscess
- Fitz-Hugh-Curtis syndrome (RUQ tenderness and elevated LFT's)
- Pregnancy
- Severe illness (severe pain and vomiting)
- Unable to tolerate PO intake
- Immunodeficiency
- Failure of outpatient therapy
- Return visit for same acute complaint
- Likely noncompliance with outpatient treatment
- Poor follow-up

Ovarian Cysts

Definition

- Fluid filled sac in ovary

Differential diagnosis

- PID
- UTI
- Ovarian torsion
- Appendicitis
- Diverticulitis
- Endometriosis
- Inflammatory bowel disease
- Ovarian cancer

Considerations

- Most asymptomatic and benign
- Cysts < 5 cm usually resolve
- Cysts > 5 cm need referral and follow-up

Evaluation

- Pelvic and abdominal exam
- UCG
- U/A
- CBC for
    - Fever
    - Tachycardia
    - Hypotension
    - Moderate to severe pain
- BMP for
    - Dehydration
    - Tachycardia
    - Hypotension
    - Diabetes

Treatment options

- Pain control if not hypotensive
- Notify physician promptly for bleeding from hemorrhagic cysts or signs of hemorrhagic volume loss
    - Heart rate ≥ 110; SBP < 90; orthostatic vital signs or hypotension
        - IV NS 500–1000 cc bolus prn
- Severe pain order pelvic ultrasound

Discharge criteria

- Simple ovarian cysts
- Stable vital signs

Discharge instructions

- Ovarian cyst aftercare instructions
- Return if pain worsens or dizziness develops

Consult criteria

- Severe pain
- Fever
- Heart rate ≥ 110; SBP < 90; orthostatic vital signs or hypotension

Endometriosis

Definition

- Endometriosis is the presence of endometrial-like tissue outside the uterine cavity, which induces a chronic inflammatory reaction

Differential diagnosis

- Appendicitis
- Ectopic pregnancy
- Diverticulitis
- Inflammatory bowel disease
- UTI
- PID
- Ovarian cysts
- Ovarian torsion
- Primary dysmenorrhea

Considerations

- Dysmenorrhea
- Heavy or irregular vaginal bleeding
- Pelvic, lower abdominal and lower back pain
- 15% of all pelvic pain
- Similar evaluation as ovarian cyst if diagnosis in doubt
- UCG if fertile

Treatment options

- Pain control with NSAID's and/or narcotics
- Provera 10–20 mg qday
- Ortho-Cyclen for one month

Discharge criteria

- Pain controlled
- Stable vital signs

Discharge instructions

- Endometriosis aftercare instructions
- Follow up with primary care provider or gynecologist within 7 days if possible

Consult physician if diagnosis uncertain

- Heart rate ≥ 110
- Orthostatic vital signs
- Fever
- Severe pain

Ectopic Pregnancy

Definition

- Pregnancy outside of uterus

Differential diagnosis

- Threatened abortion
- Inevitable abortion
- Incomplete abortion
- Missed abortion
- Appendicitis
- Diverticulitis
- Inflammatory bowel disease
- UTI
- PID
- Ovarian cysts
- Ovarian torsion
- Primary dysmenorrhea

Evaluation

- Pelvic and abdominal exam
- Rh type
- CBC
- BMP
- Pelvic ultrasound
- Type and screen if vital signs stable
- Type and cross for 2 units PRBC's if hypotensive

Treatment options

- Notify physician promptly
- Notify physician if ectopic pregnancy is possible consideration

IV NS 500–1000 cc bolus

- Heart rate ≥ 115 and rupture suspected

- Orthostatic vital signs
- Hypotension

Pelvic Pain Consult Criteria

- Dehydration
- Significant blood loss
- Ectopic pregnancy or possible ectopic pregnancy
- Suspected or diagnosed appendicitis or diverticulitis
- Acute surgical abdomen
- Moderate to severe pain of uncertain cause
- Severe pain with any diagnosis
- Return ED visit within 14 days for same acute pelvic pain complaint
- Elevated LFT's
- Any of the above subtopics consult criteria

Vital signs consult criteria

- Pelvic pain that develops hypotension or relative hypotension (SBP < 105 with history of hypertension)
- Heart rate ≥ 110

Lab consult criteria

- WBC > 15,000 or < 3,000
- Bandemia ≥ 15%
- Significant electrolyte abnormally
- Glucose ≥ 400 mg/dL in diabetic patient
- Glucose ≥ 300 mg/dL in non-diabetic patient
- Hyperglycemia with metabolic acidosis (decreased serum CO2 or elevated anion gap)
- Worsening anemia; decrease > 1 gm hemoglobin
- Metabolic acidosis

Notes

PREGNANCY COMPLICATIONS PROTOCOL

When using any protocol, always follow the Guidelines of Proper Use (page 16).

Definition

- Processes that interfere with a normal intrauterine pregnancy (IUP) progression

Differential Diagnosis

- Threatened abortion — closed cervical os, benign exam and no tissue passed
- Inevitable abortion — open cervical os
- Incomplete abortion — partial passage of products of conception (POC)
- Missed abortion — fetal death < 20 weeks without passage of POC
- Septic abortion — infection with pain, fever or foul smelling/purulent discharge
- Preeclampsia — IUP > 20 weeks gestation with hypertension, proteinuria and frequently edema
- Eclampsia — preeclampsia with seizures or altered mental status
- Hypertension is 140/90 or rise of SBP 20 and DBP 10 over prepregnancy levels
- HELLP — hemolysis; elevated liver enzymes; low platelets
- Ectopic pregnancy — occurs 1.6% of all pregnancies

Considerations

- Bleeding occurs in 20–30% of pregnancies in first 20 weeks (50% will have eventual spontaneous abortion)
- Late pregnancy (last 20 weeks) bleeding occurs 3–5%
- 11.5% are pregnant who say it is not possible to be pregnant
- 7.5% pregnant with normal LMP

General Evaluation

- History of LNMP, amount of bleeding, any POC passed
- CBC
- Serum quantitative HCG
- U/A
- Fetal heart tones – usually 120–160/minute (dependent on gestational age)
- Rh type (if there is vaginal bleeding history or findings)
- Ultrasound (usually)
- LFT's if preeclampsia/eclampsia present
- BMP if vomiting and tachycardia present
- Type and screen for significant bleeding or tachycardia
- Type and cross for 2 units PRBC's if hypotensive
- Pelvic and abdominal exam
- Complete physical examination
- Defer pelvic exam last 20 weeks of gestation if bleeding

Ectopic pregnancy

- Occurs 1.6% of pregnancies
- Missed > 40% on first visit
- 90% with pain and 50–80% with bleeding
- 30% atypical presentations
- Normal pelvic exam does not rule out ectopic
- Falling B-HCG does not exclude ectopic pregnancy
- B-HCG normally double every 2 days when < 10,000 mIU/ml with normal pregnancy
- No IUP on ultrasound is suspicious for ectopic pregnancy

Preeclampsia and eclampsia

- IUP > 20 weeks gestation with hypertension and proteinuria
- Can occur up to 4–6 weeks postpartum
- Frequently with pedal and hand edema
- Gestational hypertension is not associated with proteinuria
- Notify physician

Risk factors for preeclampsia or eclampsia

- Advanced maternal age > 35 years or young maternal age < 20 years
- Substance abuse
- PID
- Prior C-section or ectopic pregnancy
- Prior preeclampsia history
- Hypertension
- Trauma
- Multiple gestation
- Molar pregnancy
- Diabetes
- Smoking

Severe Preeclampsia

- SBP > 160 or DBP > 110
- RUQ/epigastric pain
- Hyperreflexia
- Thrombocytopenia
- Severe headache
- Eclampsia
- Dyspnea
- Elevated PT and PTT
- Visual changes
- Papilledema

Eclampsia

- Preeclampsia with seizures or altered mental status

Evaluation

- Cardiac monitoring
- CBC
- U/A
- LFT's
- BMP
- PT and PTT
- DIC panel
- Uric acid (is elevated early)

Treatment options

- Delivery is definitive treatment
- Blood pressure goal of SBP 140–155 mm Hg and DBP 90–100 mm Hg
    - Hydralazine 5–10 mg IV may repeat Q20min prn (NMT 60 mg)
    - Labetalol 50–100 mg IV q30 min prn (NMT 300 mg)

Seizure prophylaxis

- Magnesium sulfate 4–6 gms IV over 20 minutes followed by drip of 1–2 gms IV/hr
    - Stop MgSO4 (magnesium sulfate)
        - If DTR's are lost
        - For respiratory depression (calcium gluconate 1 gm IV over 10 minutes if needed to reverse magnesium toxicity)
    - Monitor magnesium levels
    - Caution if renal failure is present

Active seizures

- Give magnesium sulfate 4 gms IV over 5–10 minutes — followed by magnesium drip of 1–2 gms IV per hour
- Dilantin or Ativan can be used for magnesium sulfate failure (see Adult Seizure Protocol)

Placenta abruption

- Separation of a normally positioned placenta after 20 weeks of gestation and before birth

Signs and symptoms

- Painful vaginal bleeding 80% (dark red commonly)
    - No vaginal bleeding 20%
- Abdominal tenderness 70%
- Uterine tenderness 70%
- Uterus has frequent and hypertonic contractions 35%

- Shock out of proportion to estimated blood loss
- Fetal distress
- Premature labor
- Fetal death 15 %

Risk factors for placenta abruption

- Previous abruption
- Hypertension — most common cause
- Diabetes
- Chronic renal disease
- Abdominal trauma
- Preeclampsia
- Advance maternal age
- Cocaine use
- Cigarette smoking
- Alcohol use

Evaluation

- CBC
- BMP
- LFT's
- DIC panel
- Type and screen if not in shock
- Type and cross 4 units PRBC's if class 2 or greater hemorrhage (see Bleeding Protocol)
- Transabdominal ultrasound may or may not help
- Continuous fetal monitoring if available

Treatment

- 2 large bore IV's of NS
- If class 2 hemorrhage or greater give 1–2 liter NS bolus
- See Bleeding Protocol as needed

Consult criteria

- Notify physician and obstetrician promptly

Placenta previa

- Implantation of the placenta near or over the cervical os

- Occurs in the second and third trimesters of pregnancy
- Common cause of pregnancy bleeding

Signs and symptoms

- Painless bright red vaginal bleeding
- Fetal heart tones may be normal
- Bleeding may be intermittent
- Shock can occur

Evaluation

- **Do not** perform vaginal or rectal exam (may provoke increased bleeding)
- CBC
- Type and screen
- Serum quantitative HCG
- DIC panel
- Bedside transabdominal ultrasound
- Transabdominal or transvaginal ultrasound in radiology if vital signs stable and bleeding amounts judged not to be dangerous
- Continuous fetal monitoring if available

Consult criteria

- Consult physician and obstetrics

UTI

- **Treat all asymptomatic** and simple cystitis urinary tract infections for 7–10 days
    - Increased incidence of premature rupture of membranes and fetal death if not treated
- Send urine for culture
- No trimethoprim first trimester or sulfa antibiotic last trimester
- Consult for admission on all pyelonephritis patients that are pregnant

Bacterial vaginosis

- Most common cause of vaginal discharge
- Gardnerella vaginalis replaces normal flora

- Risk of preterm labor, premature rupture of membranes and postpartum endometritis if not treated

Criteria – has 3 of 4

- Profuse thin white discharge
- Fishy odor
- pH > 4.5
- Clue cells

Treatment

- All pregnant patients
- All symptomatic nonpregnant patients

Antibiotics

- Metronidazole options (avoid 1st trimester)
  - 250 mg PO tid × 7 days
  - Gel 0.75% 5 gm intravaginally qday × 5 days
- Clindamycin 300 mg PO bid × 7 days

Treatment Options

- Rhogam 300 microunits IM if Rh negative and vaginal bleeding has or is occurring
- IV D5NS rehydration as needed for vomiting of pregnancy (D5 decreases ketosis); No infusion with D5NS > 300 cc/hr
- IV NS bolus and drip for hemorrhagic compromise (notify physician promptly)
  - No more than 2 liters NS before starting blood transfusion and FFP if possible
  - Give blood:FFP at 1:1 or 2:1 ratio
  - Improved mortality when FFP added
- Phenergan (promethazine) 6.25 mg IV (25–50 mg IM or PO) or Zofran (ondansetron) 4 mg IV or Reglan 10 mg IV prn
- Narcotics prn (Category B, or C if commonly used in pregnancy)
- Methergine (methylergonovine) 0.2 mg IM prn postpartum or abortion (spontaneous or incomplete) related heavy bleeding

- See Preeclampsia and Eclampsia sections above

Discharge Criteria

- Benign causes of pain of pregnancy (round ligament, etc.)
- Benign pelvic pain and threatened abortion with stable vital signs
- Rehydration with heart rate < 100 in vomiting of pregnancy

Discharge instructions

- Pregnancy aftercare instructions
- Threatened abortions aftercare instructions
- Follow up with OB/GYN provider within 1–3 days
- Return if pain persists or increases
- Return if bleeding recurs or increases

Consult Criteria

- Heart rate ≥ 110
- BP ≥ 140/90
- Intractable vomiting
- Anemia
- Preeclampsia or eclampsia
- Placental abruption
- Placenta previa
- Ectopic or possible ectopic pregnancy
- Threatened abortion
- Inevitable abortion
- Incomplete abortion
- Missed abortion
- Fetal demise
- Septic abortion
- Significant vaginal bleeding or hypotension or orthostasis (notify physician promptly)
- Late pregnancy bleeding (last 20 weeks)
- Significant pelvic/abdominal pain or headache
- Pyelonephritis

Notes

Infectious Disease

Section Contents

Sexually Transmitted Disease Protocol

Human Immunodeficiency Virus (HIV) Protocol

HIV and Hepatitis B Postexposure Prophylaxis Recommendations

Endocarditis Protocol

Tetanus Protocol

When using any protocol, always follow the Guidelines of Proper Use (page 16).

Sexually Transmitted Disease Protocol

When using any protocol, always follow the Guidelines of Proper Use (page 16).

Definition

- Diseases transmitted by sexual contact

Differential Diagnosis

- Gonorrhea
- PID
- Chlamydia
- Epididymitis
- Orchitis
- Syphilis
- Hepatitis B
- Prostatitis

Considerations

- Gonococcal and chlamydial disease frequently seen together
- Syphilis — 100,000 new cases per year

Presentations

- Pelvic inflammatory disease (PID)
- Prostatitis (usually age < 35 years)
- Epididymoorchitis
- Bartholin cyst
- Venereal warts
- Urethritis
- Vaginitis

Gonococcal Disease

Definition

- Disease spectrum caused by Neisseria gonorrhoeae

Differential diagnosis

- Nonspecific urethritis
- Chlamydial infections
- Strep pharyngitis
- Leucocytoclastic vasculitis (rash)
- Septic arthritis
- Meningitis
- Orchitis
- Epididymitis
- UTI
- Cervicitis
- PID
- Proctitis
- Conjunctivitis

Considerations

- May be disseminated
    - Joints — frequently single and migratory (knee most common)
    - Skin
    - Tenosynovitis
    - Meningitis
    - Endocarditis
- Coexist 25–50% of the time with chlamydial infection
- May coexist with trichomonas and syphilis

Females

- Asymptomatic carriers
- PID — 20% has gonorrhea
    - Cervical motion tenderness
    - Usually bilateral adnexal tenderness
    - RUQ tenderness with elevated LFT's may represent Fitz-Hugh-Curtis syndrome
- Cervicitis
- Associated often with chlamydia and trichomonas

Males

- Severe dysuria
- Purulent urethral discharge

- Proctitis (homosexual sexual relations)
- Pharyngitis

Evaluation

- Sexual and reproductive/menstrual history
- Genital exam usually indicated
- Smear with intracellular gram negative diplococci can be performed
- Culture
- RPR prn

Treatment options

- Follow CDC guidelines
- May use Sanford Guide
- Analgesics prn
- Rocephin (ceftriaxone) 125 mg IM
- Doxycycline 100 mg PO bid × 7 days to cover chlamydia

Discharge criteria

- Nondisseminated gonococcal disease
- Nontoxic patient

Discharge instructions

- STD aftercare instructions
- Return if symptoms persist > 3 days
- Return if worse
- Follow up with health department within 3 days

Consult criteria

- Toxic patient
- Disseminated gonococcal disease
- See General Patient Criteria Protocol (page 20)

Pelvic Inflammatory Disease (PID)

Definition

- Spectrum of the female genital tract infections to include uterus, tubes, ovaries and peritoneum

Differential diagnosis

- Ectopic pregnancy
- Normal pregnancy
- Ovarian cyst
- Endometriosis
- Ovarian torsion
- Uterine fibroids
- Chronic pelvic pain syndrome
- UTI
- Renal colic

Considerations

- Common in females of reproductive age
- Gonorrhea and chlamydia are most common causes
- Important to treat sexual partners
- Can lead to tubo-ovarian abscess

Symptoms and findings

- Can cause peritonitis
- Usually bilateral pelvic pain and tenderness
- Associated with vaginal discharge frequently
- Dyspareunia
- Cervical motion tenderness
- Fever and chills
- Nausea and vomiting

Evaluation

- Pelvic and abdominal exam
- CBC
- UCG
- U/A
- Consider RPR
- Consider C-reactive protein
- LFT's if right upper quadrant tenderness for Fitz-Hugh-Curtis syndrome
- Cultures for gonorrhea and chlamydia; wet prep
- Consider pelvic ultrasound if TOA suspected
- CT scan if appendicitis also suspected

Treatment options

Outpatient

- Rocephin (ceftriaxone) 250 mg IM

  +

- Doxycycline 100 mg PO BID × 14 days

  +

- Flagyl (metronidazole) 500 mg PO BID × 14 days (avoid ethanol)
- Treatment for sexual partners or refer for treatment for STD
- NSAID's; narcotics prn; Phenergan (promethazine) prn
- May use Sanford Guide
- Follow CDC recommendations

Inpatient

- Cefotetan 2 gms IV

  +

- Doxycycline 100 mg IV
- Consult physician

Discharge criteria

- Mild to moderate pain
- Does not meet consult criteria

Discharge instructions

- PID aftercare instructions
- Follow up in 3 days to monitor treatment effectiveness
- Return if pain or fever worsens

Consult criteria

- Uncertain diagnosis or toxic appearance
- Suspected pelvic abscess
- Fitz-Hugh-Curtis syndrome (RUQ tenderness and elevated LFT's)
- Pregnancy
- Severe illness (severe pain and vomiting)
- Unable to tolerate PO intake
- Immunodeficiency
- Failure of outpatient therapy

- Return visit for same acute complaint
- Likely noncompliance with outpatient treatment
- Poor follow up

Urethritis and Epididymoorchitis

Definition

- Infection or inflammation of the urethra, epididymis or testicle

Differential diagnosis for epididymoorchitis

- Testicular torsion
- Mumps
- Trauma
- Hernia
- Tumor – usually painless

Considerations

- Gonorrhea and chlamydia are the main causes and coexist 25–50% of the time
- Urethral discharge
- Tender and swollen epididymis and/or testicle

Gonorrhea

- Dysuria
- Thick purulent discharge from urethra
- Gram negative intracellular diplococci

Chlamydia

- Thinner discharge from urethra
- Little to no discomfort

Evaluation

- Sexual history
- Genital exam
- Smear for intracellular gram negative diplococci can be performed
- Culture
- RPR prn

Treatment options

- Follow CDC guidelines

- May use Sanford Guide
- Analgesics prn
- Rocephin (ceftriaxone) 125 mg IM

  +
- Doxycycline 100 mg PO bid × 7 days to cover chlamydia

Discharge criteria
- Nontoxic patient

Discharge instructions
- Epididymoorchitis aftercare instructions
- Return if worse
- Follow up with PCP or urologist in 3–7 days

Consult criteria
- Systemic toxicity
- Refer to General Patient Criteria Protocol prn (page 20)

Prostatitis

Definition
- Infection or inflammation of the prostate gland

Differential diagnosis
- Prostate cancer
- Urethritis
- Mechanical back pain
- UTI

Considerations
- Gonorrhea and chlamydia are the main causes in men age < 35 years and coexist 25–50% of the time
- Prostate tender (caution with vigorous palpation if fever or toxicity present)
- Age > 35 years usual cause is bacterial
- Nonbacterial prostatitis is inflammatory condition without infection
- Chronic prostatitis
  - Increases risk of UTI and BPH

Acute bacterial prostatitis age > 35 years

- Fever
- Chills
- Perineal prostatic pain
- Dysuria
- Obstructive bladder symptoms
- Low back pain
- Low abdominal pain
- Spontaneous urethral discharge

Evaluation options

- U/A
- CBC
- RPR if STD suspected

Treatment options

Age < 35 years

- Follow CDC guidelines
- May use Sanford Guide
- Analgesics prn
- Rocephin (ceftriaxone) 125 mg IM

  +
- Doxycycline 100 mg PO bid × 10–14 days
- Treatment for sexual partners or refer for treatment for STD

Age > 35 years

- May use Sanford Guide
- Septra DS 1 PO bid × 14–28 days
- Quinolone 14–28 days
- NSAID's and/or narcotics prn

Discharge criteria

- Nontoxic patient
- Refer to General Patient Criteria Protocol prn (page 20)

Discharge instructions

- Prostatitis aftercare instructions
- Return if worse

- Follow up with PCP or urologist in 3–7 days

Consult criteria

- Systemic toxicity
- Urinary retention

Venereal Warts

- Usually condyloma acuminata
    - Painless pedunculated or sessile wart

Can be secondary syphilis (condyloma lata)

- Highly contagious (wear gloves)
- Smooth, moist flat wart
- Secondary syphilis rash is maculopapular and mimics other diseases
- Painless chancre sore history or finding
- Order RPR

Antibiotic choices for syphilis

- Bicillin LA 2.4 IM
- Doxycycline 100 mg PO × 14 days

Treatment for condyloma acuminata

- Podofilox 0.5% gel or solution bid on wart only for 3 days, rest 4 days, and another cycle of 3 days, repeat up to 4–6 cycles

Discharge criteria

- All nontoxic patients

Discharge instructions

- Venereal wart aftercare instructions
- Refer to health department or PCP within 3–7 days

Consult criteria

- Complicating comorbidities

Syphilis

Definition

- Infection caused by Treponema palladium

Differential diagnosis

- Pityriasis rosea
- Chanchroid
- Condyloma acuminata
- Psoriasis
- Lymphogranuloma venereum
- Herpes simplex

Considerations

Primary syphilis

- Painless chancre (sore) at site of infection

Secondary syphilis

- Occurs 2–10 weeks after primary infection
- Widespread mucocutaneous lesions
- Spreads to liver, joints, muscle, lymph nodes and brain

Latent syphilis

- Asymptomatic
- Can last up to 30 years
    - Early phase within one year of primary infection
    - Late phase after one year of primary infection

Tertiary syphilis

- Noninfectious at this stage
- Irreversible
- Can affect
    - Heart (coronary aneurysms)
    - Aorta
    - Eyes
    - Brain
    - Nerves
    - Bones
    - Joints
- Neurosyphilis develops in 5% of tertiary syphilis
    - Meningovascular type most common

- Tabes dorsalis (post column of spinal cord with loss of position sense)

Treatment options

Antibiotics choices for primary, secondary or early latent syphilis

- Bicillin LA 2.4 IM
- Doxycycline 100 mg PO × 14 days

Antibiotic choices for late latent syphilis

- Bicillin LA 7.2 million units IM qweek × 3 weeks

Discharge criteria

- Primary, secondary or early latent syphilis

Discharge instructions

- Syphilis aftercare instructions
- Refer to health department within 3 days

Consult criteria

- Late latent syphilis
- Neurosyphilis
- Tertiary syphilis
- Pregnancy

Notes

Human Immunodeficiency Virus (HIV) Protocol

When using any protocol, always follow the Guidelines of Proper Use (page 16).

Definition

- Infection by HIV

Differential Diagnosis

- Cytomegalovirus
- Mononucleosis
- Syphilis
- Influenza
- Meningitis
- Encephalitis
- Viral hepatitis
- Idiopathic thrombocytopenic purpura
- Candidiasis

Considerations

- Six month window between acquiring primary HIV infection and seroconversion
- Life expectancy is 24 years with HIV infection on current treatment regimens

HAART (highly active antiretroviral therapy)

- Combination of 2 NRTIs with a NNRTI or Protease Inhibitor
- CD4 counts < 350 cells/ml should be started on HAART
- Has significantly increased life expectancy
- Potential for hepatotoxicity
- May cause lactic acidosis
- May cause GI symptoms, rashes, headache and psychiatric disorders
- Pneumonia is usually caused by S. pneumoniae in patients on HAART

- Increases coronary heart disease
- Increases cerebrovascular disease
- Increases uveitis and iritis
- Increases sarcoidosis and autoimmune thyroiditis
- Osteoporosis and osteonecrosis

Drug interactions with HAART

- Increases concentrations of antiarrhythmia drugs
- Increases levels of anticonvulsants
- Increase concentrations of benzodiazepines
    - Okay to give 1 dose in ED
- Increases rhabdomyolysis risk with statin drugs
- Increases warfarin concentrations

Causes

- Unprotected sexual intercourse
- Anal receptive sexual intercourse is high risk
- Parenteral drug use and needle sharing
- Occupational needle stick
- Contaminated blood product transfusion

Signs, Symptoms, Findings or Processes

- May have no symptoms or physical findings
- Fever
- Fatigue
- Night sweats
- Oral ulcers
- Pharyngitis
- Diarrhea
- Genital ulcers
- Rashes
- Alopecia
- Weight loss
- Headache
- Myalgias
- Lymphadenopathy
- Altered mental status
- Pneumonia

- COPD
- Kidney damage
- Progressive multifocal leukoencephalopathy
- CNS lymphoma
- Anemia
- Sensory neuropathies
- Staph pyomyositis with CD4 < 50 (usually in thigh)
- Staph folliculitis
- Psychiatric disorders

Immune reconstitution inflammatory syndrome

- Immune system improves with HAART and attacks dormant opportunistic infections
- Can worsen autoimmune disorders
- Can manifest as pneumonitis, lymphadenitis, hepatosplenomegaly and hypercalcemia
- Treatment is with NSAIDs and/or corticosteroids
- Discontinuation of HAART is rarely needed

Evaluation

- History of CD4 counts if known
- Medication history
- Previous hospitalizations
- Previous infections or cancers

Testing options

- CBC
- LFT's
- U/A if fever or urinary symptoms
- BMP if abnormal vital signs or diabetic
- Stool for ova/parasites and cultures
- STD testing if indicated
- HIV testing offered to patient
- Chest x-ray if respiratory complaints or findings
- CT brain with and without contrast for neurologic complaints or findings

Treatment Options

- Treatment of associated infections

- Discuss AIDS related opportunistic infections or findings with physician
- Antiretroviral treatment per physician or experienced practitioner

Discharge Criteria

- Stable afebrile patient
- Social support systems present
- Pneumonia in HAART patients who are nontoxic, not hypoxic with normal blood pressure and heart rate may be candidates for outpatient treatment
    - Treatment is the same as for typical community acquired pneumonia
    - Discuss with physician

Discharge instructions

- HIV aftercare instructions
- Refer to primary care provider, health department or AIDS clinic for follow-up

Consult Criteria

- Toxic patient
- Altered mental status
- Neurologic deficit
- Respiratory distress
- Fever
- Unable to ambulate
- Vomiting
- Unable to self-hydrate
- Pericardial or pleural effusion
- Significant weight loss
- Acute psychiatric symptoms
- Pneumonitis

Lab consult criteria

- Adult WBC ≥ 13,000 or < 1,000 neutrophils;
- Bandemia
- Acute thrombocytopenia
- Hemoglobin < 10 (unless chronic and stable)
- O2 Sat ≤ 94% on room air if acute

- Moderate or severe dyspnea

Vital sign and age consult criteria

- Adult heart rate > 100
- Pediatric heart rate
    - 0–4 months ≥ 180
    - 5–7 months ≥ 175
    - 6–12 months ≥ 170
    - 1–3 years ≥ 160
    - 4–5 years ≥ 145
    - 6–8 years ≥ 130
    - 7–12 years ≥ 125
    - 12–15 years ≥ 115
    - 16 years or older ≥ 100

Notes

HIV AND HEPATITIS B POSTEXPOSURE PROPHYLAXIS RECOMMENDATIONS

When using any protocol, always follow the Guidelines of Proper Use (page 16).

Follow your institution's policies and procedures for postexposure prophylaxis if present. Refer to CDC links at the end of this Protocol.

General Wound Guidelines

- Irrigate and clean wound copiously with flushing 1% betadine solution
- The need for tetanus and/or hepatitis B prophylaxis is based on medical history (see Tetanus Protocol, page 580)
- Health care providers should be immunized against hepatitis B
- Hepatitis A prophylaxis may (rarely) need to be considered depending on the source-patient situation
- The need for HIV or chemoprophylaxis (antiretrovirals) is based on an assessment of the risk developed by the Centers for Disease Control and Prevention (CDC)

Testing of Source and Exposed Person

- Hepatitis profile
- HIV
- Liver function tests
- Serum anti-HBs titers on exposed person if there is a hepatitis B vaccination history

Recommended HIV Postexposure Prophylaxis (PEP) for Needlestick Injuries

Definitions of exposure type

Less severe exposure

- Solid needle

- Superficial injury

More severe exposure

- Large bore hollow needle
- Deep puncture
- Visible blood on device
- Needle used in patient's artery or vein

HIV-positive classes

Class 1

- Asymptomatic HIV infection
- Low viral load (< 1,500 RNA copies/ml)

Class 2

- Symptomatic HIV infection
- AIDS
- Acute seroconversion
- Known high viral load

HIV regimens

Basic regimen for 28 days

- Truvada 1 tablet daily (tenofovir 300 mg+ emtricitabine 200 mg) — dose q48hr if creatinine clearance 30-49 ml/min: avoid with creatinine clearance < 30 ml/min

  OR

- Combivir 1 tablet PO bid (zidovudine 300 mg + lamivudine 150 mg) — avoid use with creatinine clearance < 50 ml/minute

Basic regimen toxicity

- Nephrotoxicity
- Hepatotoxicity
- Lactic acidosis
- Read literature for all adverse reactions/contraindications of any HIV antireviral drugs used

Expanded Regimen for 28 days

- Kaletra (Lopinavir/ritonavir 400/100 mg) PO bid with food

  \+

- Combivir 1 tablet PO bid

OR

- Truvada 1 tablet once daily

Treatment recommendations

Less severe exposure + HIV-positive class 1

- Basic regimen

Less severe exposure + HIV-positive class 2

- Expanded regimen

More severe exposure + HIV-positive class 1

- Expanded regimen

More severe exposure + HIV-positive class 2

- Expanded regimen (≥ 3 drugs)

Source of unknown HIV status

- Generally no PEP
- Can consider basic regimen for HIV risk factors

Unknown source (needle from sharps container, for example)

- Generally no PEP
- Can consider basic regimen in areas in which exposure to HIV infected persons is likely

HIV negative source

- No PEP

Recommended HIV Postexposure Prophylaxis (PEP) for Mucosal Membrane and Nonintact Skin Exposures

Definitions of exposure type

Small volume

- Few drops

Large volume

- Major blood splash

Treatment recommendations

Small volume exposure + HIV-positive class 1

- Basic regimen

Small volume exposure + HIV-positive class 2

- Basic regimen

Large volume exposure + HIV-positive class 1

- Basic regimen

Large volume exposure + HIV-positive class 2

- Expanded regimen (≥ 3 drugs)

Source of unknown HIV status

- Generally no PEP
- Can consider basic regimen for HIV risk factors

Unknown source (needle from sharps container, for example)

- Generally no PEP
- Can consider basic regimen in areas in which exposure to HIV infected persons is likely

HIV negative source

- No PEP

Consultation criteria

Delayed (> 24–36 hours after exposure)

- Interval in which lack of benefit from PEP is undefined

Unknown source

- Use of PEP on case by case basis

Known or suspected pregnancy in exposed person

- Use of optimal PEP not precluded

Breastfeeding in exposed person

- Use of optimal PEP not precluded

Resistance of source virus to antiretrovirals

Toxicity of initial PEP regimen

- Adverse symptoms common with PEP (nausea and diarrhea)
- Symptoms often manageable without changing regimen with GI medications

Hepatitis B Postexposure Prophylaxis

Unvaccinated exposed worker

Source HBsAg positive

- HBIG 0.06 cc/kg IM × 1
- Initiate hepatitis B vaccine series

Source HBsAg negative

- Initiate hepatitis B vaccine series

Source unknown or not available for testing

- Initiate hepatitis B vaccine series

Previously vaccinated

Known responder

- No treatment

Known nonresponder with source HBsAg positive or high risk

- HBIG 0.06 cc/kg IM × 1
- Reinitiate hepatitis B vaccine series

  OR

- HBIG × 2

Antibody response unknown and source HBsAg positive

- Test exposed person
    - If adequate (serum anti-HBs ≥ 10 mIU/cc)
        - No treatment
    - If inadequate (serum anti-HBs < 10 mIU/cc)
        - HBIG × 1

- Vaccine booster

Antibody response unknown and source unknown or not available for testing

- Test exposed person
    - If adequate (serum anti-HBs ≥ 10 mIU/cc)
        - No treatment
    - If inadequate (serum anti-HBs < 10 mIU/cc)
        - Vaccine booster
        - Recheck titer in 1–2 months

Further Reading

http://www.cdc.gov/mmwr/preview/mmwrhtml/rr5011a1.htm#box2

http://www.cdc.gov/mmwr/PDF/rr/rr5409.pdf

http://aidsetc.org/aidsetc?page=cg-301_occupational_pep

The clinician managing the exposed person can call the National Clinicians' Post-Exposure Prophylaxis Hotline (PEPline) at 888-HIV-4911 (888-448-4911) at no charge. Service is available 7 days a week, (More information is available at the PEPline website)

Notes

ENDOCARDITIS PROTOCOL

When using any protocol, always follow the Guidelines of Proper Use (page 16).

Definition

- Infection of the endocardial surface of the heart including the heart valves

Considerations

Acute endocarditis

- Usually from Staph aureus or group B strep
- Occurs on normal valves
- More aggressive course
- Related to IV drug abuse
- Valve replacement > 60 days prior

Subacute endocarditis

- Usually from Strep viridans or enterococci
- Less aggressive course
- Valve replacement > 60 days prior

Signs and symptoms

- Fever
- Petechiae
- Heart murmur
- CHF
- Neurologic complaints or findings
- Delirium
- Pericarditis
- Neck pain
- Anemia
- Leukocytosis
- Proteinuria
- Hematuria
- Splenomegaly
- Embolic findings
    - Splinter hemorrhages on nail beds
    - Osler nodes on fingertip pads

    - Roth spots are retinal hemorrhages
    - Janeway lesions are nontender macular rash on palms and soles

Evaluation

- History and physical examination
- Consider in IV drug abuser and fever
- CBC
- Chest x-ray
    - Evaluate for septic emboli, cavitary lesions and infiltrates
- C-reactive protein and ESR (elevated > 90% of patients)
- BMP
- U/A
    - Evaluate for proteinuria and hematuria
- Blood culture q5–10 minutes × 2 sets
- EKG
    - For conduction defects (poor prognostic sign)
- Transesophageal echocardiography

Treatment

- Oxygen prn
- Treat CHF if present
- IV NS as needed

Subacute endocarditis

- Penicillin G 2–3 million units IV q4hr
- Vancomycin for suspected resistant organisms
- May use Sanford guide

Acute endocarditis

- Nafcillin 2 gms IV q4hr
- Vancomycin for suspected resistant organisms
- May use Sanford Guide

Prophylaxis

History of

- Congenital heart disease
- Prosthetic valve
- History of prior endocarditis

- Prophylaxis treatment

Procedural conditions

- Dental procedures
- Abscess I&D
- Incision of respiratory mucosa (tonsillectomy)
- Not recommended for GI or GU procedures

Antibiotic regimens

Adult options

- Amoxicillin 2 gms PO

OR

- Ampicillin 2 gms IV

OR

- Cleocin (clindamycin) 600 mg PO or IV

OR

- Cephalexin 2 gm PO

OR

- Zithromax (azithromycin) 500 mg PO

OR

- Rocephin (ceftriaxone) 1 gm IV or IM

OR

- Use Sanford Guide

Pediatric options

- Amoxicillin 50 mg/kg PO — NMT 2 gms

OR

- Ampicillin 50 mg/kg IV or IM — NMT 2 gms

OR

- Cleocin (clindamycin) 20 mg/kg PO — NMT 600 mg

OR

- Zithromax (azithromycin) 15 mg/kg PO — NMT 500 mg

OR

- Cephalexin 50 mg/kg PO — NMT 2 gm

OR

- Rocephin (ceftriaxone) 50 mg/kg IV or IM — NMT 1 gm

OR

- Use Sanford Guide

Consult criteria

- Discuss with physician all endocarditis or suspected endocarditis patients

Notes

TETANUS PROTOCOL

When using any protocol, always follow the Guidelines of Proper Use (page 16).

Tetanus infection

Definition

- Anaerobic infection caused by Clostridium tetani producing a toxin that causes muscle spasms and pain

Differential diagnosis

- Conversion disorder
- Meningitis
- Encephalitis
- Dystonic drug reaction
- Mandible dislocation
- Hypocalcemia
- Black widow spider bite
- Subarachnoid hemorrhage
- Peritonsillar abscess
- Retropharyngeal abscess
- Rabies

Considerations

- Found in soil, feces, house dust and is ubiquitous
- Tetanus spores can remain in normal tissue for months to years
- Tetanus infection may occur without apparent wound
- Incidence of tetanus infection has decreased markedly secondary to childhood immunizations and current tetanus prophylaxis recommendations
- Medium incubation period is 7 days, but can be less than 4 days or greater than 14 days
- Tetanus booster does not prevent acute tetanus disease occurrence
    - It prevents future infections

- Tetanus immune globulin prevents acute infections in under-immunized patients
- Elderly are frequently under-immunized

Signs and symptoms

- 75% have generalized muscle rigidity – "lockjaw"
- Dysphagia
- Fever
- Tachycardia
- Sweating
- Laryngospasms – can cause asphyxia
- Acute abdominal pain mimicking surgical abdomen

Evaluation

- History and physical examination
- No specific lab tests available
- Diagnosis is clinical
- Spatula test
    - Touching tongue with tongue blade causes masseter spasm and biting of the blade
    - Sensitivity 94%
    - Specificity 100%
    - No complications from procedure

Treatment

- Tetanus immune globulin 3,000–5,000 units IM with part of dose injected around infection site
- Rapid sequence intubation per physician if needed acutely
    - Needed in 2/3 of patients
- Wound debridement out to 2 cm from wound edges
- Incision and drainage of any abscesses

Medications

- Valium
    - Adult
        - Mild spasms 5–10 mg PO

            - Moderate spasms 5–10 mg IV
            - Severe spasms 40 mg/hour IV infusion
        - Pediatric
            - Mild spasms 0.1–0.8 mg/kg PO divided tid–qid (NMT 10 mg)
            - Moderate to severe spasms 0.1–0.3 mg/kg IV q4–8h (NMT 10 mg)
    - Antibiotics
        - Efficacy not proven
        - May try penicillin ,Flagyl (metronidazole) or doxycycline
    - Vecuronium per physician (if intubated)

Consult criteria

- Immediate physician notification

Tetanus prophylaxis

- Tetanus prophylaxis
    - High risk = every 5 years
    - Low risk = every 10 years
    - Tetanus IG 250–500 units IM at different site from wound if high risk and less than 3 tetanus or unknown history of immunizations previously in life — usually with the elderly

High risk wound

- More than 6 hours old
- Greater than 1 cm deep
- Exposed to saliva or feces
- Stellate wounds
- Crush wounds
- Puncture wounds
- Ischemic appearance

Tdap

- Recommended by CDC for adults
- A substitute for Td once only
- Contains pertussis in addition to tetanus toxoid and diphtheria toxoid
- Adacel is only formulation recommended for adults

    - Pediatric Td and Tdap contain 3–4 times more diphtheria toxoid than adult formulation (do not give to adults)
- Use only once, then use regular Td from then on in patients needing a tetanus booster
- May be used in second and third trimester of pregnancy

Discharge instructions

- Wound aftercare instructions
- Refer to health department or primary care provider to complete tetanus primary vaccination series if < 2 vaccines given in past

Notes

Dermatology

Section Contents

Human and Animal Bite Protocol
Spider Bite and Insect Sting Protocol
Snake Bite Protocol
Cellulitis Protocol
Soft Tissue Abscess Protocol
Henoch-Schonlein Purpura Protocol
Erythema Multiforme Protocol
Erythema Nodosum Protocol
Dyshidrotic Eczema Protocol
Atopic Dermatitis/Eczema Protocol
Psoriasis Protocol
Contact Dermatitis Protocol
Impetigo Protocol
Scabies Protocol
Tinea Capitis Protocol
Tinea Corporis Protocol
Tinea Pedis (Athlete's Foot) Protocol
Urticaria Protocol
Pityriasis Rosea Protocol
Herpes Simplex Gingivostomatitis Protocol
Herpetic Whitlow Protocol
Genital Herpes Protocol
Herpes Zoster (Shingles) Protocol
Tick Bite Protocol
Lyme Disease Protocol
Varicella (Chicken Pox) Protocol
Hand Infection Protocol

Human and Animal Bite Protocol

When using any protocol, always follow the Guidelines of Proper Use (page 16).

Human Bites

- 15–20% infection rate
- Staph aureus most common
- Usually hand wounds from fist fight

Evaluation

- Wound exploration
- X-ray
- Assess bone, joint, muscle and tendon for injury

Treatment options

- Consider closure only if all 4 criteria present:
  - Cosmetically significant (face wound)
  - Uninfected wound
  - Less than 12 hours old (< 24 hours on face)
  - Not on hand or foot
- Do not close puncture wounds
- Flush with > 250 cc of 1% betadine solution using 18 gauge angiocath (mix 1 cc of 10% betadine with 9 cc of NS)
- May rinse with NS
- Remove devitalized tissue
- ADT 0.5 cc IM if more than 5 years from last immunization
- Tetanus immune globulin 250–500 units IM different site if < 3 tetanus immunizations in the past
- Refer to health department or primary care provider to complete tetanus primary vaccination series if < 2 vaccines given in past
  - See Tetanus Protocol (page 580)
- Antibiotics prophylaxis
  - Superficial: none

Deeper wound antibiotic treatment options

- Augmentin (amoxicillin/clavulanate) 875 mg PO bid × 5 days for prophylaxis (adults > 40kg)
- Augmentin (amoxicillin/clavulanate) 15 mg/kg PO bid × 5 days for prophylaxis (pediatrics < 40 kg)
- Doxycycline 100 mg PO bid × 5 days if allergic to penicillin
- Doxycycline 1.5–2 mg/kg PO bid × 5 days if allergic to penicillin (age > 8 years and < 45 kg)
- May refer to Sanford Guide

Discharge criteria

- Superficial wounds without infection
- No bone, joint or tendon involvement

Discharge instructions

- Human bite aftercare instructions
- Return if infection occurs in bite
- Return if pain increases

Consult criteria

- Infected wounds
- Closed fist wounds penetrating to joint, tendon or bone
- Significant bites to hand
- Fever
- Toxicity

Dog Bites

- 15–20% infection rate
- Most common pathogens
  - Aerobes: staph aureus, Pasteurella multocida, streptococcus
  - Anaerobes: enterobacter, pseudomonas, bacillus
- Infection < 24 hours — Pasteurella multocida
- Infection > 24 hours — staph or strep

Evaluation

- Wound exploration
- X-ray
- Assess bone, joint, muscle and tendon for injury
- Assess for foreign body (tooth, etc.)

Treatment

- Flush with > 250 cc of 1% betadine solution (mix 1 cc of 10% betadine with 9 cc of NS using 18 gauge angiocath)
- Rinse with NS
- ADT 0.5 cc IM if more than 5 years from last
- Tetanus immune globulin 250–500 units IM different site if < 3 tetanus immunizations in the past
- Refer to health department or primary care provider to complete tetanus primary vaccination series if < 2 vaccines given in past
    - See Tetanus Protocol (page 580)
- Add viricidal 1% benzalkonium chloride if risk of rabies
- Remove devitalized tissue
- Consider closure
    - Bite < 8 hours old
    - Bite < 12 hours old on face
    - Do not close puncture wounds
- Antibiotic prophylaxis
    - Usually not needed
    - Use in high risk wounds; facial wounds
    - Use in immunocompromised or asplenic patients
    - Same antibiotic regimen as for human bites
- Consider rabies prophylaxis
- Notify rabies control

Discharge criteria

- Same as human bites

Discharge instructions

- Dog bite aftercare instructions
- Return if infection occurs in bite

- Return if pain increases

Consult criteria

- Severely infected wounds
- Wounds penetrating to joint, tendon, or bone
- Neurovascular deficit or injury
- Significant bites to hand
- Fever
- Toxicity

Cat Bites

- High infection risk
- 25–50% infection rate
- Pasteurella multocida up to 80% of infections
- Infection > 24 hours usually streptococcus — can progress rapidly
- May cause
    - Osteomyelitis
    - Septic arthritis
    - Abscess
    - Sepsis

Evaluation

- Wound exploration
- X-ray
- Assess bone, joint, muscle and tendon for injury
- Assess for foreign body (tooth, etc.)

Treatment

- Flush with > 250 cc of 1% betadine solution using 18 gauge angiocath (mix 1 cc of 10% betadine with 9 cc of NS)
- May rinse with NS
- ADT 0.5 cc IM if more than 5 years from last dose
- Tetanus immune globulin 250–500 units IM different site if < 3 tetanus immunizations in the past
- Refer to health department or primary care provider to complete tetanus primary vaccination series if < 2 vaccines given in past
    - See Tetanus Protocol (page 580)

- Add viricidal 1% benzalkonium chloride if risk of rabies
- Remove devitalized tissue (not puncture wounds)
- Closure not recommended on
    - Puncture wounds or deep bites
    - Infected wounds
    - Wounds > 24 hours

Antibiotics prophylaxis options

- Augmentin (amoxicillin/clavulanate) 875 mg PO bid-tid × 5 days for prophylaxis (adults > 40 kg)
- Augmentin (amoxicillin/clavulanate) 15 mg/kg PO bid-tid × 5 days for prophylaxis (pediatrics < 40 kg)
- Doxycycline 100 mg PO bid × 5 days if allergic to penicillin
- Doxycycline 1.5–2 mg/kg PO bid × 5 days if allergic to penicillin (age > 8 years and < 45 kg)
- Can refer to Sanford Guide

Mild infections options

- Augmentin (amoxicillin/clavulanate) 875 mg PO bid × 10–14 days (adults > 40 kg)
- Augmentin (amoxicillin/clavulanate) 15 mg/kg PO bid × 10–14 days (pediatrics < 40 kg)
- Doxycycline 100 mg PO bid × 10–14 days if allergic to penicillin
- Doxycycline 1.5–2 mg/kg PO bid × 10–14 days if allergic to penicillin (age > 8 years and < 45 kg)
- Can refer to Sanford Guide

Moderate infections options

- Augmentin (amoxicillin/clavulanate) 875 mg PO bid × 10–14 days (adults > 40 kg)
- Augmentin (amoxicillin/clavulanate) 15 mg/kg PO bid × 10–14 days (pediatrics < 40 kg)

    - Doxycycline 100 mg PO bid × 10–14 days if allergic to penicillin
    - Doxycycline 1.5–2 mg/kg PO bid × 10–14 days if allergic to penicillin (age > 8 years and < 45 kg
    - Rocephin (ceftriaxone) 1–2 gms IM qday × 10–14 days
    - Rocephin (ceftriaxone) 50 mg/kg IM qday × 10–14 days not to exceed adult dose for children
    - Can refer to Sanford Guide
- Consider rabies prophylaxis
- Notify rabies control

Discharge criteria

- Superficial wounds
- Mild to moderate infected wounds

Discharge instructions

- Cat bite aftercare instructions
- Return if infection occurs in bite
- Return if pain increases

Consult criteria

- Severely infected wounds
- Wounds penetrating to joint, tendon, or bone
- Neurovascular deficit or injury
- Significant bites to hand
- Fever
- Toxicity

Wild Animal Bites

- Similar evaluation, treatment and disposition as Dog Bites Protocol
- Notify rabies control

Notes

SPIDER BITE AND INSECT STING PROTOCOL

When using any protocol, always follow the Guidelines of Proper Use (page 16).

Brown Recluse Spider Bite

- Found in dark areas
- Envenomation can be mild if spider has recently fed
- Symptoms develop 4–8 hours after bite
- Symptoms and findings that may occur are
    - Local reaction only
    - Tissue necrosis
    - Severe pain
    - Pruritus
    - Fever
    - Nausea/vomiting
    - Headache
    - Myalgias
    - Initial papule which develops central dark area of necrosis over 48–72 hours

Evaluation

- History of bite
- Exam of lesion area

Systemic symptoms

- CBC to check for thrombocytopenia and anemia
- BMP to check for renal involvement
- PT/PTT/INR if DIC suspected
- U/A to check on dipstick for blood for hemolytic anemia

Treatment options

- Clean wound
- Benadryl (diphenhydramine) or other antihistamines for pruritus and rash

- ADT 0.5 cc IM if more than 5 years from last dose (see Tetanus Protocol, page 580)
- Antibiotics if secondary infection present
  - Augmentin (amoxicillin/clavulanate) 875 mg PO bid × 10–14 days (adults > 40kg)
  - Augmentin (amoxicillin/clavulanate) 15 mg/kg PO bid × 10–14 days (pediatrics < 40 kg)
  - Doxycycline 100 mg PO bid × 10–14 days if allergic to penicillin
  - Doxycycline 1.5–2 mg/kg PO bid × 10–14 days if allergic to penicillin (age > 8 years and < 45 kg) — NMT 100 mg per dose
- May use Sanford Guide
- Follow up with primary care provider or surgeon within 7 days if wound necrotic

Discharge criteria

- Nontoxic patient
- No systemic symptoms

Discharge instructions

- Brown recluse spider bite aftercare instructions
- Return if pain worsens
- Return if fever occurs
- Return for occurrence of systemic symptoms

Consult criteria

- Toxic patient
- Systemic symptoms
- Anemia
- Thrombocytopenia
- Acute renal insufficiency
- Significant cellulitis
- Necrotic area > 2 cm

Black Widow Spider Bites

- Red hourglass on abdomen

Grade 1 (mild envenomation)

- Immediate pain at site
- Normal vital signs

Grade 2 (moderate envenomation)

- Muscle pain in bitten extremity
- Muscle pain may extend to abdomen if lower extremity bitten
- Muscle pain may extend to chest if upper extremities bitten
- Diaphoresis at bite site
- Normal vital signs

Grade 3 (severe envenomation)

- Generalized muscular pain
- Generalized diaphoresis
- Nausea/vomiting
- Headache
- Hypertension
- Tachycardia

Evaluation

- U/A for hematuria
- CPK
- Labs and other testing to rule out other acute abdominal process if suspected

Treatment options

- IV NS
- Tetanus prophylaxis (see Tetanus Protocol, page 580)
- Cool compresses to site
- Benadryl (diphenhydramine) IV 50 mg or weight adjusted for pediatrics if antivenin to be given
- Pain control with narcotics
- Black widow antivenin (consult physician before using)

Consult criteria

- All black widow spider bites
- Before any antivenin given

Bees, Wasps, and Fire Ants

- Refer to Allergy Protocol if needed
- Remove stinger
- Cool compresses
- Can make a Adolph Meat Tenderizer paste with water and apply for 1 hour to break down proteins in venom
- NSAID's prn for pain
- Topical hydrocortisone cream may be used
- Tetanus prophylaxis if > 10 years (see Tetanus Protocol, page 580)
- Respective aftercare instructions

Local Reactions from Insect Bites or Stings

- 1–5 cm of nontender induration usually
- Light pink or red color
- Antihistamine OTC prn
- Cool compresses prn
- Steroids 1–3 day course can be considered — usually not needed (avoid in diabetes)
- If cellulitis present, refer to Cellulitis Protocol
- May use Sanford Guide
- Local reaction aftercare instructions

Notes

SNAKE BITE PROTOCOL

When using any protocol, always follow the Guidelines of Proper Use (page 16).

Considerations

- 2,000 venomous snake bites per year
- Alcohol intoxication frequently a contributing factor
- Mortality < 0.5% with advent of antivenin
- Venomous snake bites involve pit vipers (Crotalids) or coral snakes
- Eastern coral snake considered deadly
- Arizona coral snake not deadly
- Oozing at fang bite site reliable predictor of envenomation

Pit vipers (are responsible for majority of venomous bites)

- Rattlesnakes
- Cottonmouths
- Copperheads
- Water moccasins

Identification

Pit vipers

- Depressions or pits between eyes and nostrils
- Triangular head
- Elliptical eyes
- 2 fangs
- Subcaudal plates

Coral snake

- Black nose
- Colored rings
- Confused with King snake
  - "Red on yellow, kill a fellow; red on black, venom lack" denoting color rings of Coral and King snakes respectively
- Venom usually either hemotoxic or neurotoxic

Pit vipers symptoms and findings

- Local injury (swelling starts in 15–30 minutes)
- Systemic vascular damage
- Hemolysis; hematuria; hematemesis
- Fibrinolysis and coagulopathy
- Neuromuscular dysfunction
- Compartment syndrome
- Airway edema

Coral snake symptoms and findings

- No significant local injury
- Respiratory failure
- Cranial nerve dysfunction
- Tremors
- Salivation
- Seizures

Crotalid (Pit Viper) Envenomation Grading

No envenomation

- Snakebite suspected
- Minimal pain
- No systemic symptoms or lab abnormalities in first 12 hours after bite

Mild envenomation

- Local redness, swelling, ecchymosis limited to bite site

Moderate envenomation

- Local redness, swelling, and ecchymosis that extends beyond bite site
- Nausea
- Paresthesias
- Metallic taste in mouth
- Mild hypotension
- Mild tachycardia
- Mild tachypnea
- Coagulation factors normal and no active bleeding signs

Severe envenomation

- Rapidly spreading swelling, redness, and ecchymosis to involve entire limb
- Altered mentation
- Respiratory compromise
- Severe hypotension (7%)
- Extreme tachycardia
- Coagulopathy
- Active bleeding

Coral Snake Envenomation

- Coral snake bite symptoms can be delayed up to 12 hours
- Ptosis early sign
- Muscle weakness
- Salivation
- Slurred speech
- Dizziness
- Respiratory failure
- Other neurologic abnormalities

Diagnosis of Snake Bites

- Fang marks (pit vipers)
- History of snake exposure
- Local tissue injury
- Coral snake may have tiny punctures and minimal local tissue changes

Evaluation of Snake Bites

- History and physical exam
- Mark edematous area with a pen every 15 minutes – 30 minutes to assess progression
- CBC
- CMP
- PT/PTT/INR
- U/A

Moderate to severe envenomation

- EKG
- Chest x-ray

- ABG
- Troponin
- DIC panel

Treatment Options

- Clean wound with antiseptic or soap/water
- No arterial constrictive banding, no wound excisions, no ice
- Venous banding can be considered if there is a large snake bite and prolonged delay reaching hospital
- Keep limb immobilized at heart level
- Tetanus toxoid (ADT) 0.5 cc IM if > 5 years since last dose
- Tetanus immune globulin 250–500 units IM at different site if < 3 tetanus doses in life
- Refer to health department or primary care provider to complete tetanus primary vaccination series if < 2 vaccines given in past
    - See Tetanus Protocol (page 580)
- Antibiotics if infected — usually not needed otherwise
    - Augmentin (amoxicillin/clavulanate) or dicloxicillin

Pain and nausea control options prn

- Dilaudid (hydromorphone) 0.5–1 mg IV (double if IM) prn — may repeat prn × 2
- Morphine 2–5 mg IV prn — may repeat prn × 2
- Stadol (butorphanol) 0.5–1 mg IV (double if IM) — may repeat prn × 1
- Phenergan (promethazine) 6.25 mg IV or 25–50 mg IM prn
- Zofran (ondansetron) 4–8 mg IV prn

Pit viper antivenin (mainstay of treatment) — notify physician

Crofab (less allergic reactions than horse serum)

- Read package insert
- Mild or no envenomation does not require antivenin for pit vipers
- 4–6 vials IV for moderate to severe envenomation initially — give slowly for first

10 minutes at 25–50 cc/hr to observe for allergic reaction
  - 2 vials IV q6hr up to 3 doses if further doses needed after initial dosing

Coral snake (eastern) antivenin

- Read package insert
- Pretreat with Benadryl (diphenhydramine) and Pepcid (famotidine) IV
- Keep epinephrine at bedside
- 3–6 vials IV over 1–2 hours if definitely bitten
- 10 vials IV initially if systemic manifestations present

Complications of antivenin

Acute allergic reaction – see Allergy Protocol Anaphylaxis sections

- Benadryl (diphenhydramine) 50 mg adult; 1.5 mg/kg pediatrics not to exceed 50 mg
- Pepcid (famotidine) 20–40 mg IV adult
- Pepcid (famotidine) 0.25 mg/kg up to 20 mg for children
- Solumedrol (methylprednisolone) 125 mg IV for adults
- Solumedrol (methylprednisolone) 1 mg/kg IV for children not to exceed 125 mg
- If reaction is severe notify physician immediately
  - Epinephrine 0.3–0.5 SQ/IM/IV for adults depending on severity; pediatrics 0.1 mg/kg SQ/IM/IV depending on severity not to exceed 0.5 mg
- It is preferable to consult a on venomous snake bite patients

Serum sickness

- Fever
- Arthralgias
- Rash (usually occurs 7–10 days after antivenin; can occur earlier)

Treatment

- Antihistamines prn
- Steroids for 7–10 days PO

Discharge Criteria

- Pit viper bite is dry, and is asymptomatic after 8 hours of observation
- Sonoran and Arizona coral snake bite: can be discharged

Discharge instructions

- Snake bite aftercare instructions
- Refer to primary care provider or surgeon

Consult Criteria

- Notify physician promptly for all snake bites
- All eastern coral snake or suspected eastern coral snake bites (need admission)
- Pit vipers with any envenomation (need admission)
- Abnormal vital signs
- Abnormal lab; chest x-ray; EKG
- Neurologic abnormalities
- Suspected compartment syndrome

Notes

CELLULITIS PROTOCOL

When using any protocol, always follow the Guidelines of Proper Use (page 16).

Definition

- Local inflammatory reaction of the skin and subcutaneous tissue secondary to bacteria infection

Differential Diagnosis

- Erysipelas
- Osteomyelitis
- Septic arthritis
- Lymphadenitis
- Abscess
- Deep vein thrombosis
- Necrotizing fasciitis

Considerations

- Pain, tenderness, redness, swelling and warmth
- Abscess frequently co-exists

Caused by

- S. aureus (MRSA)
- Group A streptococcus
- H. influenzae
- Pseudomonas
- Anaerobes

Complications

- Bacteremia
- Osteomyelitis
- Septic joint
- Cavernous sinus spread

Higher risk

- Diabetics
- Peripheral vascular disease
- Chronic edema

- IV drug abuse
- Elderly
- Immunocompromise

Evaluation

- Complete history and physical examination
- Assess for tissue gas
- Palpate for tenderness assessment

No tests needed

- For small area of involvement
- No fever or systemic signs
- No high risk factors

Testing considerations

- CBC, BMP for high risk factors
- Possibly blood cultures if toxic or septic appearance
- Ultrasound useful to evaluate for possible abscess if suspected
- X-ray if crepitus noted or tissue gas suspected
- Bedside ultrasound frequently changes therapy if abscess found

Treatment Options

- Uncomplicated — Septra (trimethoprim /sulfamethoxazole) or doxycycline for community acquired MRSA
- Strep infection concern add cephalosporin or Augmentin (amoxicillin/clavulanate) to Septra (trimethoprim/sulfamethoxazole) or doxycycline
- Human, dog or cat bite — Augmentin (amoxicillin/clavulanate) or Sanford guide
- Preseptal ocular cellulitis — Augmentin (amoxicillin/clavulanate) or Sanford guide
- Drain associated abscesses

Discharge Criteria

- Mild cellulitis without systemic toxicity
- Low grade fever
- Available follow up

Discharge instructions

- Cellulitis aftercare instructions
- Follow up with PCP within 3–5 days if not improving
- Return if fever develops or pain increases
- Return for progressive increase in cellulitis

Consult Criteria

- Rapidly spreading
- Pain out of proportion to exam
- Crepitus or gas in tissues
- Systemic toxic appearance
- Necrotizing fasciitis or Gas gangrene
- Vital signs abnormal per General Patient Criteria Protocol
- Large abscess
- Facial cellulitis
- Orbital cellulitis
- Suspected bony involvement

Higher risk comorbidities

- Diabetics with poor control
- Peripheral vascular disease
- Chronic edema
- IV drug abuse
- Elderly
- Immunocompromise

Vital signs and age consult criteria

- Age < 6 months or ≥ 70 years old
- Hypotension or relative hypotension SBP < 105 in patient with hypertension history
- Fever > 101°F (38.3°C)

Lab consult criteria

- WBC ≥ 15,000 or < 3,000
- Bandemia ≥ 15%
- Acute thrombocytopenia
- Significant electrolyte abnormally
- Glucose ≥ 350 mg/dL in diabetic patient

- Glucose ≥ 200 mg/dL in non-diabetic patient
- Hyperglycemia with metabolic acidosis (decreased serum CO_2 or elevated anion gap)
- Worsening preexisting anemia
- Metabolic acidosis

SOFT TISSUE ABSCESS PROTOCOL

When using any protocol, always follow the Guidelines of Proper Use (page 16).

Definition

- Collection of purulent material in the soft tissues

Differential Diagnosis

- Cellulitis
- Erysipelas
- Osteomyelitis
- Septic arthritis
- Lymphadenitis
- Deep vein thrombosis
- Necrotizing fasciitis

Considerations

- Incision and drainage usually curative without antibiotics
- MRSA most common cause
- Cellulitis frequently surrounds abscess
- May be in deep areas like the buttocks
- Ultrasound useful when in doubt of an abscess being present
- Recurrent groin and axillary abscesses suggest hidradenitis suppurativa

Higher risk comorbidities

- Diabetics
- Peripheral vascular disease
- Chronic edema
- IV drug abuse
- Elderly
- Immunocompromise

Evaluation

- Assess for systemic toxicity
- Bedside ultrasound frequently changes therapy
- Examine for deeper structure involvement
- Culture Bartholin cysts for GC and Chlamydia
- Consider abscess culture
- CBC, BMP for high risk factors
- Blood cultures if toxic or septic appearance

Treatment Options

- Skin prep with betadine
- Local anesthesia with ethyl chloride and/or lidocaine
- May use 18–20 gauge needle to aspirate to confirm an abscess
- Incise with #11 scalpel maximum area of swelling and/or tenderness
- Break any deeper adhesions
- Drain pus
- Pack with gauze if large abscess present for 24–48 hours — patient can remove at home or return to see a Provider
- Do not pack facial abscesses
- NSAID's, Tylenol or narcotics short course prn

Antibiotic choices

- If significant associated cellulitis (> 2 cm adjacent to abscess) use MRSA antibiotics
  - Septra (trimethoprim/sulfamethoxazole)
  - Doxycycline
  - Clindamycin
- Consider antibiotics for higher risk patients

Discharge Criteria

- Uncomplicated abscess without toxicity
- No high risk co-morbidity
- Outpatient follow up available

Discharge instructions

- Abscess aftercare instructions

- Return if pain worsens or involved area increases in size
- Return if fever develops or worsens

Consult Criteria

- Rapidly spreading
- Pain out of proportion to exam
- Crepitus or gas in tissues
- Systemic toxic appearance
- Hypotension or relative hypotension SBP < 105 in patient with hypertension history
- Necrotizing fasciitis
- Gas gangrene
- Vital signs abnormal — see General Patient Criteria Protocol (page 20)
- Facial abscess
- Large abscess
- Perirectal or pilonidal abscess
- Suspected bony or muscle involvement

Higher risk comorbidities

- Diabetics with poor control
- Peripheral vascular disease
- Chronic edema
- IV drug abuse
- Elderly
- Immunocompromise

Vital signs and age consult criteria

- Age < 6 months or ≥ 70 years old
- Hypotension or relative hypotension SBP < 105 in patient with hypertension history
- Fever > 101°F (38.3°C)

Lab consult criteria

- WBC ≥ 15,000 or < 3,000
- Bandemia ≥ 15%
- Acute thrombocytopenia
- Significant electrolyte abnormally
- Glucose ≥ 350 mg/dL in diabetic patient

- Glucose ≥ 200 mg/dL in non-diabetic patient
- Hyperglycemia with metabolic acidosis (decreased serum CO_2 or elevated anion gap)
- Worsening anemia
- Metabolic acidosis

Notes

HENOCH-SCHONLEIN PURPURA PROTOCOL

When using any protocol, always follow the Guidelines of Proper Use (page 16).

Definition

- Henoch-Schonlein purpura (HSP) is an inflammatory disorder characterized by a generalized vasculitis involving the small vessels of the skin, kidneys, GI tract, joints, and rarely the lungs and central nervous system

Differential Diagnosis

- Disseminated intravascular coagulation
- Meningitis
- Idiopathic Thrombocytopenic Purpura
- Mononucleosis
- Rocky Mountain spotted fever
- Septic shock
- Acute renal failure
- Intussusception
- Hand-Foot-Mouth disease
- Kawasaki disease
- Acute Glomerulonephritis
- Chicken pox
- Thrombocytopenic Purpura
- Systemic Lupus Erythematosus

Considerations

- Disease of children and young adults
- Diffuse vasculitis of unknown etiology
- Often an antecedent infection history present
- Peak incidence is 4 years of age
- Typical age range 2–11 years of age
- Spring peak
- Renal involvement most serious sequelae
    - Develops within 3 months of rash

    - Renal failure can develop up to 10 years after rash
    - More common in adults
- Generally a benign self-limited condition
- 40% have reoccurrence usually with rash and abdominal pain
- Normal platelet count, PT, and PTT

Signs and Symptoms

- Palpable purpura
- Rash of erythematous papules followed by nonthrombocytopenic purpura
    - Typically on buttocks; lower extremities; can be elsewhere
- Abdominal pain — 2/3 of patients; can mimic acute abdomen
- Low grade fever
- Vomiting
- Diarrhea — can be bloody
- Arthritis — 70% of patients; transient and no permanent deformity
- Nephritis
- End stage renal disease develops in 5% of cases
- Hematuria
- Intussusception
- Intracranial hemorrhage

Evaluation

- CBC
- BMP
- U/A
- PT/PTT/INR
- CT abdomen/pelvis scan if severe abdominal pain or bleeding present

Treatment

- IV NS for signs of hypovolemia
- Ibuprofen per weight
- Prednisone 1 mg/kg qday × 5–7 days if renal or severe GI involvement

Discharge Criteria

- Normal platelet count
- Normal renal function
- Minimal or no abdominal pain
- Discuss with physician prior to discharge

Discharge instructions

- Henoch-Schonlein Purpura aftercare instructions
- Follow up within 24 hours if discharged on prednisone

Consult Criteria

- Severe abdominal pain
- Neurologic abnormalities
- Gastrointestinal bleeding
- Intussusception
- Renal involvement

Notes

ERYTHEMA MULTIFORME PROTOCOL

When using any protocol, always follow the Guidelines of Proper Use (page 16).

Definition

- Erythema multiforme (EM) is an acute, self-limited, and occasionally recurring skin condition thought to be a type IV hypersensitivity reaction associated with certain infections, medications, and other various triggers

Differential Diagnosis

- Urticaria
- Herpes simples
- Pityriasis rosea
- Secondary syphilis
- Viral exanthems
- Septicemia
- Drug eruptions
- Collagen vascular disease
- Serum sickness

Considerations

Erythema multiforme (EM) minor

- Target lesions or raised red papules
- No mortality

Erythema multiforme major

- Similar to EM minor with mucous membrane involvement
- Epidermal detachment < 10% total body surface area
- No mortality

Stevens Johnson Syndrome (SJS)

- Widespread blisters/bullae on trunk and face

- Mucous membrane involvement
- SJS — epidermal detachment < 10% BSA (body surface area)
- Mortality approximately 5%

Toxic Epidermal Necrolysis (TEN)

- Widespread blisters/bullae on trunk and face
- Mucous membrane involvement
- TEN — epidermal detachment > 30% BSA
- Mortality approximately 30%

Symptoms and Findings

Erythema multiforme: minor and major

- Burning sensation of rash
- Pruritus usually absent
- Eye involvement up to 10%; bilateral purulent conjunctivitis
- Any mucous membrane involvement is mild
- Viral type prodrome in 50%

Rash

- Target or iris lesions (red papules and macules with central clearing)
- Vesiculobullous lesions can develop in existing rash
- Sudden onset and symmetrical
- Centripetal spread
- Favors palms and soles
- Dorsal hands
- Extensor limb surfaces
- Face

SJS/TEN

- Generalized cutaneous and/or mucocutaneous vesiculobullous lesions
- Hemorrhagic bullae
- Fever
- Vomiting and diarrhea can occur
- Oral pain may be severe
- Eye pain and discharge

- Dyspnea may occur
- Dysuria
- Oral involvement may appear similar to aphthous ulcers
- Nasal pharynx, respiratory tract, GI and GU systems can be involved

Causes

- No identifiable cause in 50%
- Viral
  - Herpes simplex (10%)
  - Chicken pox
  - Various other viruses
- Bacterial
  - Mycoplasma
  - Salmonella
  - Gonorrhea
  - Various others
- Fungal
- Postvaccination
- Drugs
  - Sulfonamides
  - Hypoglycemics
  - NSAID's
  - Anticonvulsants
  - Various antibiotics
  - Malignancy
  - Hormonal
  - Autoimmune disorders

Evaluation

- Erythema multiforme
  - Testing driven by history and physical exam
  - May not need testing
- SJS/TEN
  - CBC
  - BMP
  - LFT's
  - Chest x-ray
  - Cultures prn

Treatment Options

- Remove offending agents if identified
- Erythema multiforme
    - Symptomatic treatments
    - Narcotics short course prn
    - NSAID's prn
    - Cool compresses with saline or Burrow's solution
    - Saline or Benadryl (diphenhydramine) elixir gargles prn for oral findings/symptoms
    - No oral steroids
- SJS/TEN
    - IV NS for hydration
    - Cultures prn

Discharge Criteria

- Uncomplicated erythema multiforme

Discharge instructions

- Erythema multiforme aftercare instructions
- Return immediately if signs of SJS/TEN develops

Consult Criteria

- Refer to General Patient Criteria Protocol (page 20)
- All suspected SJS/TEN

Notes

ERYTHEMA NODOSUM PROTOCOL

When using any protocol, always follow the Guidelines of Proper Use (page 16).

Definition

- Erythema nodosum (EN) is an acute, nodular, erythematous eruption that usually is limited to the extensor aspects of the lower legs, thought to be a hypersensitivity reaction

Differential Diagnosis

- Urticaria
- Nodular vasculitis
- Insect bites
- Erysipelas
- Superficial thrombophlebitis

Considerations

- Delayed hypersensitivity reaction
- Painful red tender 2–6 cm nodules on extensor lower extremities
- Usually acute and self-limited
- May last weeks to years
- More common in females age 30–50 years
- Idiopathic 50% of the time
- Often a marker for systemic disease

Causes

- Idiopathic 50% of the time
- Most commonly secondary to strep infections; sarcoidosis
- Drug reactions
    - Sulfa
    - Penicillin
    - Oral contraceptives
- Systemic infections
    - Tuberculosis
    - Fungal

- Ulcerative colitis
- Malignancy
    - Leukemia
    - Lymphoma

Evaluation

- Strep test of pharynx
- ESR or C-reactive protein (may be very high)

Treatment

- NSAID's prn
- Treat underlying infection or causes if found
- Cool compresses prn
- Elevation of legs
- Bed rest

Discharge Criteria

- All uncomplicated cases

Discharge instructions

- Erythema nodosum aftercare instructions

Consult Criteria

- Refer to General Patient Criteria Protocol (page 20)
- Serious associated comorbidities

Notes

DYSHIDROTIC ECZEMA PROTOCOL

When using any protocol, always follow the Guidelines of Proper Use (page 16).

Definition

- Vesicular eruption with pruritic deep-seated vesicles of the fingers, hands and feet of unknown etiology

Differential Diagnosis

- Scabies
- Contact dermatitis
- Irritant dermatitis

Considerations

- Related to stress; drugs; illness
- "Id" reaction from variety of stimuli; distant fungal infections
- Last approximately 3 weeks
- Is a chronic relapsing palmoplantar dermatitis
- Spring and summer prevalence
- Warm climates
- 50% have childhood atopic dermatitis, asthma or similar conditions

Treatment Options

- Moisturizing lotions (Eucerin)
- Topical steroids
- Oral antihistamines prn itching
- Ointments beneficial where increased moisture is needed
- Creams preferred in scalp and moist areas

Discharge Criteria

- Uncomplicated process

Discharge instructions

- Dyshidrotic eczema aftercare instructions

Consult Criteria

- Moderate to severe superinfection

Notes

ATOPIC DERMATITIS/ECZEMA PROTOCOL

When using any protocol, always follow the Guidelines of Proper Use (page 16).

Definition

- Poorly defined red patchy plaque-like rash with edema acutely and skin thickening chronically, mostly on flexor surfaces
- Also known as Eczema

Differential Diagnosis

- Seborrheic dermatitis
- Discoid eczema
- Contact dermatitis
- Scabies
- Insect bites
- Psoriasis

Considerations

- Can be acute or subacute
- Chronic relapsing most common
- Pruritic inflammation of epidermis or dermis
- Family history of asthma, hay fever, allergic rhinitis, allergic dermatitis
- Immune modulated
- More frequent in formula fed babies
- Manifests in infancy or early childhood usually
- Relationship to food allergies: milk, soy, eggs, wheat
- More frequent in winter
- Increased humidity contribution
- Bathing with hot water removes moisture from skin — worsening the rash

Symptoms

- Dry skin
- Erythematous patches and plaques

- Surrounding erythema and scaling may occur
- Skin excoriations frequent
- Often in skin flexures — antecubital and popliteal fossa
- May be generalized

Treatment Options

- Tacrolimus or pimcrolimus ointment
- Antihistamines
- Topical steroids
- May need oral steroids
- Avoid soap and hot water on rash as much as possible
- Topical or oral antibiotic for staph superinfection
- Eucerin
- Tar containing shampoo for scalp seborrheic dermatitis

Discharge Criteria

- Uncomplicated process

Discharge instructions

- Atopic dermatitis or eczema aftercare instructions

Consult Criteria

- Moderate to severe superinfection

Notes

Psoriasis Protocol

When using any Protocol, always follow the Guidelines of Proper Use (page 16).

Definition

- A chronic, relapsing, multisystem inflammatory condition manifested most commonly with skin rash and arthritis, with a familial predisposition

Differential diagnosis

- Seborrheic dermatitis
- Atopic dermatitis
- Tinea corporis, pedis or capitis
- Contact dermatitis
- Blepharitis
- Syphilis
- Squamous cell carcinoma
- Diaper dermatitis
- Pustular eruptions
- Various skin malignancies

Considerations

- Rash most commonly on elbows, knees, scalp, lumbosacral region, intergluteal clefts and glans penis
- Arthritis occurs in up to 30% of patients
- Plaque-type most common rash
  - Plaques are raised, red, inflamed with silvery white scaly appearance
- Ocular involvement occurs in up to 10% of patients
- Flares may be secondary to recent strep throat or viral infection, immunization or trauma

Symptoms and Findings

- Scaling red macules, papules and plaques that are frequently pruritic
- Guttate psoriasis are small pink 1–10 mm macules commonly on upper trunk frequently 2–3 weeks after strep throat
- Rash may be pustular
- Fever, chills, hypothermia and dehydration may occur when most of the body is covered with psoriasis rash

- Pits on the nails
- Arthritis is usually of hands and feet, though may include large joints
- White oral lesions and/or cheilosis
- Geographic tongue
- Blepharitis
- Uveitis
- Conjunctivitis

Evaluation options

- Usually a clinically diagnosis
- Joint x-rays may help with determining type of arthritis
- If immunologic therapy started, obtain baseline CBC, BMP, LFT's and TB screening

Treatment options

- Systemic steroids not effective and may worsen the psoriasis when discontinued
- Minimize soap exposure to rash as much as is practical
- Moisturizing lotions
- Sunlight exposure
- Sea bathing
- Topical corticosteroids for rash
    - Triamcinolone 0.025–0.1% cream is drug of choice for new treatment
    - Betamethasone 0.025–0.1% for disease resistant to triamcinolone or hydrocortisone creams
- Ocular corticosteroids for eye involvement
    - Prednisolone 1% (Pred Forte) bid
    - Dexamethasone 1% ophthalmic
- Coal tar 0.5–33% (DHS Tar, Doctar, Theraplex T)
    - Shampoo for scalp lesions
    - Topical corticosteroid in addition to coal tar preparation increases effectiveness
- Salicylic acid preparations help to remove scales
- Calcipotriene (vitamin D analogue)
- Combination therapy with tazarotene (a retinoid) or calcipotriene with a topical corticosteroid more effective than either alone
- Oatmeal baths may help symptoms

Severe cases may need treatment from some of the following

- Systemic retinoids, cyclosporine, methotrexate, azathioprine, a Biologic, or hydroxyurea — **consult dermatologist prior to using and read PDR**
  - Biologics are infliximab (Remicade), etanercept (Enbrel), adalimumab (Humira), and alefacept (Amevive) — **consult dermatologist prior to using and read PDR**
  - Psoralen with ultraviolet A light retinoids
  - Ultraviolet B
  - Anthralin preparations 0.1–1% (Drithocreme, Anthra-Derm)

Disease–modifying antirheumatic drugs (DMARD's)

Considerations

- Check CBC, creatinine, LFT's and investigate abnormalities before DMARD or Biologics medications used
- Document negative pregnancy test and discussion of contraception in fertile females before treatment
- Consider pneumovax vaccination
- Document PPD results before Biologics therapy
- Be familiar with effects and side effects of medications as listed in the Physician Desk Reference (PDR)

Biologics (tumor necrosis factor inhibitors)

Cautions

- Severe infection risk exists
- Stop all DMARDs and Biologics if infection identified or suspected until treated and resolved
- Malignancy risks may be increased

- Do not use in optic neuritis or multiple sclerosis patients or in a first degree relative of these patients
- Do not use in patients with significant heart failure
- Avoid live vaccines
- Biologics may be used with or without DMARDs
- Be familiar with effects and side effects of medications as listed in the Physician Desk Reference (PDR)

Discharge criteria

- Uncomplicated psoriasis

Discharge instructions

- Psoriasis aftercare instructions
- Referral to PCP or dermatologist

Consult criteria

- Systemic symptoms or findings
- Fever
- Systemic treatment needed for severe disease

Notes

CONTACT DERMATITIS PROTOCOL

When using any protocol, always follow the Guidelines of Proper Use (page 16).

Definition

- Hypersensitivity reaction manifested by acute or chronic inflammatory reactions to substances that contact the skin

Differential Diagnosis

- Cellulitis
- Scabies
- Atopic dermatitis/eczema
- Psoriasis
- Herpes simplex
- Erythema multiforme

Considerations

- Is 90% of workman's compensation dermatologic claims
- Rash limited to exposure area with sharp margins or linear excoriations

Some causes

- Rhus dermatitis (toxicodendron)
    - Poison ivy, poison oak, poison sumac
- Metals: nickel common
- Chemical
    - Hair dyes; paraphenylenediamine

Treatment Options

- Identify and limiting exposure
- Soothing moist dressings
- Topical steroids
- Systemic steroids with severe cases up to 10 days
- Toxicodendron or Rhus dermatitis (poison ivy, etc.) use soap and water, especially under nails

- Zanfel over the counter can be used for Rhus dermatitis acutely

Discharge Criteria

- Uncomplicated process

Discharge instructions

- Contact dermatitis aftercare instructions

Consult Criteria

- Severe superinfection

Notes

IMPETIGO PROTOCOL

When using any protocol, always follow the Guidelines of Proper Use (page 16).

Definition

- Impetigo is a highly contagious gram-positive bacterial infection of the superficial layers of the epidermis that exists in 2 forms which are bullous impetigo and non-bullous impetigo

Differential Diagnosis

- Erythema multiforme
- Fixed drug eruption
- Bullous pemphigoid
- Herpes simplex
- Herpes zoster
- Insect bites
- Stevens-Johnson syndrome
- Toxic Epidermal Necrolysis
- Varicella (Chicken pox)
- Atopic dermatitis
- Scabies

Considerations

- Contagious superficial bacterial infection of epidermis
- Crusted erosions or ulcers
- Most common in children ages 2–5 years
- Clinical diagnosis
- Predisposing factors
- Close contact with infected person
- Warm/humid climates
- Poor hygiene
- Crowding
- Poverty
- Non-bullous form most common
- MRSA most prevalent
- GABHS still occurs

Treatment Options

- Mupirocin topical for 5–10 days or until lesions gone for 2 days
- More severe cases can give systemic antibiotics — choices
    - Septra (trimethoprim/sulfamethoxazole)
    - Doxycycline
    - Clindamycin
    - Beta-lactams if strep infection suspected

Discharge Criteria

- Uncomplicated infection

Discharge instructions

- Impetigo aftercare instructions
- Return if fever develops
- Follow up with PCP if rash persists > 10 days

Consult Criteria

- Systemic symptoms
- Immunocompromise

Notes

SCABIES PROTOCOL

When using any protocol, always follow the Guidelines of Proper Use (page 16).

Definition

- Dermatitis secondary to the mite Sarcoptes scabiei, spread by direct contact with hosts or fomites

Differential Diagnosis

- Insect bites
- Atopic dermatitis
- Contact dermatitis
- Urticaria
- Psoriasis
- Lice
- Secondary syphilis
- Bedbug bites
- Dyshidrotic eczema
- Chicken pox
- Folliculitis

Considerations

- Excruciating pruritus especially at night
- Transmission primarily from skin to skin
- Transmission can occur from infected linens or clothing
- Eggs hatch in 3 days
- Mite viable 2–5 days
- Lesions are small excoriations with erythematous papules
- Burrow not always present, but pathognomonic
- Burrow is grey to red to brown thin line 2–15 mm in length
- Does not affect scalp in adults
- Can affect scalp in infants
- Diagnosis is clinical
- Can be confirmed with microscopic visualization of mite

- Itching can last 4 weeks after treatment due to hypersensitivity reaction to dead mite
- Itching lasting > 4 weeks search for another cause of the itching

Distribution

- Intertriginous areas
- Sides and webs of fingers
- Axillary folds
- Flexor wrists
- Extensor elbows
- Waist
- Genital folds
- Buttocks
- Thighs
- Extensor knees
- Posterior feet

Treatment

- Permetherin cream 5%
    - Massage cream in from neck to soles of feet
    - Leave on 8–14 hours
    - Second application may be needed one week later
- Lindane (Kwell lotion)
    - Massage cream from neck to soles of feet
    - Leave on 8–14 hours
    - Second application may be needed one week later
- Oral ivermectin 200 mcg × 1 dose
    - Not recommended in pregnant or lactating women
    - Not recommended in children < 15 kg
- Benadryl (diphenhydramine) prn itching
- Topical steroids prn once mite eradicated
- Treat all family members or close contacts
- Infected linens and clothing washed in hot water and dried with heat or ironing

Discharge Criteria

- Nontoxic patient with routine symptoms

Discharge instructions

- Scabies aftercare instructions
- Follow up with PCP as needed

Consult Criteria

- Moderate to severe topical or systemic superinfection

Notes

Tinea Capitis Protocol

When using any protocol, always follow the Guidelines of Proper Use (page 16).

Definition

- A disease caused by superficial fungal infection of the skin of the scalp

Differential Diagnosis

- Alopecia areata
- Psoriasis
- Drug eruptions
- "Id" reaction
- Contact dermatitis
- Seborrheic dermatitis
- Secondary syphilis
- Impetigo
- Systemic lupus erythematosus

Considerations

- Is a fungal superficial infection of the scalp
- Most common in younger pediatric population
- Spread by person to person contact
- Spread by shared objects such as combs and hair brushes
- Erythematous patch increasing over time
- Alopecia can occur
- May develop painful lymphadenopathy
- Kerion can develop — multiple boggy nodules of pus with associated hair loss
- Diagnosis can be clinical or confirmed with KOH prep

Treatment Options

- Adult
    - Oral griseofulvin 500 mg to 1 gm microsize PO qday for 6–8 weeks
    - Sporanox 200 mg PO qday for 4–6 weeks
- Pediatric

  - Oral griseofulvin 20–25 mg/kg microsize PO qday for 6–8 weeks (do not exceed adult doses)
  - Sporanox 3–5 mg/kg PO qday for 4–6 weeks (do not exceed adult doses)
- Monitor LFT's due to possible liver toxicity of griseofulvin
- Six weeks or more may be needed for treatment

Discharge Criteria

- Uncomplicated rash
- Children may return to school once appropriate treatment has started

Discharge instructions

- Tinea capitis aftercare instructions
- Follow up with PCP within 14 days if no improvement in rash
- Follow up with PCP in 3–4 weeks if rash persists

Consult Criteria

- Moderate to severe superinfection
- Systemic symptoms
- Immunocompromise

Notes

Tinea Corporis Protocol

When using any protocol, always follow the Guidelines of Proper Use (page 16).

Definition

- Superficial fungal infection of the body

Differential Diagnosis

- Tinea versicolor
- Cutaneous candidiasis
- Seborrheic dermatitis
- Psoriasis
- Impetigo
- Pityriasis rosea
- Secondary syphilis

Considerations

- Commonly called "ring worm"
- Erythematous lesion with central clearing
- Diagnosis usually clinical

Treatment Options

- Topical Lamisil qday for 1-4 weeks (apply on rash and 2 cm out from rash)
- Lotrimin bid for 2-6 weeks (apply on rash and 2 cm out from rash)
- Treat until no rash visible for 2 days
- Oral griseofulvin or ketoconazole for more severe infection (monitor LFT's)
    - May combine with topical treatment
    - May use in immunosuppressed patients
    - Use in tinea unguium (nails) or tinea capitis
- Avoid sharing infected objects
- Launder all possible infected linens and clothing separately
- Good hand washing
- Topical steroids can be used for initial 1-4 days to relieve symptoms

Discharge Criteria

- Uncomplicated rash
- Children may return to school once appropriate treatment has started

Discharge instructions

- Tinea corporis aftercare instructions
- Follow up with PCP within 14 days if no improvement in rash
- Follow up with PCP in 3–4 weeks if rash persists

Consult Criteria

- Moderate to severe superinfection
- Systemic symptoms
- Immunocompromise

Notes

Tinea Pedis (Athlete's Foot) Protocol

When using any protocol, always follow the Guidelines of Proper Use (page 16).

Definition

- Superficial fungal infection of the foot

Differential Diagnosis

- Cutaneous candidiasis
- Erythema multiforme
- Psoriasis
- Secondary syphilis

Considerations

- Most common superficial dermatophyte fungal infection
- Commonly called "athletes foot"
- Excessive sweating and occlusive footwear predispose to infection
- Acute and chronic states occur
- Inflammatory vesicles and bullae
- Located in toe webs — most common 4th and 5th
- Clinical diagnosis usually
- Can confirm with KOH prep if desired
- Can lead to cellulitis

Treatment Options

- Topical Lamisil qday 1–4 weeks or until rash gone for 2–4 days
- Oral griseofulvin or ketoconazole for more severe infection (monitor LFT's)
    - May combine with topical treatment
- Avoid sharing infected objects
- Launder all possible infected linens and clothing separately
- Good hand washing

- Avoid tight fitting shoes
- Keep feet dry
- May use topical steroid initial 2–4 days of treatment to relieve symptoms

Discharge Criteria

- Uncomplicated rash
- Children may return to school once appropriate treatment has started

Discharge instructions

- Tinea pedis aftercare instructions
- Follow up with PCP within 14 days if no improvement in rash
- Follow up with PCP in 3–4 weeks if rash persists

Consult Criteria

- Moderate to severe superinfection
- Systemic symptoms
- Immunocompromise

Notes

URTICARIA PROTOCOL

When using any protocol, always follow the Guidelines of Proper Use (page 16).

Definition

- Vascular reaction of the skin with transient wheals, soft papules and plaques usually with pruritus

Differential Diagnosis

- Erythema multiforme
- Angioedema
- Serum sickness
- Cutaneous vasculitis
- Toxic epidermal necrolysis
- Leprosy
- Juvenile rheumatoid arthritis
- Thrombophlebitis
- Cellulitis
- Pityriasis rosea

Considerations

- Transient wheals — soft papules and plagues
- Is pruritic
- Acute reaction lasting < 30 days usually allergic
- Chronic reaction lasting > 30 days often idiopathic
- Angioedema can occur with chronic urticaria

Causes

- Idiopathic
- Food allergies
- Infections
- Medications
- Insect bites or stings
- Sunlight
- Physical and emotional stressors
- Autoimmune diseases
- Systemic diseases
- Serum sickness

- Transfusion reaction

Treatment Options

Benadryl (diphenhydramine)

- Adult: 50 mg PO or IM
- Pediatrics: 1–2 mg/kg PO or IM (NMT 50 mg)
- May continue for 5–7 days PO

Additional treatment if needed

Pepcid (famotidine)

- Adult 20 mg IV (double for PO)
- Pediatric 0.25 mg/kg IV (double for PO) — NMT adult dose

Epinephrine (preferable to discuss with a physician)

- Do not use if history of coronary artery disease
- Adult: 0.3 SQ
- Pediatrics: 0.01 mg/kg SQ not to exceed adult dose

Consider steroids

- Prednisone 40–60 mg PO qday for 5–7 days (> 40 kg)
- Prednisone/prednisolone 1 mg/kg PO qday for 5–7 days (< 40 kg)

- Avoid offending agent if known

Discharge Criteria

- Good resolution of rash and itching

Discharge instructions

- Urticaria aftercare instructions
- Return if rash persists or worsens
- Follow up with primary care provider within 7 days

Consult Criteria

- Systemic symptoms
- Hypotension

- See General Patient Criteria Protocol (page 20)

Notes

Pityriasis Rosea Protocol

When using any protocol, always follow the Guidelines of Proper Use (page 16).

Definition

- Common skin disorder observed in otherwise healthy people, most frequently in children and young adults which manifests as an acute, bilateral, self-limiting, papulosquamous eruption with a 6-week to 8-week duration

Differential Diagnosis

- Viral exanthem
- Tinea corporis
- Erythema multiforme
- Secondary syphilis
- Drug eruption
- Tinea versicolor
- Seborrheic dermatitis

Considerations

- More common in late childhood to early adulthood
- Spring and fall prevalence
- Etiology unknown
- Not contagious
- Self-limited
- Resolves in 6–12 weeks
- Differential diagnosis considerations are secondary syphilis or drug eruption

Appearance

- Herald patch — single oval slightly raised plaque 2–5 cm, red color, on trunk usually
- Generalized eruption 1–2 weeks after herald patch
  - Fine scaling plaques and papules
  - Dark pink "Christmas tree" pattern along cleavage lines
  - Most noticeable on back

Treatment Options

- Benadryl (diphenhydramine) prn
- Aveeno or calamine prn
- UV exposure may hasten resolution
- Topical steroids

Discharge Criteria

- Self-limited disease so no consultation usually needed

Discharge criteria

- Pityriasis rosea aftercare instructions
- Follow up with PCP within 7–10 days as needed

Consult Criteria

- See General Patient Criteria Protocol as needed (page 20)

Notes

HERPES SIMPLEX GINGIVOSTOMATITIS PROTOCOL

When using any protocol, always follow the Guidelines of Proper Use (page 16).

Definition

- Grouped vesicles on erythematous base of the skin or mucous membranes usually causes by herpes simplex−1

Differential Diagnosis

- Aphthous stomatitis
- Hand-Foot-Mouth disease
- Candidiasis
- Chanchroid
- Pharyngitis
- Secondary syphilis
- Urethritis

Considerations

- Regional lymphadenopathy can occur
- Oral lesions are HSV-1 type usually
- HSV-1 type can cause genital herpes
- Recurrent outbreaks in one-third of patients; decreases over time
- Prodrome of tingling, itching or pain approximately 24 hours preceding rash
- Diagnosis clinical
- Can be confirmed with Tzanck smear

Triggers

- Skin infections
- Stress
- UV radiation

Treatment Options

- Avoid contact with infected individuals

- Antiviral treatment within 48–72 hours of onset of lesions

Antiviral choices

- Acyclovir ointment 5% 5 times a day for 5 days
- Acyclovir 400 mg PO qid × 7 days for severe infection
- Pediatric acyclovir oral dosing 15 mg/kg 5 times a day for 7 days (do not exceed adult doses)
- Valtrex (valacyclovir) 500–1000 mg PO bid × 7 days for adults

Discharge Criteria

- Benign local disease

Discharge instructions

- Herpes simplex–1 aftercare instructions
- Follow up with PCP within 7–10 days as needed
- Return if rash increases or spreads

Consult Criteria

- Encephalitis
- Altered mental status
- Disseminated infection
- Severity of symptoms enough to cause dehydration
- Immunocompromise
- Ocular involvement
- Refer to General Patient Criteria Protocol (page 20) as needed

Notes

HERPETIC WHITLOW PROTOCOL

When using any protocol, always follow the Guidelines of Proper Use (page 16).

Definition

- Herpes simplex infection of the digits manifested as painful grouped vesicles

Differential Diagnosis

- Felon
- Paronychia
- Cellulitis

Considerations

- Patients usually less than 20 years of age
- Usually caused by HSV-1
- Incision not recommended

Treatment Options

- Avoid skin contact with uninfected individuals
- Antiviral treatment within 48–72 hours of rash onset
- **Do not incise**

Antiviral choices

- Acyclovir ointment 5% 5 times a day for 5 days
- Acyclovir 400 mg PO qid × 7 days for severe infection
- Pediatric acyclovir oral dosing 15 mg/kg 5 times a day for 7 days (do not exceed adults doses)
- Valtrex (valacyclovir) 500–1000 mg PO bid × 7 days for adults

Discharge Criteria

- Most patients without severe superinfection

Discharge instructions

- Herpetic whitlow aftercare instructions
- Follow up with PCP within 7–10 days

Consult Criteria

- Moderate to severe superinfection
- Immunocompromise

Notes

GENITAL HERPES PROTOCOL

When using any protocol, always follow the Guidelines of Proper Use (page 16).

Definition

- Sexual transmitted disease by skin to skin contact caused by herpes simplex type 2 usually and occasionally by herpes simplex type 1 virus

Differential Diagnosis

- Candidiasis
- Syphilis
- Chanchroid
- Herpes zoster

Considerations

- May be transmitted during asymptomatic periods
- Recurrent outbreaks less frequent over time
- May cause systemic complaints

Treatment Options

- Avoid sexual contact with infected individuals
- Antiviral treatment within 48–72 hours of rash onset
- Analgesics prn

Antiviral choices

- Acyclovir ointment 5% 5 times a day for 5 days
- Acyclovir 400 mg PO qid × 7 days for severe infection
- Pediatric acyclovir oral dosing 15 mg/kg 5 times a day for 7 days (do not exceed adults doses)
- Valtrex (valacyclovir) 500–1000 mg PO bid × 7 days for adults

Discharge Criteria

- Immunocompetent patient without systemic symptoms

Discharge instructions

- Genital herpes aftercare instructions
- No sexual relations during prodrome and until lesions healed
- Follow up with PCP within 7–10 days
- Return if unable to void
- Return if rash worsens

Consult Criteria

- Systemic symptoms
- CNS infection
- Severe local symptoms
- Immunocompromise
- Urinary retention secondary to severe pain or sacral nerves involvement
- Refer to General Patient Criteria Protocol (page 20) as needed

Notes

HERPES ZOSTER (SHINGLES) PROTOCOL

When using any protocol, always follow the Guidelines of Proper Use (page 16).

Definition

- Acute dermatomal reactivation of varicella virus (chickenpox) in dorsal nerve roots ganglia

Differential Diagnosis

- Herpes simplex virus infection
- Varicella (chickenpox)
- Impetigo
- Cellulitis
- Folliculitis
- Contact dermatitis
- Prodromal pain thought to be
    - Biliary colic
    - Appendicitis
    - Angina

Considerations

- Seen with increasing age and decreasing immunocompetence
- Many patients have normal immune systems
- 10–20% of the general population will eventually develop herpes zoster
- Can have mild symptoms
- Immunosuppression increases risk of occurrence
- Prodrome of pain 3–5 days before rash occurs in 75% of cases
- Rash may be pruritic
- Rash crusts over in 7–10 days
- Prodrome frequently causes medical evaluation for unrelated diseases
- Pain duration is usually < 1 month
- Pain > 1 month is defined as post-herpetic neuralgia

- Recurrence is rare
- Herpes zoster can cause varicella (chickenpox) in exposed non-immunized patients

Findings

- Initially a vesicular patchy dermatomal rash on a red base that may involve 1 or more adjacent dermatomes
- Usually no more than 2–3 adjacent dermatomes involved with normal hosts
- Thoracic dermatomes followed by lumbar dermatomes are the most commonly involved areas
- Fever, malaise, headache and fatigue occur in < 20% of patients
- Can involve cranial nerves and visceral organs
- Pain is usually described as burning, stabbing or throbbing

Post-herpetic neuralgia (PHN)

- Pain > 1 month is defined as post-herpetic neuralgia
- Increases with increasing age, rash severity and severity of pain
- Occurs in 10–15% of cases
- Most debilitating symptom of disease
- May be difficult to control pain
- Antiviral therapy early in disease may help prevent PHN

Treatment choices

- Capsaicin ointment
- Narcotics
- NSAID's
- Amitriptyline
- Desipramine
- Dilantin
- Valproic acid
- Carbamazepine
- Gabapentin
- SSRI's limited usefulness

Treatment Options

- Antiviral treatment started within 72 hours of rash
- Valtrex (valacyclovir) 1,000 mg PO tid × 7 days
- Consider varicella immune globulin in elderly or pediatric patients
- Analgesics prn
- Steroids may help quality of life in patients at risk for PHN — controversial
  - Prednisone 40–60 mg qday × 1 week; taper over following week

Discharge Criteria

- Uncomplicated infection

Discharge instructions

- Herpes zoster aftercare instructions
- Return for systemic symptom develop
- Follow up with PCP within 7–10 days

Consult Criteria

- Immunosuppression
- Severe or disseminated disease
- 3 or more dermatomes affected
- Ophthalmic disease or ophthalmic dermatomal involvement
- Involvement of trigeminal nerve
- Visceral involvement
- Intractable pain
- Ramsey Hunt syndrome (7–8th cranial nerve involvement)
- Acute altered mental status
- Meningitis or encephalitis

Tick Bite Protocol

When using any protocol, always follow the Guidelines of Proper Use (page 16).

Definition

- Various disease processes transmitted by tick bites

Differential Diagnosis

- Lyme disease
- Rocky Mountain spotted fever
- Babesiosis
- Ehrlichiosis
- Measles
- Meningococcemia
- Rubella
- Varicella
- Mononucleosis
- Disseminated gonorrhea
- Typhus
- Kawasaki disease
- Toxic shock syndrome
- Secondary syphilis
- Gastroenteritis
- Allergic vasculitis
- Collagen vascular disease
- Juvenile rheumatoid arthritis
- Heat illness

Considerations

- Many patients with tick borne disease do not recall a tick bite
- Degree of tick engorgement is a marker for length of attachment
- Most tick borne illness occurs after attachment for 24-48 hours
    - Low risk of infection within 36 hours of tick attachment
- Hard body ticks cause most disease

- Ticks are found in brushy or wooded areas usually
- Lifecycle over 2–3 years
- Have to brush against where tick is (they do not jump, fly, or drop on to people)
- Spring and summer time when most tick borne diseases are transmitted
- "Summer fever" or "summer virus" check CBC for thrombocytopenia
- Can cause DIC (disseminated intravascular coagulation)
- Can cause acute renal failure

Tick removal

- Grasp head and mouth parts at skin and pull with gentle pressure for several minutes until tick is removed
- Can inject skin at site with lidocaine 1% to see if tick will release on its own
- Any mouth parts left in skin are not infectious

Tick types

Deer tick

- Lyme
- Ehrlichiosis
- Babesiosis

Dog tick

- Rocky Mountain spotted fever (RMSF)

Lone Star tick

- Lyme
- RMSF
- Ehrlichiosis
- Tularemia

Tick-borne diseases

- Lyme disease
- Rocky Mountain spotted fever (RMSF)
- Babesiosis
- Relapsing fever
- Tularemia

- Ehrlichiosis
- Q-fever
- Colorado Tick fever
- Tick paralysis

Lyme Disease

- See Lyme Disease Protocol

Rocky Mountain Spotted Fever

Symptoms and findings

- Fever and chills
- Up to 30–40% of patients report no tick bite within the past 14 days
- Headache
- Photosensitivity
- Nausea and vomiting
- Diarrhea
- Myalgias
- Maculopapular rash on extremities 3–5 days after fever onset spreading to rest of body
    - 10–20% do not get rash
    - 40–60% gets petechial rash 6 days after illness onset

Lab testing for

- Leukopenia
- Anemia
- Thrombocytopenia
- Elevated LFT's and creatinine
- Single titer of 1:64 supportive; 4 fold rise diagnostic
- PCR can be ordered

Treatment

- Adult: doxycycline 100 mg PO bid for 7 days continuing until afebrile for 2 days
- Children > 45 kg: doxycycline 100 mg PO qday for 7 days continuing for 2 days until afebrile
- Children < 45 kg: doxycycline 2–4 mg/kg PO qday for 7 days continuing until afebrile for 2 days

- Age < 8 consult physician (usually can use doxycycline for the treatment course needed in rickettsial infections)
- Macrolides (erythromycin or Zithromax (azithromycin) do not work

Babesiosis

Malarial like disease

- Diffuse weakness is hallmark of disease
- Fever and chills
- Nausea and vomiting
- Headache
- Cough
- Diarrhea
- Splenomegaly
- Jaundice
- Petechiae

Lab findings

- Hemolytic anemia
- Thrombocytopenia
- Elevated LFT's
- Organisms can be seen on a slide smear prep

Treatment

- Adults — Zithromax (azithromycin) 600 mg qday for 7–10 days plus Atovaquone 750 mg PO bid for 7–10 days
- Children — Zithromax (azithromycin) 12 mg/kg qday for 7–10 days plus Atovaquone 20 mg/kg PO bid for 7–10 days (do not exceed adult doses)

Ehrlichiosis

Symptoms and findings

- Appear toxic
- Fever, chills and rigors
- Headache
- Nausea and vomiting
- Rare maculopapular rash 5–10% of patients
- Arthralgias

Lab testing for

- Leukopenia
- Anemia
- Thrombocytopenia
- Elevated LFT's and creatinine

Treatment

- Adult: doxycycline 100 mg PO bid for 14 days
- Children > 45 kg: doxycycline 100 mg PO qday for 14 days
- Children < 45 kg: doxycycline 3 mg/kg PO qday for 14 days
- Age < 8 consult physician (usually can use doxycycline for the treatment course needed in rickettsial infections)

Discharge Criteria

- Mild disease in healthy patient
- Sanford Guide can be used

Discharge instructions

- Tick bite aftercare instructions
- Follow up with primary care provider within 1–2 days
- Return if symptoms worsens or rash develops

Consult Criteria

- Ill appearing patient
- Thrombocytopenia
- Hepatitis
- Splenectomy
- Immunocompromise
- Hemolytic anemia
- Significant comorbidities
- Refer to General Patient Criteria Protocol (page 20)

Notes

Lyme Disease Protocol

When using any protocol, always follow the Guidelines of Proper Use (page 16).

Definition

- Infection caused by the spirochete Borrelia burgdorferi

Differential Diagnosis

- Rocky Mountain spotted fever (RMSF)
- Babesiosis
- Relapsing fever
- Tularemia
- Ehrlichiosis
- Q-fever
- Colorado Tick fever
- Rheumatic fever
- Viral meningitis
- Septic arthritis
- Juvenile rheumatoid arthritis
- Brown recluse spider bite
- Fibromyalgia
- Reiter syndrome

Considerations

- Transmitted by bite of infected tick
- Most common tick infection in North America
- Peak April and November prevalence
- Transmitted by deer tick most commonly
- 1/3 of patients recall a tick bite
- Can cause hepatitis
- Ocular involvement — keratitis, iritis, optic neuritis
- No person-to-person transmission

Symptoms

Stage 1

Erythema migrans (EM)

- Is initial rash

- "Bull's eye" rash
- Macule with distinct red border that enlarges with central clearing
- Diameter > 5 cm
- Occurs in 90% of patients
- May be multiple in 10–20% of patients
- May have central induration, vesiculation or necrosis

Other symptoms/findings

- Headache
- Regional lymphadenopathy
- Myalgias
- Arthralgias
- Fatigue and malaise

Stage 2

- Days to weeks after tick bite
- Aseptic meningitis
- Cranial neuritis
- Radiculoneuritis
- Bell's palsy most common nerve involvement
- May present without rash
- Prognosis generally good

Cardiac

- Tachycardia
- Bradycardia
- AV block
- Myopericarditis

Stage 3

- Onset > 1 year after tick bite
- Acrodermatitis (resembles scleroderma)
- Arthritis
    - Brief attacks
    - Monoarthritis or oligoarthritis
    - Occasionally migratory
    - Most common joints: knee, shoulder, elbow

Evaluation

- CBC — leukocytosis, anemia, thrombocytopenia
- ESR > 30 seconds
- BMP
- LFT's
- Serology

Treatment

- Remove tick
- NSAID's prn
- ASA for cardiac involvement
- Vaccine (LYMErix) for prevention
- May use Sanford Guide
- Doxcycline 100 mg PO within 72 hours of a deer tick bite effective in preventing Lyme disease

Stage 1 choices

- Amoxicillin or doxycycline or cefuroxime for 21 days
- Zithromax (azithromycin) for 14–21 days

Stage 2 choices

- Amoxicillin with probenecid for 30 days
- Doxycycline for 10–21 days
- Consult physician

Stage 3

- Consult physician

Discharge Criteria

- Patients treated with oral therapy

Discharge instructions

- Tick bite aftercare instructions
- Follow up with primary care provider within 3–7 days
- Return if symptoms worsens

Consult Criteria

- Stage 2 or 3

- Immunocompromise
- Systemic symptoms
- Meningeal signs

Notes

Reference:

Nadelman RB, et. al. Prophylaxis with single-dose doxycycline for the prevention of Lyme disease after an *Ixodes Scapularis* tick bite *NEJM*July 12, 2001

Mayo Clin Proc, 4/10,e13

VARICELLA (CHICKEN POX) PROTOCOL

When using any protocol, always follow the Guidelines of Proper Use (page 16).

Definition

- Successive crops of pruritic vesicles evolving to pustules and crusts caused by varicella zoster virus primarily in childhood

Differential Diagnosis

- Herpes simplex infection
- Herpes zoster
- Impetigo
- Hand-Foot-Mouth disease
- Henoch-Schonlein Purpura
- Erythema multiforme
- Stevens-Johnson syndrome
- Toxic Epidermal Necrolysis
- Scabies
- Toxic shock syndrome

Considerations

- Fever and malaise may occur
- Primarily childhood disease
- Older patients may have more severe disease — pneumonia or encephalitis
- Transmission by airborne droplets or direct contact
- Infectious period is from first vesicle to when all vesicles are crusted
- Diagnosis is clinical
- "Dew drop" vesicle is initial finding
- Palms and soles spared
- Self-limiting

Treatment and Prevention

- Supportive

- Vaccination
- Antivirals may decrease duration of infection
- No aspirin (can cause Reyes syndrome)
- Antibiotic choices for secondary bacterial infection
    - Mupirocin topical for 5–10 days
    - Septra (trimethoprim/sulfamethoxazole)
    - Doxycycline
    - Clindamycin
    - Beta-lactams

Discharge Criteria

- Uncomplicated infection in children
- Trim nails

Discharge instructions

- Varicella aftercare instructions
- Return if systemic symptoms worse

Consult Criteria

- Encephalitis
- Altered mental status acutely
- Pregnancy
- Immunocompromise
- Systemic symptoms
- Moderate to severe secondary superinfection
- Adult infection

Notes

HAND INFECTION PROTOCOL

When using any protocol, always follow the Guidelines of Proper Use (page 16).

Definition

- Local inflammatory reaction of the skin and/or subcutaneous tissue of the hand secondary to bacteria or viral infection

Paronychia

Definition

- Cellulitis or abscess of nail margins and/or nail bed

Differential diagnosis

- Felon
- Draining osteomyelitis
- Herpetic whitlow
- Neoplasm

Considerations

- Secondary to trauma, nail biting, chemicals, incorrect nail trimming or chronic moist environment (dishwashers, bartenders, etc.)
- Acute infection: staph or strep
- Chronic infection: C. albicans or other fungi
- Vesicles suggest herpes infection
- Do not incise herpes infection (herpetic whitlow)

Evaluation

- CBC, BMP if signs of systemic infection present
- X-ray if chronic or recurrent to check for osteomyelitis

Treatment

No abscess

- Warm soaks and antibiotics

Subcuticular Abscess

- Local 1% plain lidocaine digital block (without epinephrine); may add 5% marcaine
- Elevate eponychial fold at the nail plate
- Incise at maximal swelling and tenderness to allow drainage
- If pus extends below nail, remove lateral ¼–½ of nail
- Give antibiotics for any associated cellulitis — MRSA coverage (see Soft Tissue Abscess Protocol) or Sanford Guide

Discharge criteria

- Noncomplicated paronychia without systemic symptoms/findings or bony involvement

Discharge instructions

- Paronychia aftercare instructions
- Refer to primary care provider or hand surgeon within 7–10 days as needed

Consult criteria

- Osteomyelitis
- Systemic symptoms/findings
- Associated proximal hand or tendon infection

Felon

Definition

- Infection/abscess of the pulp space of the distal finger

Differential diagnosis

- Paronychia
- Draining osteomyelitis
- Herpetic whitlow

Considerations

- Wooden splinters, minor cuts or diabetic testing methods are the common causes
- Paronychia spreading to pulp
- Staph aureus most common infection

- Can lead to osteomyelitis

Evaluation

- X-ray if osteomyelitis is suspected
- Neurovascular and tendon examination

Treatment

- Discuss with physician unless experienced
- Digital block with 1% plain lidocaine ± marcaine
- Lateral incision 5 mm distal to DIP joint on the dorsal 1/3 avoiding the neurovascular bundle, extending not past the distal nail corner
- Avoid incising the ulnar thumb side, and the radial side of index or middle finger to avoid a scar that interferes with pinching
- Pack with gauze
- Splint and elevate finger
- Cefazolin IV, then cephalexin or dicloxicillin PO × 10 days

Discharge instructions

- Felon aftercare instructions
- Follow up in 24 hours
- NSAID's or narcotic short course

Consult criteria

- Osteomyelitis
- Flexor tenosynovitis
- Systemic symptoms or findings

Herpetic Whitlow Protocol

Definition

- Herpes simplex infection of the digits manifested as painful grouped vesicles

Differential diagnosis

- Felon
- Paronychia
- Cellulitis

Considerations

- Patients usually less than 20 years of age
- Usually caused by HSV-1
- Do not incise

Treatment options

- Avoid contact with infected individuals
- Antiviral treatment within 48–72 hours

Antiviral medication choices

- Acyclovir ointment 5% 5 times a day for 5 days
- Acyclovir 400 mg PO qid × 7 days for severe infection
- Pediatric acyclovir oral dosing 15 mg/kg 5 times a day for 7 days (do not exceed adult doses)
- Valtrex (valacyclovir) 500–1000 mg PO bid × 7 days for adults

Discharge criteria

- Most patients without severe superinfection

Discharge instructions

- Herpetic whitlow aftercare instructions
- Follow up with PCP within 7–10 days

Consult criteria

- Moderate to severe superinfection
- Immunocompromise

Closed (Clenched) Fist Infection or Injury

Definition

- Laceration or skin injury from a clenched fist striking human teeth

Differential diagnosis

- Cellulitis
- Osteomyelitis
- Abscess

Considerations

- Assumed to be from human teeth
- High risk for infection
- All bite wounds with evidence of infection require physician consultation
- Usually over the MP dorsal joint

Evaluation

- Neurovascular and tendon examination
- X-ray
- CBC if fever present
- Assess for infection

Treatment

- No suturing of wound
- Irrigate with > 250 cc of 1% betadine with 18 gauge angiocath. (1% betadine: mix 1 cc of 10% betadine with 9 cc NS)
- If no infection present, and no neurovascular or tendon acute deficits or injuries, then prescribe Augmentin (amoxicillin/clavulanate) or follow Sanford Guide for prophylaxis treatment
- Pain treatment prn
- See Human and Animal Bite Protocol

Discharge criteria

- Noninfected wound
- No bony, tendon or neurovascular acute abnormality
- Reliable follow up

Discharge instructions

- Human bite aftercare instructions
- Return if infection occurs in bite
- Return if pain increases

Consult criteria

- Infected wound
- Bony, tendon or neurovascular acute abnormality
- Hand surgeon preferred if available

Deep Space Infection

- Consult physician

Flexor Tenosynovitis

Definition

- Infection or inflammation of the flexor tendon sheath

Differential diagnosis

- Noninfectious flexor tenosynovitis
- Fracture
- Septic joint
- Tendon rupture
- Gout
- Rheumatoid arthritis
- Endocarditis

Considerations

- Usually penetrating injury history to volar surface; frequently cat bites
- Kanavel's signs
    - Pain on passive extension
    - Finger held in flexed position
    - SEVERE tenderness along tendon sheath
    - Symmetric swelling (sausage finger)
    - May see with ultrasound using linear probe in water bath as dark fluid collections around tendon

Consult criteria

- All patients
- Admission
- Surgical treatment
- IV antibiotics

Notes

Hematology and Oncology

Section Contents — one protocol

Venous Thromboembolic Disease Protocol

Sickle Cell Anemia Protocol

Cancer Emergency Protocol

When using any protocol, always follow the Guidelines of Proper Use (page 16).

VENOUS THROMBOEMBOLIC DISEASE PROTOCOL

When using any protocol, always follow the Guidelines of Proper Use (page 16).

Definition

- Formation of thrombus within veins that may or may not propagate toward the central circulation

Differential diagnosis

- Cellulitis
- Hematoma
- Superficial thrombophlebitis
- Varicose veins
- Contusion or muscle strain/tear
- Arterial insufficiency
- Postphlebitic syndrome
- Dependent edema
- Lymphedema
- Baker's cyst

Considerations

- Deep vein thrombosis (DVT) and pulmonary embolism (PE) are manifestations of the same disease process
- DVT involves the legs most commonly, followed by the arms
- Early recognition and treatment are very important in decreasing morbidity and mortality
- Thrombus damages vein valves causing reflux of blood and postphlebitic syndrome — chronic edema and venous stasis ulcers
- Most DVT's develop complete or partial recanalization and collaterals over time
- Proximal large vein thrombosis can cause pulmonary embolism
- PE occurs in ~ 10% of DVT
- Calf DVT may produce 1/3 of PE
- Most DVT is occult and resolves spontaneously

- Up to 40% of DVT patients when diagnosed have a silent PE
- Paradoxic emboli may pass through an atrial septal defect and cause a CVA or distal arterial occlusion
- D-dimers remain elevated for 7 days after thrombus formation

Risk factors

- Cancer
- Advanced age
- Immobilization > 3 days
- Major surgery in the prior 4 weeks
- Clotting disorders are common risk factors for venous thromboembolism (VTE)
    - 5–10% of VTE is from protein C, protein S or antithrombin III disorders
    - Factor V Leiden mutation
- Most common risk factor is prior VTE
- CHF
- AMI
- CVA
- Sepsis
- Estrogens
- IV drug abuse
- Pregnancy and postpartum period
- Thrombocytosis and polycythemia vera

Virchow triad for formation of thrombus

- Venous stasis
- Activation of the coagulation system
- Vein damage

Goals of DVT treatment

- Reduce morbidity
- Prevent postphlebitic syndrome
- Prevent pulmonary embolism

Signs and symptoms

DVT

- Extremity pain

- Involved area red and swollen
- May be asymptomatic

Severe DVT

Phlegmasia alba dolens

- Blanched leg appearance
- Massive iliofemoral thrombotic occlusion

Phlegmasia cerulea dolens

- Follows phlegmasia alba dolens
- Associated with arterial spasm
- Risk of gangrene
- Shock may occur
- Mortality 20–40% if venous gangrene develops
- Notify or consult promptly a physician for phlegmasia of any type
- May be treated conservatively with heparin and elevation if no ischemia present

Pulmonary embolism

- Hypoxemia
- Chest pain
- Shock or hypotension
- May have no symptoms or findings

EKG

- Sinus tachycardia most common
- Nonspecific STT wave changes or with ischemic appearing biphasic T waves in V2 and V3
- New right bundle branch block
- S1Q3T3 pattern in 19%
- Right axis deviation in 5%
- Left axis deviation in 10%
- New onset atrial fibrillation
- EKG may be normal in 13%

Evaluation options

- Chest x-ray

- CBC if fever or tachycardia present
- BMP if diabetic or tachycardia present
- D-dimer (if negative with Well's criteria 0–1 makes PE unlikely)
- CT chest (see below)
- Apply Well's pulmonary embolism and DVT criteria and chart Well's score as indicated
- Extremity venous ultrasound for moderate to high probability Well's criteria as indicated
    - CT abdominal/pelvis scan for suspected intra-abdominal or pelvic DVT
- Record positive or negative calf tenderness and Homan's sign

Evaluation with D-dimer

D-dimer (LIA method) — some methods currently in use not reliable

- Useful if negative at cutoff value to rule out DVT or PE
- Negative D-dimer with low to moderate probability Well's DVT or PE score largely excludes venous thromboembolic disease
- Well's DVT criteria high probability: order ultrasound scan regardless of D-dimer result
- If positive — not as useful as a negative result which usually rules out VTE (venous thromboembolic) disease
- Frequently positive with
    - Hospitalization in past month
    - Chronic bedridden or low activity state
    - Increasingly positive with age without significant acute disease process
    - CHF
    - Chronic disease processes
    - Edematous states

Well's DVT criteria

- One point each:
    - Active cancer
    - Paralysis/recent cast immobilization
    - Recently bedridden > 3 days or surgery < 4 weeks

  - Deep vein tenderness
  - Entire leg edema
  - Calf swelling > 3 cm over other leg
  - Pitting edema > other calf
  - Collateral superficial veins
- Two points — alternative diagnosis less likely

High probability: ≥ 3 points

Moderate probability: 1–2 points

Low probability: 0 points

Well's PE criteria score 3 or greater consider D-dimer and CT chest PE protocol

- Suspected DVT = 3
- Alternative diagnosis less likely than PE = 3
- Heart rate > 100 = 1.5
- Immobilization/surgery past 4 wks. = 1.5
- Previous DVT/PE = 1.5
- Hemoptysis = 1
- Cancer past 6 months = 1

Well's score ≥ 6: order CTA chest PE protocol

Document positive or negative Homan's sign or calf tenderness regardless of Well's scores

Document PERC and/or Well's scores when appropriate

Pulmonary Embolism Rule-out Criteria (PERC Rule)

(Reportedly decreases significantly the likelihood of pulmonary embolism if all 8 criteria met)

- Age < 50
- Pulse oximetry > 94%
- Heart rate < 100
- No history of DVT or VTE
- No hemoptysis
- No estrogen use
- No unilateral leg swelling

- No recent surgery or trauma hospitalization past 4 weeks

Treatment options

DVT

May be treated as outpatient if none of the following present

- Pulmonary embolism
- Significant cardiopulmonary comorbidities
- Pregnancy
- Morbid obesity
- Homeless
- Creatinine > 2 mg/dL
- No follow up
- Inherited bleeding disorder
- Iliofemoral DVT
- Contraindications to anticoagulation
- Disorder of coagulation
- Patient does not want to be discharged

- Enoxaparin (Lovenox) 1 mg/kg SQ q12hr (1 mg/kg SQ q24hr if creatinine clearance<30 ml/minute)

OR

- Heparin (unfractionated) 80–100 U/kg IV loading dose and 15–18 U/kg/hour IV (keep PTT 2–2.5 times normal

OR

- Fondaparinux (Arixta) – no INR or PTT monitoring needed
    - < 50 kg: 5 mg SQ qday
    - 50–100 kg: 7.5 mg SQ qday
    - > 100 kg: 10 mg SQ qday

Stop all heparins if platelet count drops to 100,000, or a 50% decrease in baseline platelet count occurs, or 30% decrease in platelet count with new thrombus formation development (heparin induced thrombocytopenia) — a life threatening immune process

- Warfarin (Coumadin)

  - 2–10 mg PO qday to achieve INR 2–3
  - Treatment for 3–6 months
  - Can cause initially a transient hypercoagulable state if started without heparin treatment
  - Has a myriad of drug and other substances interactions
  - Can cause life threatening hemorrhage
  - Read drug information before using to determine interactions and patient risks
- Thrombin inhibitors
  - Argatroban for heparin-induced thrombocytopenia
- Thrombolytics
  - Use under direction of physician
  - For severe iliofemoral DVT (Phlegmasia cerulea dolens) — catheter directed
- Mechanical extraction
  - Consult vascular surgeon or interventional physician with appropriate skill set

Pulmonary embolism

- Same medication treatment as DVT
- Oxygen
- IV NS 500–1,000 bolus if hypotensive and notify physician promptly
  - Thrombolytics may be considered if PE caused hypotension is present

DVT prophylaxis

- Enoxaparin (Lovenox) 40 mg SQ q24hr

OR

- Heparin (unfractionated) 5,000 units SQ q8–12h

For admitted patients with any of the following

- Age > 60 years
- CHF
- Systemic infection
- History of DVT or PE
- Inflammatory disorders
- Cancer

    - ICU admission
    - Hypercoagulable state
    - Immobilization ≥ 3 days or severely compromised ambulation

Discharge criteria

- DVT not meeting exclusionary criteria above
    - Discuss with physician

Consult criteria

- All DVT and PE patients, or suspected DVT/PE diagnosis
    - Tachycardia
    - Hypotension or relative hypotension (SBP < 105 with history of hypertension)
    - Dyspnea

Notes

SICKLE CELL ANEMIA PROTOCOL

When using any protocol, always follow the Guidelines of Proper Use (page 16).

Definition

- Inherited disorder of hemoglobin synthesis causing sickling and destruction of RBC's with resulting vascular obstruction and tissue ischemia

Differential Diagnosis

- Appendicitis
- Cholecystitis
- Pneumonia
- Pulmonary embolism
- Acute myocardial infarction
- Priapism
- Anemia from other causes
- Hemorrhage
- Pancreatitis
- Osteomyelitis
- CVA
- Meningitis
- Hepatitis

Considerations

- Has increased incidence of life threatening infections
- Functional asplenia
- Chronic hemolysis
- Hand-foot syndrome — ages 6–24 months
- Aseptic necrosis of bone and osteomyelitis may occur
- Vascular occlusion pain most common presentation
- Stroke common
- Pulmonary embolism increased risk
- Mean survival: females 48 years; males 42 years from SS disease
- WBC elevated; platelet count elevated; reticulocyte count averages > 2–3%
- Precipitants

- Infection
- Cold exposure
- Dehydration

Crises types

Vaso–occlusive crises

- Bones
- Lungs (acute chest syndrome)
- Musculoskeletal pain most common complaint
- Abdominal pain 2nd most common complaint

Acute chest syndrome (ACS)

- Pulmonary infiltrates with one of the following:
    - Chest pain
    - Cough
    - Fever
    - Tachypnea
    - Wheezing
- Leading cause of death
- 50% of ACS cases develop in patients admitted for other sickle cell disease diagnoses

Aplastic Crises

- Severe anemia from cessation of erythropoiesis; can be related to parvovirus B19 infection
- Low reticulocyte count

Acute splenic sequestration crises

- Sudden hemoglobin decrease ≥ 2 gms
- Syncope
- Abdominal distension

Priapism

- Sickle cell patients may need exchange transfusion
- Consult physician and urologist immediately
- See Male Genitalia Protocol

Evaluation of sickle cell anemia

- Complete physical exam
- CBC
- BMP
- U/A
- Reticulocyte count (should be elevated)
- Chest x-ray
- ABG if significant dyspnea
- LFT's for abdominal pain
- Blood cultures if febrile
- O2 saturation measurement

History for

- Prior episodes
- Transfusion history
- Dyspnea
- Fever
- Cough
- Headache
- Neurologic deficits
- Previous hemoglobin level

Treatment Options

- D5½NS at maintenance rate if not hypotensive or hypovolemic — otherwise IV NS as needed for hypovolemia or hypotension
- Pain control
- Toradol (ketorolac) 10 mg PO or 30 mg IV prn (avoid IM)
  - Do not use Toradol (ketorolac) if creatinine is elevated

Narcotics IM or IV options prn

- Dilaudid (hydromorphone) 0.5–1 mg IV or 1–2 mg IM — may repeat × 2 prn
- Morphine 2–5 mg IV or 5–10 mg IM — may repeat × 2 prn
- Phenergan (promethazine) or Zofran (ondansetron) with narcotics
- Hydrocodone or oxycodone PO prn if discharged

- Supplemental oxygen if hypoxic or O2 saturation < 95%
- Albuterol aerosol if dyspneic without CHF
- IV 1/2NS or NS at 125–150 cc/hour or 150% maintenance
- Folic acid PO as outpatient if not already taking it

Exchange transfusion indicated for

- Significant cardiopulmonary decompensation
- Priapism
- Acute nervous system event

Transfusion indicated for

- Severe anemia (hemoglobin < 5 gms)
- Symptomatic anemia (consult physician)

Discharge Criteria

- Resolution of the painful crises to the satisfaction of provider and patient
- No indications for admission

Discharge instructions

- Sickle cell anemia aftercare instructions
- Return if pain persists or worsens
- Return if fever develops
- Follow up with PCP in 1–2 days

Consult Criteria

- Refractory pain crises
- Signs of bacterial infection
- Fever
- Acute chest syndrome
- Acute splenic sequestration crises
- Aplastic crises (reticulocyte count not elevated)
- CVA or TIA
- Refractory priapism
- Symptomatic anemia

Notes

CANCER EMERGENCY PROTOCOL

When using any protocol, always follow the Guidelines of Proper Use (page 16).

Definition

- Cancer conditions and treatments resulting in urgent and emergent symptoms and findings

Considerations

- There is an increase in the amount of cancer patients surviving longer
- Cancer is the second most common cause of death in the U.S.

3 most common categories of cancer emergencies

- Neutropenic fever (most common)
- Mechanical complications
- Metabolic derangements

Neutropenic fever

Definition

- WBC (white blood count) < 500 cells/μL
- WBC < 1000 cells/μL with anticipation of WBC < 500 cells/μL
- Temperature > 101°F (38.3°C) on one reading or 100.4°F (38.0°C) > 1 hour

Considerations for neutropenic fever

- May have minimal symptoms besides fever
    - Pneumonia patients may have no infiltrates on chest x-ray and or any cough
    - CT chest may be needed to make diagnosis
- UTI patients may not have much frequency, dysuria or pyuria
- Progression of symptoms may be rapid
- Staphylococcus aureus and coagulase negative staphylococcus are the most common pathogens

Evaluation

- CBC

- BMP
- Chest x-ray
- Blood cultures 5 minutes apart x 2
- Blood culture from any venous central catheters
- U/A
- Urine culture and sensitivity
- Lactic acid level if hypotensive or evidence of tissue hypoperfusion

Treatment

- Early empiric antibiotic monotherapy with
  - Ceftazidime 1 gm IV q8–12hr or cefepime 1 gm IV q12hr

    Or

  - Imipenem-cilastatin 500–1000 mg IV q6hr or meropenem 1 gm IV q6hr

<u>Add</u>

- Vancomycin 1 gm IV q12hr for the following
  - Suspected central catheter related infection
  - History of MRSA colonization
  - Preliminary blood culture growth of gram positive bacteria
  - Hypotension or cardiovascular compromise
- Neupogen (filgrastim) may be added per physician or oncologist
- Reverse isolation room if admitted and available

Discharge criteria

- Per physician consultation
- Most patients will be admitted

Consult criteria

- All febrile neutropenic patients
- Notify physician promptly if patient is hypotensive (or recent history of hypotension) or appears toxic, or signs/symptoms of hypoperfusion present

Mechanical cancer emergencies

- Spinal cord compression
- Superior vena cava syndrome
- Neoplastic cardiac tamponade
- Hyperviscosity syndrome
- Leukostasis

Spinal cord compression

Definition

- Compression of the spinal cord by tumor

Considerations

- Back pain with history of cancer is a Red Flag
- Patient outcomes improved with rapid detection
- Very important to consider this as a possible diagnosis

Symptoms and findings

- Back pain worsened by cough, worse at night or in supine position
- Numbness and paresthesia
- Loss of proprioception
- Bowel or bladder incontinence
- Bladder retention with overflow incontinence
- Decreased rectal tone
- New onset radicular pain on occasion may be caused by nerve root compression by tumor
- Back pain and tenderness may or may not be midline

Evaluation

- Complete history and physical exam with detailed neurologic and rectal tone exam
- MRI scan is preferred imaging modality
- CBC, BMP, U/A as indicated
- Plain spine films for vertebral lesions

Treatment

- Decadron (dexamethasone) 0.1 mg/kg IV when suspected or diagnosed
- Radiation therapy may be needed

Discharge criteria

- Per physician and/or oncologist

Consult criteria

- All suspected or diagnosed spinal cord compression patients to be discussed with physician or oncologist and neurosurgeon

Superior vena cava syndrome

Definition

- Obstruction of the superior vena cava

Considerations

- More of an urgency than emergency unless
    - Cerebral edema or laryngeal edema present

Common causes are

- Lung cancer
- Lymphoma
- Central line related DVT (deep vein thrombosis) of superior vena cava

Symptoms or findings

- May be vague
- Venous distension of neck, chest or upper extremities
- Facial or neck swelling
- Chronic cough
- Hoarseness
- Supine facial cyanosis (rare but pathognomonic)
- Dyspnea
- Fatigue
- Headache

Evaluation options

- Thorough history and physical exam
- CBC and BMP
- Chest x-ray
- CT scanning with contrast may be considered

Treatment options

- Elevate head of bed
- Radiation therapy
- Corticosteroid therapy with dexamethasone 0.1 mg/kg IV or IM (NMT 10 mg)
- Diuretic therapy
- Outpatient management

Discharge criteria

- No cerebral edema or airway impairments/ concerns

- Diagnosis firm

Discharge instructions

- Follow up with PCP or oncologist within 1–2 days
- Return if worsening symptoms

Consult criteria

- Discuss all patients with suspected or diagnosed superior vena cava syndrome with physician

Neoplastic cardiac tamponade

Definition

- Pericardial effusion with impairment of cardiac filling and function

Considerations

- May present with stable vital signs or hypotension
- Beck's triad of hypotension, muffled heart sounds and jugular venous distension may not present

Symptoms and findings (may or may not be present)

- Beck's triad
- Cardiomegaly on chest x-ray
- Low EKG voltage
- Dyspnea
- Pulsus paradoxus present up to 60% of patients (decrease in blood pressure > 10 mm Hg with inspiration — may be seen with COPD and asthma patients also)
- Volume depletion may mask findings
- Associated malignant pleural effusion may occur

Evaluation

- Chest x-ray
- CBC and BMP
- EKG
- Echocardiogram (diastolic collapse diagnostic)

Treatment

- Needle pericardiocentesis per physician
- Pericardial window per cardiothoracic surgeon

Consult criteria

- All suspected or diagnosed cardiac tamponade patients

Hyperviscosity syndrome

Definition

- Elevation of blood viscosity from increase in plasma proteins or blood component cells causing impaired circulation to tissues

Considerations

- Symptoms related to degree of hyperviscosity

Symptoms and findings (variable)

- Mental status changes (may be only manifestation)
- Unexplained dyspnea
- Headache
- Total serum protein minus albumin > 4
- Vision changes
- Somnolence
- Epistaxis
- Vertical nystagmus
- Hearing impairment
- Ataxia
- Retinal hemorrhages
- Paresthesias
- Congestive heart failure
- Low anion gap may be seen with multiple myeloma
    - Low anion gap may also be seen with lithium treatment or low serum albumin

Evaluation

- Serum viscosity measurement
- CBC and BMP
- Other tests as dictated by symptoms or findings

Treatment options

- Per physician

- Phlebotomy of 2–3 units of blood
- IV NS hydration

Consult criteria

- All suspected or diagnosed hyperviscosity syndrome patients

Leukostasis

Definition

- Tissue hypoperfusion secondary to elevated WBC

Considerations

- Seen with acute leukemias
- Typically seen when WBC > 100,000 cells/μL
- Can be seen with monoblastic leukemia of 25,000–50,000 cells/μL
- Watch out for tumor lysis syndrome with leukemia chemotherapy
    - Hyperkalemia
    - Hyperuricemia
    - Hyperphosphatemia
    - Renal failure

Evaluation

- CBC
- BMP
- Chest x-ray
- Uric acid needed for tumor lysis syndrome

Treatment

- Chemotherapy
- Tumor lysis syndrome treated with
    - Aggressive IV fluid hydration
    - Allopurinol 300 mg PO
    - Amphojel 30–60 cc PO for hyperphosphatemia
    - Hemodialysis
- Blood transfusion can cause hyperviscosity and rapid patient deterioration
- Supplemental oxygen for dyspnea or O2 saturation < 92%

Consult criteria

- All patients with leukostasis or tumor lysis syndrome

Metabolic emergencies

Syndrome of Inappropriate Antidiuretic Hormone Secretion (SIADH)

Definition

- Excess release of ADH (antidiuretic hormone) causing hyponatremia with water retention in euvolemic patient

Considerations

- Less than maximally dilute urine
- Urine sodium > 30
- Normal renal, adrenal and thyroid function
- Absence of diuretic therapy

Symptoms and findings

- Hyponatremia
- As in above **Considerations**
- Frequently chronic and stable
- Anorexia
- Weakness
- Confusion

Evaluation

- CBC
- BMP
- Urine sodium
- Chest x-ray

Treatment options

- Depends on degree of hyponatremia and associated symptoms or findings
- Demeclocycline 250 mg PO q6hr
- See Hyponatremia Protocol
    - Hypertonic saline 3% IV
    - Fluid restriction 500–1,000 cc of water per day
    - Be cautious of rapid hyponatremia correction

Consult criteria

- Discuss all suspected or diagnosed SIADH patients with a physician

Notes

Psychiatric and Social

Section Contents

Adult and Adolescent Psychiatric Protocol

Alcohol Intoxicated Patient Protocol

Withdrawal Protocol

Sexual Assault Protocol

Domestic Violence Protocol

Child Abuse Protocol

Elder Abuse Protocol

When using any protocol, always follow the Guidelines of Proper Use (page 16).

ADULT AND ADOLESCENT PSYCHIATRIC PROTOCOL

When using any protocol, always follow the Guidelines of Proper Use (page 16).

Considerations

- Suicide 9th leading cause of death
- Actively suicidal patient or patient dangerous to others is not competent to refuse evaluation and treatment, and may not depart from the department until psychiatrically and medically cleared by an evaluation to do so
- Patients with depression, substance abuse or schizophrenia are at higher risk of suicide
- Evaluation of medical causes of psychiatric symptoms important
- Evaluation for patient being dangerous to self or others very important

Restraints used when all interventions to reduce patient's dangerous behavior fail

- Placed without discussion or negotiation
- Carries risk of injury and death

Indications

- Prevent harm to patient or staff
- Prevent disruption of treatment
- Decrease stimulation of patient
- Honor patient's request for them to be applied to keep patient from harming themselves

Relative contraindications

- Delirium
- Dementia

General guidelines

- Team of at least 4 persons
- Leather restraints recommended
- Explain to patient need for restraints

- Staff member should be visible to patient at all times
- Placed so an IV is accessible
- Remove potentially dangerous objects from patient
- Raise patient's head to reduce aspiration
- Use verbal or chemical restraints after physical restraints placed if needed
- Check of circulation and limb swelling by nursing staff q15 minutes
- Remove restraints one at a time until 2 left, then last 2 together
- Never leave only one limb restrained
- Place in private area assessable and visible to staff
- Provide bedpan and nursing call light

Contraindications

- Organic brain syndrome
- Sepsis
- Cardiac illness
- Fever or hypothermia
- Metabolic disturbance
- Orthopedic problems

Restraints Time Rules

- Not to exceed 4 hours in adults
- Not to exceed 1 hour children < 9 years of age
- New order needed when time expires

Evaluation

- Directed by history and physical examination
- Routine lab tests are low yield and need not to be performed frequently unless indicated by history and physical exam
- Routine drug screens in alert, awake, and cooperative need not to be routinely performed
- Consider use of observation period to determine if psychiatric symptoms are from intoxication when substance abuse has occurred

Mental Status Examination

OMI HAT (OMI = organic disease; HAT = psychiatric or functional)

- O – Orientation
- M – Memory
- I – Intellect
- H – Hallucinations
- A – Affect disorder
- T – Thought disorder

Suicidal Ideation or Attempt

- All patients with significant psychiatric symptoms need to be asked about suicidal ideation or attempt
- Need acute psychiatric evaluation
- Cannot leave until cleared of acute suicide risk or a risk of danger to others
- Treat injuries or ingestions as per appropriate protocols

Thought Disorders

- Acute psychosis
- Brief reactive psychosis
- Schizophrenia
- Delusional

Acute psychosis

- Loss of contact with reality
- Hallucinations (usually auditory)
- Fixed delusions (a fixed false belief)
- Rule out organic conditions or drug causes

Treatment

- Treat any organic causes
- No acute treatment besides an outpatient referral if stable, chronic and not dangerous to self or others

Agitation treatment — alone or combination therapy (combination more effective)

- Lorazepam 2–4 mg IM or Versed 3–5 mg IM prn

- Haldol 5–10 mg (in elderly use 1–2 mg) IM or Droperidol 5 mg IM (works faster) prn (read droperidol's black box warning about fatal arrhythmias)
- Geodon (ziprasidone) 10–20 mg IM
- Cooperative patient — Lorazepam 4 mg PO with Risperdal (risperidone) 3 mg PO prn

Brief reactive psychosis

- Acute psychosis caused by a marked stressor
- One day to < 1 month
- Treatment same as acute psychosis

Schizophrenia (present for 6 months)

- Same as acute psychosis
- Disorganized speech and behavior, and a flat affect may be present

Treatment

- No acute medication therapy if not dangerous to self or other
- Outpatient antipsychotics and referral

Delusional disorder

- Non-bizarre delusions (jealousy or persecutory)
- Other schizophrenia symptoms not present
- Assess for organic brain syndrome
- Treatment as outpatient

Mood Disorders

Anxiety disorder

- Evaluate for organic cause
- Benzodiazepines useful if symptoms are severe
- Outpatient referral if not dangerous to self or others

Depression

- Evaluate for organic cause
- Consider antidepressant if symptoms are severe
- Outpatient referral if not dangerous to self or others and can care for self

Personality Disorder

- Outpatient referral if not dangerous to self or others and can care for self

Pain Management in Psychiatric Patients

- Treat with analgesics as indicated in limited amounts prn
- Antidepressants for chronic pain prn
- Pain clinic and psychiatric referral prn
- Refer to primary care provider prn

Discharge Criteria

- Cleared by psychiatric evaluation or provider medical evaluation
- Not dangerous to self or others
- Able to care for self or has support systems to care for self
- No suspected organic cause of psychiatric symptoms
- See General Patient Criteria Protocol (page 20)

Discharge instructions

- Respective psychiatric aftercare instructions
- Return if suicidal or homicidal

Consult Criteria

- Agitated patients requiring chemical or physical restraints
- Dangerous to self or others
- Cannot care for self and no support systems
- Organic causes of symptoms
- Delirium
- See General Patient Criteria Protocol (page 20)

Notes

ALCOHOL INTOXICATED PATIENT PROTOCOL

When using any protocol, always follow the Guidelines of Proper Use (page 16).

Definition

- Blood level over legal limit by State Statute, causing impairment of cognition or function

Differential Diagnosis

- Subdural hematoma
- CVA
- Coexisting intoxicating substances
- Meningitis
- Encephalitis
- Delirium
- Withdrawal syndromes
- Hepatic encephalopathy
- Postictal state

Considerations and comorbidities

- Alcohol metabolized around 20–30 mg% per hour
- Neurologic disorders
    - Altered mental status
    - Nystagmus
    - Pupillary dilation
    - Ataxia
- Minor head trauma from
    - Seizures
    - Falls
    - Altercations
    - Assaults
- Increased traumatic brain injury (coagulopathy common)
    - Intracerebral hemorrhage
    - Subdural hematoma
    - Epidural hematoma

- Embolic stroke
  - Atrial fibrillation
- Hemorrhagic stroke
- Alcohol related seizures
  - Withdrawal seizures
  - Usually single
  - Treat with Ativan 2–4 mg IV Q15–30 minutes prn
  - Occur within 6–12 hours of withdrawal
  - No other anticonvulsant treatment besides Ativan needed usually
  - May continue any existing seizure medication in addition to Ativan
- Increased infections
  - Altered immune system
  - Fever not uniformly present
  - WBC not necessarily increased
- Hypoglycemia
  - Alcoholic ketoacidosis
  - Mild lactic acidosis
- Thiamine deficiency
- Hypomagnesemia
  - Contributes to withdrawal symptoms
  - Can be present despite normal blood levels
- Rhabdomyolysis
  - Complication of chronic alcoholism and binge drinking
  - Impaired gluconeogenesis
  - Compartment syndrome incidence increased

Evaluation

- Complete history and physical examination
- BMP; Magnesium level prn
- Bedside glucose check if hypoglycemia suspected
- CBC — if infection suspected
- U/A — ketosis, infection or rhabdomyolysis if suspected
- CPK if rhabdomyolysis or compartment syndrome suspected
- Blood alcohol level

- LFT's if chronic alcoholic and mental status worse than expected from blood alcohol level
- CT head scan
  - Evidence of head trauma with:
    - Significant headache
    - Nausea
    - Vomiting
    - Evidence of skull fracture
    - Neurologic acute abnormalities
    - Altered mental status changes worse than expected from degree of alcohol intoxication
    - New onset seizure
- Chest x-ray
  - Fever
  - Respiratory finding or complaints
  - O2 saturation decreased from patient's baseline or < 94%
- Evaluation for other injuries or comorbidities as indicated

Osmolol gap > 10–20 suspect substance ingestion (Normal < 10)

- Gap = Osmolality measured – Osmolality calculated (calculation equation: 2(Na+K) + glucose/18 + BUN/2.8; normal 280–300mOsm/L)
- Ethanol mg%/4.6 is added to osmolol gap equation if present
- Gap > 50 carries high specificity for toxic alcohol such as methanol, ethylene glycol, or isopropyl alcohol
- Normal gap < 10

Treatment Options

- IV D5NS hydration as indicated
- Ativan IV for seizures
- Feed awake patient without acute neurologic deficits
- Thiamine 100 mg IM or slow IV
- MgSO4 (magnesium sulfate) 2 gms IM or IV unless in renal failure
- Appropriate antibiotic treatment

Discharge Criteria

- Clinically sober or blood alcohol < 300 and decreasing, and patient alert
- Unlikely to acutely decompensate
- Has support system

Discharge instructions

- Alcohol abuse aftercare instructions
- Follow up with PCP or local alcohol treatment center

Consult Criteria

- Fever
- Significant infectious process
- Acute neurologic deficits
- Acute imaging abnormalities
- Poor support system
- Hypoglycemia
- Acute hepatitis
- Mental status changes not attributable to intoxication
- Osmolol gap > 20 if checked
- Alcoholic ketoacidosis
- Metabolic acidosis
- Pneumonia
- Seizure
- Suicidal or dangerous to others
- Refer to General Patient Criteria Protocol (page 20)

Notes

WITHDRAWAL PROTOCOL

When using any protocol, always follow the Guidelines of Proper Use (page 16).

Definition

- Acute systemic manifestations of withdrawal from a substance to which the patient is addicted

Differential Diagnosis

- Subdural hematoma
- CVA
- Coexisting intoxicating substances
- Meningitis
- Encephalitis
- Delirium
- Withdrawal syndromes
- Hepatic encephalopathy
- Postictal state

Considerations for Ethanol Withdrawal

- Mild ethanol withdrawal resolves in 1–2 days
- Need to determine cause of altered mental status in alcoholic patients
- Determine degree of intoxication
- Seizures have increased occurrence
- Postictal state as a cause of altered mental state
- Infection risk increased
- Head trauma incidence increased
- Wernicke's encephalopathy may occur
- Hepatic encephalopathy from chronic alcoholism can be caused by upper gastrointestinal bleeding if hepatic cirrhosis present
- Fluid and electrolyte abnormalities increased incidence

Ethanol Withdrawal Signs and Symptoms

- Tachycardia
- Fever
- Hypertension

- Diaphoresis
- Tremor
- Anxiety
- Agitation
- Seizures
- Hallucinations
- Delirium tremens
- Each successive withdrawal occurrence can have more severe symptoms

Early withdrawal symptoms

- Occurs within hours after alcohol intake reduction
- Can occur without a total cessation of alcohol intake
- Headache
- Insomnia
- Vivid dreams
- Malaise
- Hand tremor
- Hallucinations

Ethanol related seizures

- Can occur from intoxication
- Can occur from ethanol withdrawal
- Lifetime risk is 5–10%
- Withdrawal seizures progress to delirium tremens 30% of the time
- May occur within 7 hours following decreased ethanol intake
- Ativan seizure prophylaxis may be given as 2–4 mg IV or IM
- Ativan is seizure treatment of choice: 2–6 mg IV prn (NMT 10 mg)
- Dilantin not effective
- Usually there is a single seizure; not focal usually

Delirium tremens

- Severe autonomic dysfunction plus delirium
- Rarely occurs before 48–72 hours of decreased ethanol intake

- Can start magnesium replacement in withdrawal patients with normal or low serum levels

Comorbidities

- Pneumonia
- Pancreatitis
- Hepatitis
- Hepatic cirrhosis
- Intracranial hemorrhage

Wernicke's encephalopathy

- Thiamine deficiency
- Confusion
- Oculomotor abnormalities
- Ataxia
- Korsakoff's psychosis has long term sequelae

Alcoholic ketoacidosis

- Can occur after binge drinking
- Free fatty acids metabolized from adipose tissue as a starvation ketosis
- Suppressed gluconeogenesis and insulin release occurs
- Usually occurs 24–72
- Beta-hydroxybutyrate is most common ketone which is not measured
  - Serum ketones may be minimal or negative
  - Acetone is the ketone that is measured in lab

Symptoms and findings

- Nausea and vomiting
- Abdominal pain
- Dehydration
- Confusion
- Tachycardia and tachypnea
- Arterial pH usually > 7.2

Evaluation Options

- Cardiac monitor and O2 saturation for moderate to severe withdrawal
- Complete history and physical examination

- BMP; magnesium level
- Bedside glucose check
- CBC
- U/A
- CPK
- Blood alcohol level
- LFT's
- CT head scan for
  - Evidence of head trauma with:
    - Headache
    - Nausea
    - Vomiting
    - Evidence of skull fracture
    - Neurologic acute abnormalities
    - New onset seizure
    - Acute altered mental status not attributed to withdrawal
- Chest x-ray
  - Fever
  - Respiratory finding or complaints
  - O2 saturation decreased from patient's baseline
- Evaluation for other injuries or comorbidities as indicated

Treatment Options

- IV D5NS hydration as indicated (rate 50–250 cc/hr) if not hypotensive
- IV NS 500–1000 bolus if hypotensive (notify physician immediately)
- Ativan 2–4 mg IV q 15–30 minutes prn for moderate to severe withdrawal symptoms or findings (monitor for respiratory depression)
- Feed awake patient without acute neurologic deficits besides intoxication
- Thiamine 100 mg IM or slow IV
- MgSO4 (magnesium sulfate) 2 gms IM or IV unless in renal failure
- Potassium as needed PO or IV
- Appropriate antibiotic treatment if infection present
- Avoid antipsychotic medications

Discharge Criteria

- Mild withdrawal
- Good social support
- Next day follow-up preferred
- Consider valium 10 mg qid taper by 25% every 2 days for 7–10 days of treatment

Discharge instructions

- Withdrawal aftercare instructions
- Return if withdrawal symptoms worsen
- Referral to addiction program

Consult Criteria

- Symptoms do not respond to 3 doses of benzodiazepines
- Moderate to severe withdrawal
- Alcoholic ketoacidosis
- Vomiting
- Delirium tremens
- Fever
- Pneumonia
- Significant infectious process
- Acute neurologic deficits
- Acute imaging abnormalities
- Poor acute support system
- Hypoglycemia
- Acute hepatitis
- Mental status changes not attributable to intoxication or withdrawal
- Osmolol gap > 20 if checked
- Metabolic acidosis
- Refer to General Patient Criteria Protocol (page 20)

Opioid Withdrawal

- Symptoms
    - Restlessness
    - Dilated pupils
    - Lacrimation
    - Nausea and vomiting

    - Abdominal cramps
    - Diarrhea
    - Muscle cramps
- Mental status remains normal
- Not life threatening except in neonates

Evaluation

- Complete history and physical examination
- CBC optional
- BMP optional
- U/A optional
- Other testing as indicated by history, examination or findings

Treatment Options

- Supportive
- Clonidine 0.1 mg q8hr for 3–10 days prn withdrawal if not hypotensive
- Consider lorazepam 1–2 mg PO q4–6h prn for 3–5 days
- Loperamide 2 mg PO tid prn diarrhea (NMT 6 qday)
- Rehydration if needed
- Inpatient treatment program if available and patient agreeable

Discharge Criteria

- Stable patient without significant comorbidities
- Support systems available

Discharge instructions

- Withdrawal aftercare instructions
- Return if withdrawal symptoms worsen
- Referral to addiction program

Consult Criteria

- Refer to General Patient Criteria Protocol (page 20)
- Suicidal ideation
- Significant comorbidities

Notes

SEXUAL ASSAULT PROTOCOL

When using any protocol, always follow the Guidelines of Proper Use (page 16).

Definition

- Defined as carnal knowledge of victim with force or threat against will of patient and varies state to state

Considerations

- Assess for nonsexual injuries
- 5–6% of victims are male
- Preexisting STD rate of victims are higher than the rate of what is acquired from the sexual assault
- Sexual assault exam and evidence collection is up to 72–96 hours post assault
- Notify police

Infection and pregnancy risks

- Gonorrhea: 4%
- Chlamydia: 1.5%
- Trichomonas: 12%
- Syphilis: 0.1%
- HIV: 0.1% if assailant HIV positive
- Pregnancy: 1–5%

Evaluation

- Be compassionate
- Evaluate for other injuries
- UCG or serum pregnancy tests in fertile female patients

History

- Date, time and location of event?
- Areas of body involved?
- Number of assailants?
- Is assailant known to victim?
- Weapons, threats, restraints and foreign bodies used?
- Type of sexual acts?

- Did ejaculation occur?
- Was condom used?
- What clean-up occurred by victim: shower, defecation, or douche?
- Were clothes changed?
- Conception prophylaxis used?
- Last menstrual period?
- Date of last consensual sexual intercourse?

Examination

- Performance of "rape kit" by provider or SANE personnel
- Activate SANE nurse program if available to perform "rape kit" and protocols
- Pelvic exam
- Rectal exam
- GC and chlamydial cultures
- RPR
- Hepatitis B testing
- Offer HIV testing
- X-rays as indicated by comorbid trauma
- Document trauma to genital and rectal areas, along with rest of body

Treatment Options

Sexual transmitted disease (STD) prophylaxis options

- Rocephin (ceftriaxone) 125 mg IM
- Flagyl (metronidazole) 2 gms PO × 1
- Zithromax (azithromycin) 1 gms PO × 1

  OR
- Doxycycline 100 mg PO bid × 7 days
- Offer hepatitis B vaccination if none previously; repeat in 1 and 6 months in no history of prior hepatitis B vaccination
- Offer HIV prophylaxis if assailant known positive HIV status or of moderate risk, or victim requests it

Pregnancy prophylaxis if patient agreeable

- Ovral 2 tablets PO now and 2 tablets PO in 12 hours

  OR

- Preven 2 tablets PO now and 2 tablets PO in 12 hours

- Offer sexual assault counseling by trained counselor

Discharge Criteria

- No comorbid conditions needing admission
- Safe home environment or shelter

Discharge instructions

- Sexual assault aftercare instructions
- Refer to primary care provider and counseling resources

Consult Criteria

- Comorbid conditions needing admission
- Refer to General Patient Criteria Protocol (page 20)

Notes

DOMESTIC VIOLENCE PROTOCOL

When using any protocol, always follow the Guidelines of Proper Use (page 16).

Definition

- Pattern of assaultive or coercive behaviors including physical, sexual, and/or psychological attacks

Considerations

- Intimate partner abuse (IPV) occurs not infrequently in pregnancy
- Economic coercion occurs
- Barriers exist to leaving a relationship — economic; religious; children
- Reported statistic of 7 attempts to leave before actually leaving
- IPV patients often present with injuries — frequently central body or defensive areas (arms and feet used for protection)
- History can be vague and evasive
- Can present with a STD from abuser
- Increased incidence of depression, anxiety and PTSD
- 60% increase in physical disorders
- 4–6 times increase in depression
- Children frequently abused also
- Most dangerous time for the abused is in disclosure of abuse and in attempting to leave relationship

Evaluation

- Evaluation for injuries
- Establish IPV diagnosis
- For emotional disorders

SAFE questions

S – Stress/safety: Do you feel safe in your relationship? What stress do you experience?

A – Afraid/abused: Have you or your children been abused? Have you ever felt afraid in your relationship?

F – Family: Does your family or friends know of your abuse? Can you tell them? Will they help?

E – Emergency plan: Do you have one? Do you have a safe place to go? Enough money available?

Treatment

- Provide safe environment
- Develop a safety plan
- Referral to abuse counseling and shelter
- Provide community IPV/domestic violence resources and contact numbers
- Do not prescribe sedatives (can interfere with ability to flee)

Discharge instructions

- Domestic abuse aftercare instructions

Consult Criteria

- Patients that need admission for injuries
- Patient that need admission for safety
- Suicidal or homicidal ideation
- Refer to Psychiatric Protocol
- Refer to General Patient Criteria Protocol (page 20)

Notes

CHILD ABUSE PROTOCOL

When using any protocol, always follow the Guidelines of Proper Use (page 16).

Definition

- Physical and/or psychological abuse of children, or neglect of children

Considerations

- Types of child abuse
  - Physical
  - Psychological
  - Sexual
  - Neglect
- Bruises most common abuse finding
- Bruises may be in various stages of healing
- Nonambulatory infants rarely bruise themselves
- Inflicted visceral injury usually is of hollow viscera
- Head injury most common cause of mortality
- More common where mother is also abused
- Mother's boyfriend who is not the father is common suspect
- Injuries with no plausible explanation

Head injury symptoms or finding in abused infants (increasing in seriousness)

- Extreme fussiness
- Inconsolable crying
- Irritability
- Lethargy
- Hypotonia
- Poor feeding
- Vomiting
- Tachypnea
- Bradycardia
- Hypothermia
- Seizures
- Gaze preferences

- Unequal pupils
- Unreactive pupils
- Stupor
- Coma
- Death

Shaken baby syndrome

- Usually < 1 year of age
- Retinal hemorrhages commonly present

Triad — some or all may be present

- Subdural or subarachnoid hemorrhage
- Cerebral edema
- Retinal hemorrhages

CT head scan best diagnostic approach for brain injury

Fractures with higher abuse association

- Posterior rib fractures
- Metaphyseal fractures
- Bilateral or multiple fractures
- Multiple fractures in various stages of healing
- Digit fractures
- Scapular fractures
- Complex skull fractures

Evaluation

- Maintain high index of suspicion
- Is directed toward injuries
- CBC
- U/A
- LFT's
- Skeletal survey
- CT head if suspected head or brain injury

Treatment

- Aimed at injuries
- Child protection actions

Disposition

- Discuss with physician
- Contact Child Protective Services or DHS if abuse diagnosed or suspected
- Do not discharge patient until cleared to do so by physician
- Admission if patient safety is in question
- Report to police if crime occurred
- Contact primary care physician to discuss case for similar previous concerns and if discharged to arrange close follow up

Notes

ELDER ABUSE PROTOCOL

When using any protocol, always follow the Guidelines of Proper Use (page 16).

Definition

- Pattern of assaultive or coercive behaviors including physical, sexual, psychological attacks

Considerations

- 3% of elderly have been abused
- Increased incidence of cognitive impairment

Signs may include

- Injuries in various stages of healing
- Unexplained injuries
- Delay in seeking treatment
- Injuries inconsistent with history
- Contradictory explanations given by the patient and caregiver
- Laboratory findings indicating under dosage or over dosage of medications
- Bruises, welts, lacerations, rope marks, burns
- STD's
- Dehydration, malnutrition, decubitus ulcers, poor hygiene
- Signs of withdrawal, depression, agitation, or infantile behavior
- Abuser may not leave Provider alone with patient
- Abuser more concerned about medical bill
- Abuser displays anger or indifference toward patient

Evaluation

- High index of suspicion
- Complete history and physical exam
- Pelvic exam for STD (may need "rape kit")
- Aimed at injuries and home situation
- CBC prn
- BMP prn

- U/A prn
- Drug levels of medications prn
- UDS (urine drug screen) prn
- Blood alcohol prn
- Relevant x-rays
- CT head, abdomen or chest as indicated

Treatment

- Directed toward injuries and comorbidities
- Protection of patient

Disposition

- Discuss with physician
- Contact DHS if abuse diagnosed or suspected
- Do not discharge patient until cleared to do so by physician
- Admission if patient safety is in question
- Report to police if crime occurred

Notes

Environmental

Section Contents

Heat Illness Protocol

Hypothermia Protocol

Frostbite and Exposure Skin Injury Protocol

Altitude Illness Protocol

Near Drowning Protocol

When using any protocol, always follow the Guidelines of Proper Use (page 16).

HEAT ILLNESS PROTOCOL

When using any protocol, always follow the Guidelines of Proper Use (page 16).

Definition

- Heat induced metabolic derangements with possible tissue injury

Differential Diagnosis

- Meningitis
- Encephalitis
- Serotonin syndrome
- Thyroid storm
- Thyrotoxicosis
- Sepsis
- Septic shock
- Neuroleptic malignant syndrome
- Tetanus
- Delirium
- Delirium tremens
- Heat stroke
- Infection in elderly without sepsis
- Malignant hyperthermia
- Intracerebral hemorrhage
- CVA
- Drugs

Considerations

- Normal temperature range is 97°F–100.4°F or 36.1°C–38°C

Excessive heat causes damage to multiple organ systems

- Heart
- Liver
- Kidneys
- Lungs
- Muscles

- Central nervous system

Heat regulation mainly by

- Radiation
- Evaporation
- Conduction
- Convection

Risk Factors for Heat illness

Age

- Elderly
- Neonates

Medical Illness

- Alcoholism
- Hyperthyroidism
- Obesity

Medications

- Anticholinergics
- Beta-blockers
- Diuretics
- MOA inhibitors
- Phenothiazines
- Tricyclic antidepressants

Illicit drugs

- Amphetamines
- Cocaine

Social

- Bedridden
- Living alone
- Lack of air conditioning
- Unable to care for self

Mild Forms of Heat illness

Heat edema

- Swollen hands and feet after prolonged sitting/standing in hot temperatures

Heat rash ("prickly heat")

- Sweat glands become blocked

Heat cramps

- Electrolyte imbalance; volume depletion; hyperventilation
- May be hyponatremic and hypochloremic
- No rhabdomyolysis

Heat tetany

- Carpopedal spasm from hyperventilation secondary to hyperthermia

Heat syncope

- Benign syncope from prolonged standing in hot environment

Severe Forms of Heat illness

Heat exhaustion

- Water or salt depletion
- Fatigue
- Weakness
- Hyperventilation
- Headache
- Dizziness
- Vertigo
- Nausea
- Vomiting
- Muscle cramps
- No CNS dysfunction
- Temperature usually < 104°F (40°C)
- Sweating present

Heat stroke

- Hyperthermia with CNS dysfunction:
    - Confusion
    - Delirium
    - Ataxia
    - Seizures
    - Coma
- Temperature usually > 104°F (40°C)
- May or may not have sweating present
- Mortality 30–80%
- Fatigue
- Weakness
- Hyperventilation
- Headache
- Dizziness
- Vertigo
- Nausea
- Vomiting
- Muscle cramps
- Rhabdomyolysis
- Compartment syndrome
- Multi-organ dysfunction
- Lactic acidosis

Evaluation

Heat illness excluding heat stroke

- CBC prn
- BMP prn
- U/A in elderly; diabetics; immunocompromised

Heat stroke

- CBC
- BMP
- LFT's
- Lactic acid level
- CPK
- Chest x-ray
- EKG

Treatment

Mild forms of heat illness

- Oral or IV rehydration and sodium replacement

Heat exhaustion

- Remove from hot environment
- No antipyretic medication (may impair heat dissipation)

Rapid cooling as needed

- Remove clothing
- Ice packs to axilla, groin and/or behind neck all prn
- Spray with tepid water and fanned prn
- IV NS rehydration prn

Heat stroke

- Remove from hot environment
- No antipyretic medication (may impair heat dissipation)
- Place foley

Rapid cooling

- Remove clothing
- Ice packs to axilla; groin; behind neck
- Spray with tepid water and fanned
- Ativan or valium to control shivering, treat seizures and sedate patient prn
- IV NS rehydration
    - NS 500 cc bolus if hypotensive in adults
    - NS 20 cc/kg bolus if hypotensive in children
        - Avoid too rapid IV NS replacement — may cause cerebral edema (free water deficit corrected over 48 hours)
    - Water deficit in liters = Total body water [0.6 × Kg] – Total body water [desired Na+ / measured Na+] (For hypernatremic patients)

Discharge Criteria

- All heat illness patients without heat stroke or severe heat exhaustion with good response to therapy
- Not hypotensive
- Refer to General Patient Criteria Protocol

Discharge instructions

- Heat illness aftercare instructions
- Return if symptoms worsen

Consult Criteria

- Heat stroke
- Severe heat exhaustion
- Significant electrolyte disturbances
- Refer to General Patient Criteria Protocol (page 20)
- Age ≥ 70 years

Notes

HYPOTHERMIA PROTOCOL

When using any protocol, always follow the Guidelines of Proper Use (page 16).

Definition

- Pathologic state in which core body temperature falls below 35°C (95°F)

Differential Diagnosis

- Cerebrovascular accident
- Toxicity
- Alcohols
- Barbiturates
- Benzodiazepines
- Carbon monoxide
- Narcotics
- Ethylene glycol
- Gamma-hydroxybutyrate
- Sedative hypnotics

Considerations

- Core temperature regulated in thermoneutral zone of 36.5°C and 37.5°C (97.7°F and 99.5°F)
- Heat production a function of metabolism
- Hypothermia affects all organ systems
- Afterdrop in core temperature can occur after rewarming started due to peripheral cold blood return perfusing the body
- Most hypothermia patients will by dehydrated

Heat loss occurs by

- Radiation – most rapid (50% of heat loss)
- Conduction
- Convection
- Evaporation

Hypothermia severity

- Mild = 32–35°C or 89.6–95°F

- Moderate = 28–32°C or 82.4–89.6°F
- Severe = 20–28°C or 68–82.4°F
- Profound < 20°C or 68°F

Risk Factors

- Burns
- Environmental cold exposure or immersion
- Toxicological causes
- Extremes of age
- Hypoadrenalism
- Hypothyroidism
- Hypoglycemia
- Hypopituitarism
- Malnutrition
- Spinal cord injury
- Sepsis
- Uremia

Findings as Temperatures Decrease

Mild hypothermia progression

- Shivering, impaired judgment, confusion
- Tachycardia, tachypnea, cold diuresis
- Bradycardia, respiratory depression, hyperglycemia, ataxia, dysarthria

Moderate hypothermia progression

- Stupor, lethargy, arrest of shivering
- Atrial arrhythmias, Osborn J-waves on EKG (upward deflection of terminal S wave), increased bradycardia
- Insulin ineffective, decreased oxygen utilization
- Progressive decreased level of consciousness, bradycardia, respiratory rate

Severe hypothermia progression

- Ventricular fibrillation susceptibility increased
- Pulse decreased by 50%
- Oxygen consumption decreased by 50%
- Loss of reflexes and voluntary movement
- Acid-base abnormalities

- No pain response
- Decreased cerebral perfusion by 2/3
- Pulmonary edema
- Apnea
- Hypotension

Profound hypothermia progression

- Lowest level for resumption of cardiac activity, pulse 20% of normal
- Asystole

Evaluation

- Complete history and physical examination (auscultate up to 45 seconds if needed)
- CBC
- BMP
- Chest x-ray
- EKG
- ABG (temperature correction not needed)
- PT/PTT/INR (coagulation panel)
- CPK
- Blood alcohol and toxicology panel as indicated
- Cardiac, oxygen saturation and vital sign monitoring

Treatment Considerations and Options

- IV fluid resuscitation as needed with NS or D5NS (avoid lactated ringer's solution)
    - Do not give D5 IV containing fluids as a bolus (too high tonicity)
- Immunocompromised patients should receive empiric antibiotics
- Intubation as needed
- NG tube if intubated
- Most cardiac dysrhythmias correct with rewarming alone
- Malignant ventricular dysrhythmias use amiodarone (avoid lidocaine and procainamide)
- Defibrillation likely ineffective with core temperature < 30°C (86°F)

Passive rewarming

- Increases temperature 0.3–1.2°C/hour
- For mild hypothermia where shivering is present and patient is healthy
- No external heat added
- Patient covered with blankets
- Remove wet garments
- Cover patient's head except face

Active external rewarming

- Increases temperature 0.3–1.2°C/hour
- For mild hypothermia with impaired thermogenesis due to illness, intoxication, medications or comorbidities
- For moderate hypothermia
- Forced warmed air systems used
- Warmed blankets
- Heat packs
- Heat lamps

Active core rewarming

- Increases temperature approximately 3°C/hour
- For severe hypothermia
- Warmed IV fluids (44°C or 111°F) — may be warmed for 1 liter for approximately 2 minutes in microwave
- Warmed humidified air or oxygen in addition to passive and active external rewarming

Extracorporeal rewarming

- Increases temperature approximately 1–18°C/hour
- Indicated for severe or profound hypothermia
- Hypothermia unresponsive to other rewarming methods
- Completely frozen extremities
- For no signs of perfusion
- Hemodialysis (can increase temperature 1–4°C/hour)
- Cardiopulmonary bypass (can increase temperature 18°C/hour)

Discharge Criteria

- Mild hypothermia that responds to passive rewarming in healthy patient

Discharge instructions

- Hypothermia aftercare instructions

Consult Criteria

- Discuss all hypothermia patients with physician

Admission Criteria

- Hypothermia < 32°C or 89.6°F

Notes

Frostbite and Exposure Skin Injury Protocol

When using any protocol, always follow the Guidelines of Proper Use (page 16).

Definition

- Cold related injury or death of tissue from freezing secondary to prolonged cold exposure

Differential Diagnosis

- Hypothermia
- Frostnip
- Trench foot
- Pernio
- Chilblains (3–6 hours of cold moist exposure without freezing)

Frostbite

Considerations

- Extremities, head, and nose most commonly affected
- Initial appearance of injury often fails to predict depth or eventual outcome

Degrees of Injury

First-degree injury

- Erythema, edema, waxy appearance, hard white plaques, and loss of sensation

Second-degree injury

- Erythema, edema, and formation of blisters filled with clear or milky fluid
- Form within 24 hours of injury

Third-degree injury

- Blood-filled blisters
- Progressing to a black eschar in several weeks

Fourth-degree injury

- Full-thickness damage affecting muscles, tendons, and bone, with necrosis of tissue

Evaluation

- Assess for hypothermia
- No lab needed in mild cases
- Assess for severe frostbite
  - CBC
  - BMP
  - U/A for evidence of myoglobin
  - CPK
  - Cultures if infection suspected
  - Technetium-99 scintigraphy 2–7 days after injury is helpful in decision making about amputation

Treatment

- Remove wet clothing
- Ibuprofen 400 mg PO prior to rewarming to improve tissue salvage
- Protect from refreezing
- Rapid rewarming for more severe cases
- Put affected area in warm water (40–42°C or 104–108°F) for 20–30 minutes
- Elevate extremity after rewarming
- Separate damaged digits with dry gauze
- Apply aloe vera (without alcohol, salicylates or other additives) after thawing
  - May be used for debridement also
- Tetanus prophylaxis (see Tetanus Protocol, page 580)
- Antibiotics not indicated unless infection present
- Liberal use of analgesics up to 7–10 days
- Leave hemorrhagic blisters intact
- Debride clear fluid filled blisters
- Physical therapy post discharge or admission
- Avoid massaging frostbite area (may increase injury)
- Splinting prn

Discharge Criteria

- First degree injury

Discharge instructions

- Frostbite aftercare instructions

Consult Criteria

- Second, third and fourth degree frostbite injuries

Admission Criteria

- Greater than first degree frostbite
- Risk of refreezing exists

Non-freezing Environmental Injuries

Trench foot

- Non-freezing injury from prolonged exposure to cold, wet environment
- May cause gangrene
- Rewarm in water if needed
- Elevate to reduce edema
- Keep warm and dry
- Ibuprofen prn
- Tetanus prophylaxis (see Tetanus Protocol, page 580)

Pernio

- 12-hour to 3-day exposure to cold moist environment without freezing
- Scaling skin and edema
- Cyanotic and red skin lesions
    - Occasionally deep seated
- Use protective clothing for prevention and emollient creams for treatment
- Tetanus prophylaxis (see Tetanus Protocol, page 580)

Chilblains

- 3–6 hours of cold moist exposure without freezing
- Chronic form from recurrent Pernio
- Swelling, tender SQ vesicles with or without bluish discoloration

- Hemorrhagic bullae and skin ulcers in severe cases
- Gently rewarm, dress with dry protective bandages
- Tetanus prophylaxis (see Tetanus Protocol, page 580)

Frostnip

- Superficial and reversible ice crystal formation without tissue destruction
- Transient numbness and paresthesia that resolves after rewarming

Disposition

- Discuss with physician trench foot, Pernio and chilblains patients

Discharge instructions

- Respective cold or moisture environment aftercare instructions

Notes

ALTITUDE ILLNESS PROTOCOL

When using any protocol, always follow the Guidelines of Proper Use (page 16).

Definition

- Syndromes resulting from lack of oxygen

Differential Diagnosis

- Anxiety
- Encephalitis
- Diabetic ketoacidosis
- Meningitis
- Migraine
- Hyponatremia
- Hypoglycemia
- Hypothermia
- Cerebrovascular accident
- Transient ischemic attack
- Transient global amnesia
- Subarachnoid hemorrhage
- Subdural hemorrhage
- Carbon monoxide poisoning
- Reyes syndrome
- Nonspecific headache
- Brain tumors
- Dehydration
- Viral syndrome

Syndromes

- Acute mountain sickness (AMS)
- High-altitude cerebral edema (HAPE)
- High-altitude pulmonary edema (HACE)

Considerations

Hypoxia is primary insult

- Degree of injury dependent on rate of hypoxia onset and magnitude

- Increase minute ventilation occurs acutely with a resultant respiratory alkalosis
- Renal compensation to respiratory alkalosis occurs more slowly than compensation to respiratory acidosis
- Increased cerebral perfusion occurs
- Symptoms occur 4–10 hours after ascent
- Incidence affected by sleeping altitude
- Physical fitness not protective
- Occurs more commonly in age < 50 years

Acute Mountain Sickness (AMS)

Definition

Headache plus one of following:

- Nausea/vomiting
- Fatigue
- Dizziness
- Insomnia

Considerations

- Mild form of high altitude illness
- Generally benign
- Occurs around 6,000 feet altitude or higher with incidence of 10–40%, increasing as altitude increases
- Usually self-limited and improves over 1–3 days if no further ascent untaken
- Continued ascent will worsen AMS and can result in HACE
- O2 saturation not helpful in diagnosing or managing AMS or HACE

Findings and symptoms

- Patients appear ill
- Normal neurologic examination
- Heart rate and blood pressure can vary
- May have rales, but oxygen saturation normal or near normal
- Fever is absent
- May have retinal hemorrhages

- Peripheral edema may be present

Treatment options

- Halt ascent
- Acetazolamide 250 mg PO q12hr
  - Prophylaxis — 125 mg PO q12hr starting 24 hours before ascent and continuing during ascent to at least 48 hours after arrival at highest altitude (or descent)
- Dexamethasone 4 mg PO/IM q6hr for 2 doses
- Ibuprofen or Tylenol for headache
- Phenergan (promethazine) prn for nausea
- Oxygen for more severe cases (4L/min to keep O2 saturation > 92%)
- Descent for more severe symptoms

Discharge criteria

- Usually discharged

Discharge instructions

- Acute mountain sickness aftercare instructions

Consult criteria

- Discuss high altitude illness with physician

High-altitude Cerebral Edema (HACE)

Definition

- Acute Mountain Sickness with gait ataxia and altered mental status

Considerations

- Usually normal exam except for gait ataxia
- Focal neurologic deficits rare
- Continued ascent with AMS can lead to HACE
- Papilledema can occur
- Retinal hemorrhages occur
- Coma can occur

Evaluation options

- CBC

- BMP
- ABG
- CT brain
- MRI brain

Treatment

- Immediate evacuation to lower altitude
- Oxygen 4L/min to keep O2 saturation > 92%
- Dexamethasone 8 mg PO/IM, followed by 4 mg PO/IM q6hr
- Elevate head of bed 30 degrees

Discharge criteria

- Dependent on severity

Discharge instructions

- High-altitude cerebral edema aftercare instructions if discharged

Consult criteria

- Discuss with physician

High-altitude Pulmonary Edema

Definition

- Noncardiogenic pulmonary edema from increased capillary hydrostatic pressure and pulmonary hypertension

Considerations

- Exercise at high altitude increases risk
- Fever common
- Orthopnea common
- Frothy pink sputum is a late finding
- Cyanosis can occur
- May occur with HACE

History and physical examination criteria

2 of the following:

- Weakness or decreased exercise tolerance
- Cough
- Dyspnea at rest

- Chest tightness or congestion
  PLUS

2 of the following:

- Rales or wheezing
- Central cyanosis or O2 saturation is lower than expected from elevation
- Tachycardia
- Tachypnea

Evaluation

- Chest x-ray
- Ultrasound shows comet tails
- CBC
- BMP
- BNP
- EKG
- Troponin

Treatment options

- Oxygen 6–8 liters by mask until improved then 4L/min to keep O2 saturation > 92%
- Albuterol aerosol prn
- Immediate descent
- Bed rest
- Nifedipine 10 mg PO q6hr if oxygen not available and not hypotensive
- Cialis (tadalafil) 10 mg bid to decrease pulmonary hypertension
- Dexamethasone 8–10 mg PO/IM/IV initially then 4 mg PO/IM/IV q4hr
- Narcotic or non-narcotic cough suppressants prn
- Phenergan (promethazine) prn nausea or vomiting, and may increase respiratory stimulation

Discharge criteria

- Normal O2 saturation (≥ 95%) breathing room air
- Significant clinical improvement
- No dyspnea at rest

Discharge instructions

- High-altitude Pulmonary Edema aftercare instructions

Admission criteria

- O2 saturation < 95%
- Dyspnea at rest
- Inability to descend

Consult criteria

- Discuss all HAPE and high altitude illness patients with physician

Notes

NEAR DROWNING PROTOCOL

When using any protocol, always follow the Guidelines of Proper Use (page 16).

Definition

- Survival from a submersion occurring within the past 24 hours of sufficient submersion duration to warrant medical attention or survival beyond 24 hours of a submersion

Differential Diagnosis

- Child abuse
- Child neglect
- Suicide attempt
- Hypothermia
- Seizure
- Drug or toxin ingestion
- Hypoglycemia
- Head and neck trauma

Considerations

- Classified either cold water (< 20°C or 68°F) or warm water (≥ 20°C or 68°F) injury
- Very cold water injury is with water temperature ≤ 5°C (41°F)
- Most patients have an aspiration of water < 4 cc/kg
- Blood imbalances occur with aspiration > 11 cc/kg
- Electrolyte imbalances occur with aspiration > 22 cc/kg
- PO ingestion more likely to cause electrolyte imbalances
- Primary injury is hypoxemia
- Survival mainly determined by amount of brain hypoxemia and injury
- Laryngospasm can prevent aspiration
- Heimlich maneuver not effective in removing aspiration water
- Differences between freshwater and salt water submersions not clinically significant

Orlowski score 1 point for each item

- Age 3 years or older
- Submersion time of more than 5 minutes
- No resuscitative efforts for more than 10 minutes after rescue
- Comatose on admission to the emergency department
- Arterial pH of less than 7.10
- Score of 2 or less = 90% complete recovery
- Score of 3 or more = 5% survival

History of event includes

- Submersion time
- Water temperature
- Symptoms
- Associated injuries
- Type of rescue
- Response to treatment
- Cough or shortness of breath
- Concomitant drug or alcohol use
- Past medical history (seizures, cardiac, diabetes, etc.)

Physical findings categories

- Asymptomatic
- Symptomatic
  - Abnormal vital signs
  - Dyspnea
  - Neurologic deficit
  - Altered level of consciousness
  - Anxiety
- Cardiopulmonary arrest
- Dead

Evaluation Options Depending on Severity of Presentation

- Chest x-ray – all patients
- O2 saturation – all patients
- ABG
- CBC

- BMP
- LFT's
- U/A
- PT/PTT/INR
- Fibrinogen, D-dimer, fibrin split products
- Troponin useful in severe presentations for prognosis
- Toxicology as indicated
- C-spine imaging as indicated
- CT head as indicated for trauma or altered mental status
- Evaluate for associated injuries
- Core temperature
- Cardiac and O2 saturation continuous monitoring prn

Treatment Options

- Notify physician immediately for altered mental status, neurologic abnormalities, hypoxia or hypotension
- Oxygen up to 100% FiO2 depending on symptoms and findings
- Correct any hypothermia (see Hypothermia Protocol)
- IV NS prn hypotension
- Vasopressors prn hypotension
- Intubation prn severe respiratory distress
- Steroids are of no benefit
- Hypothermia patients should be resuscitated while aggressive attempts to restore normal body temperature ensue
- Antibiotics can be given for submersion in sewage or contaminated water

Discharge Criteria

- Patients with normal examination, normal vital signs and normal chest x-ray and lab, and trivial history may be discharged after 6 hours observation
- Immersion history with mild symptoms, normal lab and chest x-ray, may be discharged after 6–12 hours of observation

Discharge instructions

- Near drowning aftercare instructions

- All discharged patients should be rechecked in 24–48 hours
- Return or see primary care provider promptly if cough, fever or shortness of breath occurs

Admission Criteria

- Hypoxia
- Acute neurologic findings
- Symptomatic patients
- Acute chest x-ray findings
- Prolonged submersion history

Consult Criteria

- Discuss all near drowning patients with physician

Notes

Medications

Section Contents

Pain Management Protocol

Drug Interactions

When using any protocol, always follow the Guidelines of Proper Use (page 16).

PAIN MANAGEMENT PROTOCOL

When using any protocol, always follow the Guidelines of Proper Use (page 16).

Considerations

- Pain is the most frequent complaint for seeking care in the emergency department or acute care settings
- Many studies have demonstrated the under-treatment of pain by Providers
- Abuse of prescription narcotics has increased in the recent past
- Under-treatment of pain can lead to pseudoaddiction — a condition where the patient actively seeks over time pain control
  - This is frequently perceived by Providers as drug seeking behavior
- JCAHO has standards regarding pain assessment and the right of the patient to adequate control of pain
  - This can cause the perception that the policy contributes to abuse of narcotic prescriptions
- Chronic pain is not managed well in the acute care settings
- Degree of chronic pain is not always reflected in the Provider's observation of the patient's degree of discomfort or in abnormal vital signs
  - Acute pain is reflected more so in patient's signs of discomfort and abnormal vital signs

Evaluation

- Urine and serum drug screens are not particular routinely useful in evaluating patients
  - Drug screens may be useful if patient states they have not used controlled substances for the past 10 days to determine patient truthfulness
  - Drug screens may be useful if patient states they are taking prescription narcotics currently and the drug screen is negative, perhaps indicating that they are selling the narcotics
- If a pattern of abuse is suspected, check controlled substance prescription databases where available

- Take a history of pain treatment
- Patients who request a specific controlled substance may be more suspect for abuse behavior

Treatment Options

- Patients with chronic pain that come to the emergency department or urgent care setting should be tactfully informed that chronic pain is best managed long term by one Provider in the clinic setting
- If the Provider assesses a reasonable need to prescribe controlled pain medications, it should be of a short course and limited number of pills (≤ 20) without refills usually
    - Exceptions are situations where a terminal cancer patient or other similar type patients with significant pain considerations that will have a delay in treatment in the outpatient office setting
- Pain amenable to local injections, such as dental pain etc., in patients with frequent repeat visits, can be treated with marcaine local blocks depending on skill level of Provider and referred to an outpatient settings for further care
- It is appropriate to express concern for the patient's dependence on controlled substances where the Provider feels it may be productive
- There are situations where a noncontrolled substance is more effective, such as in migraine therapy, and it should be used instead
- It may be necessary to decline controlled substance treatment of pain in patients with a history of troublesome behavior of controlled substance use where appropriate
- Effective chronic pain treatment decreases visits, use of resources, improves patient care and improves patient satisfaction

Disposition

- Refer chronic pain or frequent recurrent pain patients to their primary care provider
- Referral to a Pain Clinic is appropriate in many situations

- Short courses of controlled pain medications with limited amount of pills and no refills is encouraged depending on the clinical situation
- Chronic or acute pain aftercare instructions

Notes

DRUG INTERACTIONS

When using any protocol, always follow the Guidelines of Proper Use (page 16).

Considerations

- Geriatric patients have a 20–30% hospitalization rate from drug effects or interactions
- Drug interactions diagnosed 25% of the time

QT Interval Prolongation

Symptoms that may occur ***(not very common)***

- Syncope
- Sudden death

Drug causes

Antipsychotics	Antiarrhythmics	Antibiotics	Antidepressants
Pimozide	Amiodarone	Macrolides	Tricyclics
Olanzapine	Quinidine	Fluoroquinolones	Trazodone
Ziprasidone			
Haldol			
Droperidol			

Digoxin (digitalis) Levels

Increased by

- NSAID's
- Verapamil
- Quinidine
- Amiodarone

CYP2C9 Cytochrome Inhibition Drugs that Increase Warfarin, Sulfonylureas, Dilantin Effects or Levels

- Septra (trimethoprim/sulfamethoxazole)
- COX-II inhibitors
- Aspirin; salicylates
- ACE inhibitors

- Macrolides
- Phenobarbital
- Isoniazid
- SSRI's
- Amiodarone
- Prilosec
- Cimetidine

Serotonin Syndrome

- Caused by 2 serotonergic drug's interaction

Drugs

- Amitriptyline — Demerol (meperidine) — SSRI's
- Citalopram — Tramadol — Amphetamine
- Anafranil — Effexor — Buspar
- Robitussin — Nardil — Most antidepressants
- Fenfluramine — MAO inhibitors
- Prozac — Zoloft

Signs and symptoms

Cognitive abnormalities	Autonomic dysfunction	Neuromuscular
Confusion	Hyperthermia	Myoclonus
Agitation	Diaphoresis	Hyperreflexia
Coma	Sinus tachycardia	Rigidity
Anxiety	Hypertension	Tremor
Lethargy	Tachypnea	Hyperactivity
Seizures	Dilated pupil	Ataxia

Evaluation

- CBC
- BMP
- CPK

Treatment

- Discontinue offending drugs
- Periactin 4–8 mg PO initially prn; 4 mg PO qid prn
- Ativan or valium prn

Consult criteria

- All suspected serotonin syndromes

Notes

Disease Management

Section Contents

Hypertension Management

Coronary Artery Disease Management

Heart Failure Management

Type 1 Diabetes Mellitus Management

Type 2 Diabetes Mellitus Management

Cholesterol Management

Stroke Prevention Management

Obesity Management

Asthma Management

COPD Management

Ventilator Management

Adult Septic Shock Management

Depression Management

Headache Management

Seizure Management

Arthritis Management

When using any management guideline, always follow the Guidelines of Proper Use (page 16).

HYPERTENSION MANAGEMENT

When using any management guideline, always follow the Guidelines of Proper Use (page 16).

Definitions

- In adults ≥ 18 years of age, hypertension classifications are the following with 2 or more averaged seated BP measurements over 2 or more office visits (initial BP may be elevated due to anxiety)
    - Normal
        - SBP < 120 mm Hg
        - DBP < 80 mm Hg
    - Prehypertension
        - SBP 120–139 mm Hg
        - DBP 80–89 mm Hg
        - Some controversy exists if this label should be given to patients without diabetic, cardiac or stroke histories
    - Stage 1 hypertension
        - SBP 140–159 mm Hg
        - DBP 90–99 mm Hg
    - Stage 2 hypertension
        - SBP ≥ 160 mm Hg
        - DBP ≥ 100 mm Hg

Considerations

- SBP > 140 mm Hg in age > 50 years is more important cardiovascular disease (CVD) risk factor than diastolic pressure
- Risk doubles for CVD for each SBP/DBP increase of 20/10 mm Hg starting at 115/75 mm Hg blood pressure (BP)
- Thiazide diuretics should be used initially or in combination with other antihypertensive medications in uncomplicated hypertension
- Most patients will require 2 or more antihypertensive medications to achieve target blood pressure of < 140/90 mm Hg in patients without diabetes or chronic

renal disease, or < 130/80 mm Hg for diabetic or chronic renal disease patients

- If blood pressure is > 20/10 mm Hg over target BP, consideration should be given to initiating 2 antihypertensive drugs, one of which should be a thiazide diuretic usually
- Clinician's judgment remains paramount in using guidelines
- Self-measured averaged blood pressures at home > 135/85 mm Hg are considered hypertensive

High risk conditions that have indications for initiation of other antihypertensive medications besides a diuretic

- Heart failure
- Postmyocardial infarction
- High coronary disease risk
- Diabetes
- Chronic renal disease
- Recurrent stroke prevention in patients with history of stroke

Evaluation

- U/A
- CBC
- BMP and calcium level
- EKG
- Lipid profile
- Bilateral arm blood pressures
- Optic fundus examination
- Body mass index (BMI) calculation
- Auscultation for carotid, abdominal and femoral bruits
- Thyroid gland palpation
- Heart and lung examination
- Abdominal examination for masses and abdominal aortic pulsation
- Check legs for edema and arterial pulses
- Neurologic examination

Goals of Therapy

- Target blood pressure of < 140/90 mm Hg in patients without diabetes or chronic renal disease, or <130/80 mm Hg for diabetic or chronic renal disease patients with focus on lowering SBP in both groups

Treatment Options without High Risk Conditions

Prehypertension

- Lifestyle modification with
    - Weight loss diet rich in potassium and calcium (DASH eating plan)
    - 2400 mg sodium diet
    - Increased physical activity
    - Moderation of alcohol consumption

Stage 1 hypertension

- Lifestyle modification
- Thiazide diuretic for most patients
- May also consider
    - Angiotensin converting enzyme inhibitor (ACEI)
    - Angiotensin receptor blocker (ARB)
    - Beta-blocker (BB)
    - Calcium channel blocker (CCB)

      OR
- Combination of above medications

Stage 2 hypertension

- Lifestyle modification
- Two drug combination of stage 1 hypertension medications usually (caution if risk of orthostatic hypotension–usually elderly)

Treatment Options with High Risk Conditions

Prehypertension

- Lifestyle modification

- Drugs as applicable in conditions below

Heart failure

- If asymptomatic give ≥ 1 medication
  - Angiotensin converting enzyme inhibitor
  - Beta-blocker
- If symptomatic give ≥ 1 medication with a loop diuretic — Lasix (furosemide) or Bumex (bumetanide)
  - Angiotensin converting enzyme inhibitor
  - Beta-blocker
  - Angiotensin receptor blocker
  - Aldosterone antagonist

Ischemic heart disease (stable angina)

- Beta-blocker

  OR
- Long acting calcium channel blocker such as Norvasc (amlodipine)

Post myocardial infarction options

- Beta-blocker
- ACEI
- Aldosterone antagonist
- Lipid management
- Low dose aspirin 160-325 mg PO qday

High risk for coronary disease options

- Thiazide diuretic
- Beta-blocker
- ACEI
- CCB
- Lipid management
- Low dose aspirin 160-325 mg PO qday

Diabetic hypertension options

Combination of ≥ 2 drugs usually needed

- Thiazide diuretic
- Beta-blocker
- ACEI or ARB (reduces diabetic nephropathy)
- CCB

Chronic renal disease options

Definition of chronic renal disease

- Glomerular filtration rate (GFR) < 60 cc/min
- Creatinine > 1.5 mg/dL in men and creatinine > 1.3 mg/dL in women
- Albuminuria > 300 mg/day or 200 mg of albumin/gm creatinine

Medications

- ACEI
- ARB
- Loop diuretic such as Lasix (furosemide) may be needed with creatinine > 2.5 mg/dL
- Target BP is < 130/80 mm Hg
- Limited rise of up to 35% of creatinine with ACEI or ARB therapy is acceptable as long as hyperkalemia does not develop

Recurrent stroke prevention options

- Thiazide diuretic
- ACEI
- Lipid management
- Low dose aspirin (160–325 mg PO qday) if hypertension reasonably controlled

African Americans

- Thiazide diuretics or CCB more effective than beta-blockers, ACEIs or ARBs
- ACEI induced angioedema occurs 2–4 times more frequently than in other groups

Elderly patients

- Initial lower drug doses may be needed, though standard doses and multiple drugs are needed eventually in the majority to achieve BP control
- They are at risk of postural hypotension due to the frequent use of multiple medications

Follow Up and Achieving Blood Pressure Control

- Monthly follow up till blood pressure control is achieved
- Follow up every 3–6 months when blood control is achieved
- Serum creatinine and potassium should be checked 1–2 times per year
- Heart failure, diabetes and other comorbidities influence frequency of visits and tests needed
- Addition of a second drug should be in a different class if a single drug regimen was started initially and failed to achieve control
- Do not use 2 drugs in the same class at the same time (exception is Maxzide or Dyazide which are combination diuretic drugs)

Consult Criteria

- Unable to achieve target blood pressure reductions over several visits
- Blood pressure ≥ 180/110 mm Hg on 2 or more medications
- Symptomatic high risk conditions or comorbidities (CHF, progressive renal insufficiency, hyperkalemia, angina, stroke, etc.)

Antihypertensive Medications (refer to PDR or medication inserts)

Thiazide diuretics

- Chorothiazide (Diuril) 125–250 mg PO qday-bid
- Chorthalidone 12.5–25 mg PO qday
- Hydrochlorothiazide (HCTZ) 12.5–50 mg PO qday

Loop diuretics

- Lasix (furosemide) 20–40 mg PO bid
- Bumex (bumetanide) 0.5–1 mg PO bid
- Torsemide 2.5–10 mg PO qday

Potassium sparing diuretics

- Triamterene 25–50 mg PO qday-bid
- Amiloride 5 mg PO qday-bid

Aldosterone receptor blockers

- Aldactone 25–50 mg PO qday

Beta–blockers

- Atenolol 25–100 mg PO qday
- Metoprolol 50–100 mg PO qday-bid
- Corgard (Nadolol) 40–120 mg PO qday
- Toprol XL (metoprolol) 50–100 mg PO qday
- Propranolol 20–80 mg PO bid

Beta-blockers with intrinsic sympathomimetic activity

- Sectral (acebutolol) 200–400 mg PO bid
- Pindolol 5–10 mg PO bid

Combined alpha and beta-blockers

- Coreg (carvedilol) 6.25–25 mg PO bid increase every 1–2 weeks as tolerated and needed up to 25 mg bid
- Labetalol 100–400 mg PO bid

Angiotensin converting enzyme inhibitors (ACEI)

- Lisinopril 5–40 mg PO qday
- Captopril 12.5–50 mg PO bid
- Accupril (quinapril) 10–80 mg PO qday

Angiotensin receptor blockers

- Atacand (candesartan) 8–32 mg PO qday
- Cozaar (losartan) 25–50 mg PO qday-bid
- Diovan (valsartan) 80–320 mg PO qday

Calcium channel blockers—non-Dihydropyridines

- Cardizem CD (diltiazem) 180–420 mg PO qday
- Cardizem LA (diltiazem) 120–540 mg PO qday
- Calan (verapamil) SR 120–240 mg PO qday-bid

Calcium channel blockers—dihydropyridines

- Norvasc (amlodipine) 2.5–10 mg PO qday
- Procardia XL (nifedipine) 30–60 mg PO qday

Alpha-1 blockers (not first line drugs)

- Cardura (doxazosin) 1–16 mg PO qday
- Cardura (doxazosin) XL 4–8 mg PO qday
- Minipres (prazosin) 1–5 mg PO bid-tid
- Caution for orthostatic hypotension — give first dose and any increases at bedtime

Central alpha-2 agonists

- Clonidine 0.1–0.3 mg PO bid-tid
- Catapres -TTS (clonidine) patch 0.1–0.3 mg qweek

Combination drugs

- ACEI+CCB (Lotrel) amlodipine and benazepril 2.5/10–10/20 mg PO qday
- ACEI+HCTZ (Zestoretic) Lisinopril and HCTZ 10/12.5–20/25 mg PO qday
- ARBs+diuretic (Diovan-HCT) valsartan and HCTZ 80/12.5–160/50 mg PO qday
- Beta-blocker+diuretic (Tenoretic) atenolol and HCTZ 50/25 to 100/25 PO qday
- Diuretic and diuretic (Aldactazide) 25/25 to 50/50 mg PO qday-bid

Notes

Reference:

http://www.nhlbi.nih.gov/guidelines/hypertension/express.pdf

JNC 7 — The Seventh Report of the Joint National Committee on Prevention, Detection, Evaluation and Treatment of High Blood Pressure

Coronary Artery Disease Management

When using any management guideline, always follow the Guidelines of Proper Use (page 16).

Definitions

- Atherosclerotic changes in the walls of coronary arteries resulting in plaque formation and vascular remodeling

Differential diagnosis

- GERD
- Esophageal spasm
- Pulmonary embolism
- Musculoskeletal truncal pain
- Pleurodynia
- Anxiety disorder
- Panic disorder
- Aortic stenosis
- Aortic dissection
- Coronary artery vasospasm
- Cocaine abuse
- Pericarditis
- Myocarditis
- Peptic ulcer disease
- Gastritis
- Hiatal hernia
- Cholecystitis
- Biliary colic

Considerations

- Can cause diminished blood flow to cardiac muscle
- 14 million Americans have coronary artery disease (CAD)
- 1.5 million myocardial infarctions per year
- Greater than 500,000 deaths per year

- Patient education very important

Risk factors

- Smoking
- Male sex
- Age
- Hypertension
- Hyperlipidemia
- Dyslipidemia
- Diabetes mellitus
- Family history
- Sedentary lifestyle
- Obesity
- Metabolic syndrome
- Rheumatoid arthritis/SLE (females > males)

Acute coronary syndrome (unstable angina or AMI)

- Unstable plaque rupture causing thrombus formation obstructing vessel lumen leading to angina and/or AMI
- May have less than 50% blockage of artery by plaque alone
- Decreased incidence with statin and ACE inhibitor treatment
  - ACE inhibitors improve endothelial function
- Decreased incidence with antiplatelet agents

Signs and symptoms

- May be asymptomatic
- Chest pain centrally or in various locations
  - May occur at rest, from exertion or from emotional stress
- Arm pain
- Jaw pain
- Shortness of breath
  - Dyspnea on exertion
- Diaphoresis
- Nausea
- Vomiting
- Syncope

- Sudden cardiac arrest or ventricular fibrillation (sudden death)
- Congestive heart failure

Physical Examination

- Usually normal
- S3/S4 heart sounds may be heard during anginal episode
- Levine sign — clenched fist over central chest during chest pain suggest of angina
- Xanthelasma or xanthoma as hyperlipidemia stigmata
- Carotid or aortic bruit
- Pulmonary rales from heart failure

Evaluation options

Initial tests

- EKG
- CBC
- BMP
- HbA1c if diabetic or glucose intolerant
- Fasting lipid profile
- Thyroid function tests
- Chest x-ray
- BNP (B-type natriuretic peptide) if heart failure considered
- C-reactive protein
- Urinary albumen to creatinine ratio
- Troponin for prolonged chest pain (≥ 10 minutes) in the past week that has resolved (if angina occurring in office that appears unstable — send to ER)

Imaging or stress testing

- Exercise with EKG monitoring
    - Initial procedure of choice without ST segment baseline resting abnormalities
    - ≥ 1 mm ST segment depression 80 msec from J point most characteristic change with positive test for ischemia
    - Withhold beta-blockers for 48 hours before test if possible

    - Dobutamine, adenosine and dipyridamole stress testing may be performed in patients unable to exercise
  - Stress echocardiogram — sensitivity 78% and specificity 86%
    - Localizes ischemia and severity
    - Assists in evaluating left ventricle wall motion, cardiac chamber size and for valvular disease
    - May be technically difficult to get good images
  - Myocardial perfusion scintigraphy — sensitivity of 83% and specificity of 77%
  - Do not perform exercise stress testing with symptomatic arrhythmias, aortic stenosis or recent AMI
  - Stop exercise stress testing with development of
    - Chest pain
    - Drop in systolic blood pressure > 10 mm Hg
    - Severe shortness of breath, fatigue, dizziness or near syncope
    - ST segment depression > 2 mm
    - ST segment elevations > 1 mm without diagnostic Q waves
    - Ventricular tachyarrhythmia
  - 64 slice CT angiogram which has nearly 100% negative predictive value
  - Coronary angiography

Treatment options

- Treat risk factors (see specific management sections)
- Statins
- ACE inhibitors and angiotensin receptor blockers
- Platelet inhibitors
  - Aspirin (ASA) 81–325 mg PO qday
  - Clopidogrel (Plavix) 12 months after ACS episode, then ASA qday
- Beta-blockers
  - Stable or exertional angina
  - Heart failure
- Calcium channel blockers
- Nitrates (may cause hypotension with IHSS/ASH — hypertrophic cardiomyopathy)

- Ranolazine — reserved usually until after standard therapy has failed to control symptoms (not a first-line drug)
- Diet
  - Reduced fats
- Weight reduction as appropriate
- Increased physical activity as tolerated
- Cardiac rehabilitation

Medication treatment for stable angina

Anginal episode/week ≤ 1

- ASA
- NTG SL prn — may repeat q5minutes x 2 prn

Anginal episode/week ≥ 2

- ASA
- NTG SL prn — may repeat q5minutes x 2 prn
- Long acting NTG

May add as needed

- Beta-blocker
- ACEI or ARB to a beta-blocker
- Add calcium channel blocker when symptoms persist on beta-blocker or beta-blocker cannot be used (do not use verapamil with beta-blocker)

High risk patient

- ASA or clopidogrel
- ACEI or ARB added to nitrates and beta-blockers

Angina persists or not controlled on 3 medications

- Coronary angiography

Medication selections

Statins

- May causes liver and muscle disease
- Stop if CPK becomes elevated
- Read drug information for adverse reactions, cautions and contraindications
- Avoid in heavy alcohol use

Atorvastatin (Lipitor)

- 10–20 mg PO qday initially
- 10–80 mg PO qday maintenance
- Stop if LFT's > 3 times normal

Pravastatin (Pravachol)

- 10–40 mg PO qday — not to exceed 80 mg/day
- Hepatic and renal impairment — 10 mg PO qday
- Do not use in active liver disease

Simvastatin (Zocor)

- 10–20 mg PO qday in the evening
- If high risk for CAD — 40 mg PO qday in the evening
- Stop if LFT's > 3 times normal or renal failure develops
- Myopathy risk greater at 80 mg PO qday dosing

Rosuvastatin (Crestor)

- 10–20 mg PO qday initially — may titrate but not to exceed 40 mg PO qday
- Caution in liver disease
- Start at 5 mg PO qday in Asians

Lovastatin (Altoprev)

- 10–60 mg PO qhs
- Reduce if creatinine clearance < 30 mL/minute
- Stop if LFT's > 3 times normal, renal failure or myopathy with elevated CPK develops
- Avoid in heavy alcohol use

Fluvastatin (Lescol, Lescol XL)

- Start 20–40 mg PO qhs
- Dose range 20–80 mg PO qday
    - Divide bid if 80 mg used
- Stop if LFT's > 3 times normal, renal failure or myopathy with elevated CPK develops

Nitrates

- Decreases preload, afterload, myocardial work and oxygen consumption
- Dilates coronary arteries
- Long-acting nitrates used continuously throughout the day will develop tolerance in 24–48 hours and lose effectiveness, so a nitrate free period for 8–12 hours each day with no long-acting nitrates is needed, frequently performed during sleep periods

Short-acting nitrates

- NTG 0.3–0.6 SL prn — may repeat x 2 q5minutes prn continued ischemic cardiac pain
- May use before anginal provoking activities
    - Comes in tablets or spray
    - Tablets need refrigeration and last 3–6 months, and should tingle tongue when used
    - NTG spray lasts 2–3 years

Long-acting nitrates for stable angina

- Timing — taken at time of day that anginal symptoms or anginal equivalent symptoms (i.e., dyspnea) are most prevalent
- NTG 2.5 mg or 6.5 mg PO bid
- Isosorbide mononitrate
    - Standard dose — 20 mg PO bid given 7 hours apart
    - Smaller patients start 5 mg PO bid given 7 hours apart and increase to 10–20 mg PO bid given 7 hours apart over 2-3 days
    - Take on empty stomach 30 minutes prior to a meal or 1 hour after a meal
- Isosorbide mononitrate ER (extended release)
    - 30-120 mg PO qday
- Transdermal nitroglycerin (Nitro-Dur)
    - 0.2–0.4 mg/hr qday — remove for 10–12 hours each day
    - Max dose 0.4-0.8 mg/hr qday

- Starts acting in 30 minutes and lasts 8–14 hours

Nitrate side-effects (some)

- Headache
- Hypotension
- Tachycardia
- Nausea

Nitrate contraindications

- Shock or hypotension
- SBP < 90 m Hg or ≥ 30 mm Hg below baseline SBP in ACS
- Bradycardia < 50 beats per minute
- Tachycardia in absence of heart failure (> 100 beats per minute)
- Acute right ventricular myocardial infarction
    - Caution in inferior myocardial infarction
- Use of erectile dysfunction medications (sildenafil, tadalafil, or vardenafil)
- Severe anemia

Beta-blockers

- Reduce heart rate, blood pressure and cardiac contractility which decreases cardiac work and oxygen needs
- First choice usually in stable angina
- Prolongs survival and decreases second AMI incidence

Selective beta–1 blocker

- Metoprolol (Lopressor) initially 50 mg PO bid and may be increased to 200 mg PO bid
- Metoprolol (Toprol XL) 100 mg PO qday — NMT 400 mg PO qday
- Atenolol (Tenormin) 50 mg PO qday — NMT 200 mg PO qday

Non-selective beta–blocker

- Propranolol (Inderal) 80–120 mg PO bid — may increase at weekly intervals as needed
- Inderal LA 80–160 mg PO qday
- NMT 320 mg PO qday

Beta–blocker side effects (some)

- Bradycardia
- Hypotension
- Worsening of asthma and COPD
- Depression
- Heart failure
- Exacerbation of angina and hypertension on abrupt withdrawal (Black Box Warning)
- Worsening of peripheral arterial disease symptoms

Contraindications (some)

- Pre-existing sinus bradycardia (< 60 beats/minutes)
- Moderate to severe left ventricle failure and pulmonary edema
- SBP < 100 mm Hg
- Signs of poor peripheral perfusion
- 2nd and 3rd degree heart block
- Asthma and COPD
- Sick sinus syndrome without pacemaker
- Untreated pheochromocytoma

ACE inhibitors

- Reduces death, AMI, stroke, coronary stents revascularization and CABG
- May use in high risk patients even if no hypertension or heart failure present
- Start at low dose and titrate upward as tolerated

Ramipril (Altace)

- 2.5–10 mg PO qday

Lisinopril (Zestril)

- Start at 10 mg PO qday — usual range 20–40 mg PO qday

Quinapril (Accupril)

- Initially 5–10 mg PO qday — maintenance 20–80 mg PO qday

Side effects

- ACE inhibitor induced angioedema (may be treated with fresh frozen plasma and discontinue the ACEI or ARB)
- Renal impairment
- Hyperkalemia
- Hypotension
- Do not use in pregnancy, bilateral renal artery stenosis, hypersensitivity and history of angioedema

Calcium channel blockers

- Dilate vessels, lowers blood pressure and decreases cardiac workload
- Not as effective in decreasing angina frequency as beta-blockers, but similar as beta-blockers in reducing need for NTG and improving exercise tolerance
- Use calcium channel blocker when symptoms persist on beta-blocker or beta-blocker cannot be used (do not use verapamil with beta-blocker)

Amlodipine (Norvasc)

- 5–10 mg PO qday initially
- 10 mg PO qday maintenance
- Elderly 5 mg PO qday
- With hepatic impairment start with 5 mg PO qday

Diltiazem (Cardizem)

- Start 30 mg PO qid and increase every 1–2 days to control angina as needed up to 90 mg PO qid

Diltiazem (Cardizem CD)

- Start 120–180 mg PO qday and increase as needed over 1–2 weeks — NMT 480 mg PO qday

Calcium channel blocker side effects (some)

- Heart failure
- AV block
- Hypotension

- Erythema multiforme
- Peripheral edema
- Headache
- Elevated LFT's

Contraindications (some)

- Pre-existing sinus bradycardia
- 2nd and 3rd degree heart block
- Sick sinus syndrome without pacemaker
- Hypersensitivity

Ranolazine (Renexa)

- Antianginal agent (not first–line treatment)
- May be used in addition to other antianginal medications when angina is uncontrolled
- 500 mg PO bid initially — NMT 1,000 mg PO bid

Cautions and contraindications

- Do not use in hepatic cirrhosis patients
- Contraindicated with strong CYP3A inhibitors or inducers
    - Ketoconazole, itraconazole, clarithromycin, rifampin, carbamazepine, phenytoin, St. John's wort, nelfinavie, ritonavir, indinavir among others
- Not for acute anginal episodes
- Avoid grapefruit products
- Lower dose to 500 mg PO bid with aprepitant, diltiazem, erythromycin, fluconazole, grapefruit juice or products, verapamil — read literature for all drug interactions

Referral criteria

- Angina not controlled with 2–3 antianginal medications
- Acutely worsening angina

Notes

Reference:
Circulation 2010;122:S787-S817

HEART FAILURE MANAGEMENT

When using any management guideline, always follow the Guidelines of Proper Use (page 16).

Definition

- Inability of the heart to pump enough blood to meet the metabolic needs of the body, or only able to do so at an elevated diastolic filling pressure

Differential diagnosis

- COPD
- Pneumonia
- Asthma
- Acute myocardial infarction
- Pulmonary embolism
- Pulmonary fibrosis
- Adult respiratory distress syndrome
- End-stage renal disease

Considerations

- Fastest growing cardiac disease in the U.S.
- Systolic heart failure has decreased left ventricle (LV) pump function (decreased ejection fraction)
- Diastolic heart failure has normal or slightly reduced left ventricle ejection fraction
    - Impaired relaxation and stiffness of the LV causes decreased filling and amount of blood pumped per contraction
    - Has increased LV diastolic filling pressure
    - Associated with low mortality but high morbidity
- Most common cause of decompensation is decrease in therapy (medical or dietary noncompliance)
- Mortality following hospitalization for heart failure is 10% at 30 days, 20% at 1 year, 42% at 5 years
- Mortality for cardiogenic shock is ~80%
- ACE inhibitors and beta-blockers decrease mortality and are the recommended cornerstone of treatment

B-type natriuretic peptide (BNP)

- < 100 pg/mL – 90% do not have heart failure
- > 500 pg/mL – 90% have heart failure

Cardiorenal syndrome

- Worsening heart failure
- Decreasing renal function
- Increasing diuretic resistance
- Treatment involves combination diuretics, vasodilators, inotropes and possibly ultrafiltration
- May be mistaken for the creatinine increase that may occur after initiation of diuretic therapy

Causes of heart failure

- Coronary artery disease
- Hypertension
- Diabetes mellitus
- Valvular heart disease
- Cardiomyopathy
  - Idiopathic
  - Alcoholic
  - Cocaine
  - Chemotherapy
  - Postpartum
  - Myocarditis
- Arrhythmia (i.e., atrial fibrillation)
- Congenital heart disease

Signs and symptoms (some or all)

Left or biventricular heart failure

- Tachycardia
- Rales
- S3 gallop
- Nocturnal cough
- Pleural effusion
- Dyspnea at rest or with exertion
- Orthopnea
- Paroxysmal nocturnal dyspnea
- Tachypnea

- Bilateral pitting pedal or pretibial edema
- Jugular venous distension
- Hypotension in late or preterminal stages

Isolated or predominant right heart failure

- Ascites
- Bilateral leg edema or anasarca
- Hepatomegaly
- Nausea
- Constipation
- Absence of pulmonary congestion
- Pleural effusion (increase in death rate when right heart failure causes pleural effusion as compared to right heart failure without pleural effusion)
- S3 gallop

New York Heart Association classification

- Class 1 – no limitations of physical activity
- Class 2 – slight limitation of physical activity
- Class 3 – marked limitation of physical activity
- Class 4 – symptoms at rest and unable to do physical activity without discomfort

Evaluation options

- History and physical examination
- EKG
- Chest x-ray
- CBC (for anemia or infection)
- U/A for proteinuria
- BMP
- BNP
- LFT's
- Lipid profile
- TSH and thyroid function tests
- 2-D echocardiogram
- Exercise testing to determine suitability for exercise training
- Coronary angiography for suspected angina

Treatment options

- Patient education
- 2 to 3 gram sodium diet
- Avoid NSAID's, class 1 antiarrthymia drugs (amiodarone and dofetilide OK) and calcium channel blockers (if LV function is decreased)
- Fluid restriction to 2 liters/day if serum Na < 130 mEq/dL and if sodium restriction and loop diuretics (furosemide etc.) do not control fluid status
- Acute CHF exacerbation see Congestive Heart Failure Protocol

Long term therapy

Stage A patient

- At risk for heart failure without structural heart disease and without symptoms
    - Hypertension
    - Atherosclerotic disease
    - Diabetes
    - Obesity
    - Metabolic syndrome

Treatment

- Hypertension control
- Smoking cessation
- Treat lipid disorders
- Regular exercise
- Discourage alcohol intake
- Control metabolic syndrome
- ACEI or ARB for diabetes or vascular disease

Stage B patient

- Structural heart disease without signs or symptoms of heart failure
    - AMI
    - Left ventricular hypertrophy and low ejection fraction (EF)
    - Asymptomatic valvular disease

Treatment

- Stage A patient treatment
  Plus
- ACEI or ARB as appropriate

and/or

- Beta-blocker (BB) as appropriate

Stage C patient

- Structural heart disease with existing heart failure or history of heart failure

Treatment

- Routinely used
  - Diuretics for fluid retention
  - ACEI or ARB
  - Beta-blocker
- Selected patients
  - Aldosterone antagonist
  - ARB's
  - Digoxin
  - Hydralazine/nitrates
- Devices in selected patients
  - Biventricular pacing
  - Implantable defibrillator

Stage D patient

- Refractory heart failure despite maximal medical therapy requiring specialized interventions

Treatment

- Stage A, B and C treatments
- Hospice optional
- Extraordinary measures
  - Heart transplant
  - Chronic inotropes
  - Permanent mechanical support
  - Experimental surgery or drugs

Medications

ACE inhibitors (ACEI)

Used as first line therapy to decrease mortality

- Lisinopril (Zestril) 2.5–5 mg PO qday initially — target dose of 20 mg PO qday if needed
- Captopril (Capoten) 6.25 mg PO tid initially — target dose of 50 mg PO tid if needed
- Enalapril (Vasotec) 2.5 mg PO bid initially — target dose of 10 mg PO bid if needed

Angiotensin receptor blockers

May be used as first line therapy for heart failure and LV dysfunction or as add-on therapy

- Losartan (Cozaar) 12.5–254 mg PO qday initially — target dose of 150 mg PO qday if needed
- Valsartan (Diovan) 40 mg PO bid initially — target dose of 160 mg PO bid if needed

Beta–blockers (BB)

All patients with chronic heart failure and systolic dysfunction unless contraindicated

- When patients are euvolemic and on afterload reduction such as ACEI's/ARB's
- Carvedilol (Coreg) 3.125 mg PO bid initially — target dose of 25 mg PO bid if needed
- Moderate afterload and slight preload reduction
- Metoprolol CR/XL (Toprol XL) 12.5–25 mg PO qday initially — target dose of 200 mg PO qday if needed
- Reduces heart rate and blood pressure
- Beta–blockers may be continued or decreased by 50% with acute heart failure exacerbations if possible

Aldosterone antagonists

Recommended for heart failure patients who are hospitalized frequently or have moderate to severe symptoms and are on ACEI's and BB

- Spironolactone (Aldactone) 12.5–25 mg PO qday initially — target dose of 25 mg PO qday if needed
- Start at low dose in elderly and in patients with chronic renal insufficiency
- May cause hyperkalemia — avoid if potassium > 5 mEq/L or creatinine > 2.5 mg/dL
  - Check potassium ≤ 1 week after starting
  - Stop potassium supplements

Vasodilators

Reduces afterload — can be used especially for African Americans already on optimal therapy with ACEI's/ARB, BB and diuretics for moderate to severe symptoms

- Hydralazine/isosorbide (Bidil) 37.5 mg hydralazine/20 mg isosorbide PO tid — with double of that as the target dose if needed
- Hydralazine (Apresoline) 37.5 mg PO qid initially with target dose of 75 mg PO qid if needed

Nitrates

Reduces preload and to a lesser extent afterload — may be used as first line agent when hypotension is not present or a concern

- NTG SL prn for acute heart failure with mild to severe hypertension

Loop diuretics

Used for fluid retention prn

- Furosemide (Lasix) 20 mg PO qday up to 40 mg PO tid (NMT 600 mg PO qday)
- Torsemide (Demadex) 10 mg PO qday prn (NMT 200 mg PO qday)

Inotropic agents

Decreases hospitalizations and heart failure symptoms but does not improve survival long term

- Digoxin (Lanoxin) 0.125–0.5 mg PO qday — usual daily dose is 0.125 mg (elderly) to 0.25 mg PO
    - Initial loading dose is 0.375–0.625 mg PO bid x 1 day
    - Therapeutic range is 0.8–2.0 ng/mL
    - Can also be used for atrial fibrillation control in addition to heart failure treatment
    - Monitor digoxin levels 24 hours after starting, then weekly until stable — trough or 1 hour before scheduled dose
    - Hypokalemia and hypomagnesemia may potentiate toxicity
    - Can cause AV block, severe bradycardia, vomiting, etc. (read literature for cautions and contraindications)

Anticoagulation

- Aspirin 81 mg PO qday recommended in ischemic cardiac disease
    - Not recommended if atherosclerotic disease not present
- Warfarin
    - Heart failure with atrial fibrillation (INR target is 2.0–3.0)
    - Ischemic cardiomyopathy and recent large anterior MI or documented LV thrombus
    - Can be used as alternative to aspirin
- Clopidogrel (Plavix) 75 mg PO qday
    - Can be used as alternative to aspirin

Implantable cardiac defibrillators

- May be considered in patients with ejection fraction < 35% , NYHA Class 2 and 3 and estimated survival > 1 year
    - Treatment for sudden cardiac death

Consult criteria

- Refractory heart failure
- Heart failure requiring multiple medications
- New York Heart Association class 3 and 4

Notes

TYPE 1 DIABETES MELLITUS MANAGEMENT

When using any management guideline, always follow the Guidelines of Proper Use (page 16).

Definition

- Disease process that is dependent on exogenous insulin to sustain life

Differential diagnosis

- Type 2 diabetes mellitus
- Alcoholic ketoacidosis (for DKA)

Considerations

- Insulin levels are very low or absent
- Strong genetic predisposition
- Frequently presents with diabetic ketoacidosis (DKA)
- Increase incidence of infections
- Education is the most important aspect of treatment
    - Requires dietician, nurse, diabetic counselor and medical provider in a team approach
- HbA1c > 6% but < 6.5% commonly need lifestyle modification, nutruition counseling, and increased physical activity
- HbA1c levels reflects the previous 3 months of glycemia
- Fasting C-peptide level greater than 1 mg/dL is associated more with type 2 diabetes mellitus

Latent autoimmune diabetes of adults (LADA)

- Commonly confused with type 2 diabetes mellitus
- Islet cell antibiotics slowly destroy ß–cell function
- Not insulin requiring for at least the first 6 months of onset

- Most patients will require insulin within 6 years
- Insulin therapy is treatment of choice when diagnosis is made
- Will ultimately require insulin and the treatment is similar to type 1 diabetes mellitus
- May take up to 12 years in some patients to have complete failure of ß–cell function
- 10% of patients over age 35 years and 25% of patients under age 35 years diagnosed with type 2 diabetes mellitus will actually have LADA
- Pancreatic islet cell antibodies testing is used to diagnose and differentiate LADA from type 2 diabetes mellitus as needed

Diagnostic criteria

- Hb1Ac level ≥ 6.5%
    - HbA1c is the diagnostic test of choice for diabetes mellitus
- Fasting serum glucose ≥ 126 mg/dL on 2 occasions
- Random serum glucose ≥ 200 mg/dL and classic diabetic symptoms (polyuria, polydipsia, polyphagia and weight loss)
- 2 hour oral glucose tolerance test (75 gm glucose PO load) — serum glucose ≥ 200 mg/dL at 2 hours post ingestion of glucose load

Symptoms

- Polydipsia
- Polyuria
- Increased appetite
- Weight loss
- Blurred vision
- Yeast infections
- Paresthesias

DKA (See DKA section)

- Polydipsia
- Polyuria

- Blurred vision
- Tachypnea (Kussmaul respirations)
- Tachycardia
- Nausea and vomiting
- Abdominal pain
- Altered mental status
- Metabolic acidosis
- Elevated serum ketones

Long term complications

- Macrovascular complications
    - Coronary arterial disease (CAD)
    - Cerebrovascular disease
    - Peripheral arterial disease (PAD)
- Microvascular disease
    - Renal insufficiency
    - Retinal neovascularization
        - May occur in pre-diabetes
- Neuropathic disease
    - Peripheral neuropathy
    - Autonomic neuropathy
    - Gastroparesis (may respond to erythromycin or metoclopramide)
- Gestational diabetes complicates 4% of pregnancies
- Congestive heart failure

Evaluation

- Physical examination
    - Assess vital signs
    - Funduscopic exam
    - Foot exam for ulcers, impaired circulation and decreased sensation
- Fasting serum glucose
- Random serum glucose
- HbA1c level
    - Screening with Hb1Ac in obese patients with BMI > 25 kg/m² or that have cardiovascular risk factors
- BMP (glucose, electrolytes, creatinine and BUN)

- Creatinine level should be monitored at least yearly
- U/A
  - Evaluate for microalbuminuria which is 30–200 mg/day
  - Ratio of spot urine albumin(mg) to creatinine(gm) ≥ 30 indicates need for a timed collection of urine, either an overnight or 10 hour or 24 hour urine collection
    - Linked to increase in coronary artery disease
    - Microalbuminuria is weaker predictor of future renal disease in type 2 diabetes mellitus than in type 1 diabetes mellitus
- Autoantibodies to islet cells, insulin and glutamic acid decarboxylase are absent in type 2 diabetes

General treatment

- Dietary counseling
- Appropriate weight loss
- Increased activity regimen
- Hypertension management
- Hyperlipidemia management
  - Statin therapy to reduce cholesterol in males age > 40 years and females age > 45 years by 30–40% with LDL cholesterol target of < 100 mg/dL
  - Younger diabetic patients with risk factors or longstanding disease treat with statins
  - Target of LDL < 70 mg/dL in diabetic patients with known cardiovascular disease
- Manage vascular complications

Diabetic treatment

- Tight glycemia control decreases long term complications but must be individualized to minimize hypoglycemic reactions
  - Recurrent and chronic hypoglycemia has been linked to cognitive impairment
  - A "honeymoon" period may occur with DM type 1 patients initially where they do not require insulin after initial diagnosis and treatment, only to develop insulin dependence after weeks to months later, sometimes up to 1–2 years

Diet per dietician

- Caloric intake
    - 20% at breakfast
    - 35% at lunch
    - 30% at dinner
    - 15% late evening snack
    - Fat intake ≤ 30% of total calories
- Protein 1–1.5 gm/kg/day — and less than that in renal insufficiency or failure

Exercise

- Routine exercise sessions for 30 minutes or more — patient may need to decrease insulin 10–20% or have an extra snack (>150 minutes/week recommended if tolerated)

Insulin therapy initiation

- Calculate based on patient weight
- Usually new diabetics can be started on a total daily insulin dose of 0.2–0.4 units/kg SQ initially, but will ultimately need 0.6–0.7 units/kg SQ as the total daily dose
- ½ dosed before breakfast, ¼ before dinner and ¼ at bedtime
- Adjust dose to maintain pre-prandial serum glucose 80–150 mg/dL
- Dosing is adjusted usually 10% at a time and assessed over a 3 day period before making further adjustments
- Children with moderate hyperglycemia without ketonuria or metabolic acidosis may be started with qday SQ injection of 0.3–0.5 U/kg of intermediate insulin
    - Children with ketonuria without metabolic acidosis or dehydration may be started on 0.5–0.7 U/kg SQ of intermediate insulin qday and 0.1 U/kg SQ at 4–6 hour intervals

Insulin maintenance schedules

- Usually ½ of the daily insulin dose is given as a long acting basal dose
- Multiple injections per day needed to maintain glucose levels in desired range

- ¼ of daily insulin given at bedtime as intermediate insulin
- Additional insulin given as short-acting insulin before meals based on home glucose monitoring

Insulin types administered subcutaneously

- Rapid-acting — onset in 15 minutes, peak in 1–3 hours and lasts 3–5 hours
    - Novolog (insulin aspart)
    - Apidra (insulin glulisine)
    - Humalog (insulin lispro)
- Short-acting — onset in 30–60 minutes, peak in 2–4 hours, and lasts 6–12 hours
    - Humulin R and Novolin R (regular insulin)
- Intermediate-acting — onset in 1–2 hours, peak in 4–14 hours, and lasts 16–24 hours
    - Humulin N, Novolin N (insulin NPH)
- Long-acting — onset 1 hour and lasts 24 hours
    - Lantus (insulin glargine)
    - Levemir (insulin detemir) duration 6 hours with low dose to 24 hours with high dose
- Premixed — rapid-acting mixed with intermediate-acting insulin
    - NovoLog 50/50 and 70/30 (insulin aspart protamine/insulin aspart
    - Humalog 50/50 and 75/25 (insulin lispro protamine/insulin lispro

Other treatment

- Symlin (pramlintide)
    - Delays gastric emptying
    - Decreases glucagon secretion
    - Helps to control appetite
    - May be used with type 1 and 2 diabetes mellitus along with insulin
    - Used to improve control when needed

Hypoglycemia management

- Caused by missed meals, vomiting, exercise, or excess insulin

Symptoms

- Confusion, light-headiness, diaphoresis or headache

Treatment

- Patient consumes or family gives patient sugar or candy if alert enough to control PO intake
- D50W 25 ml IV — adults
- D25W 1 ml/kg IV — young children
- Glucagon 1 mg SQ, IM or IV
- Adjust medications as needed

Glucose monitoring

Home monitoring

- Daily before meals and at bedtime
- May need to perform 2 hours before meals prn
- Patients should adjust their insulin according to patient education and glucose levels
- Patients should test every week for several weeks with initiation of insulin therapy at 0200–0400 in the morning, and as indicated afterward
- Patients should test for urine ketones with dipstick when illness develops or very high blood glucose levels occur

Office monitoring

- HbA1c every 3 months

Consult criteria

- HbA1c > 10% after therapy maximization
- Metabolic acidosis
- Progressive renal insufficiency
- Baseline creatinine ≥ 2 mg/dL
- Hypoglycemia complications
- Blood glucose > 450 mg/dL
- New diagnosis

Notes

Reference: Latent Autoimmune Diabetes in Adults Definition, Prevalence, β-Cell Function, and Treatment doi: 10.2337/diabetes.54.suppl_2.S68 Diabetes December 2005 vol. 54 no. suppl 2 S68–S72

TYPE 2 DIABETES MELLITUS MANAGEMENT

When using any management guideline, always follow the Guidelines of Proper Use (page 16).

Definition

- Hyperglycemia disorder resulting from insulin resistance and decreased insulin secretion

Differential diagnosis

- Type 1 diabetes mellitus

Considerations

- Does not require exogenous insulin treatment to sustain life
- Can present with DKA in young adults, Hispanics and African-Americans initially
- Gestational diabetes complicates 4% of pregnancies
- 90% of patients are obese
- Genetic predisposition is common
- Diagnostic criteria
  - Hb1Ac level ≥ 6.5%
    - HbA1c is the diagnostic test of choice for diabetes mellitus
  - Fasting serum glucose ≥ 126 mg/dL on 2 occasions
  - Random serum glucose ≥ 200 mg/dL and classic diabetic symptoms (polyuria, polydipsia, polyphagia and weight loss)
  - 2 hour oral glucose tolerance test (75 gm glucose PO load) serum glucose ≥ 200 mg/dL at 2 hours post ingestion of glucose load
- HbA1c > 6% but < 6.5% commonly need lifestyle modification, nutruition counseling, and increased physical activity
- HbA1c levels reflects previous 3 months of glycemia

- Fasting C-peptide level more than 1 mg/dL is associated more with type 2 diabetes mellitus
- Impaired fasting glucose is serum glucose of 100–125 mg/dL
- Impaired glucose tolerance
    - Plasma glucose ≥ 140 mg/dL-199 mg/dL 2 hours after 75 gm oral glucose load
- Prognosis strongly influenced by disease control
- Linked to depression
- Tight control yielding HbA1c ≤ 7% is valuable in new onset diabetes mellitus in reducing complications
    - Less beneficial in complication reduction in diabetic patients ≥ 15 years in duration
- Hypertension and hyperlipidemia control important also to decrease vascular complications in diabetes
- Patient education should be intensive and comprehensive with multiple health care professionals involved:
    - Practitioner
    - Nutritionist
    - Diabetes educator
    - May require individual education in certain cases
- At time of diagnosis, patients are estimated to have had diabetes for 4–7 years
- Pre-diabetes
    - Fasting blood glucose 100–125 mg/dL
    - Blood glucose 140–200 mg/dL in a 2 hour oral glucose tolerance test (OGTT)
    - Associated with macrovascular disease and development of frank diabetes
- Metabolic syndrome (Syndrome X) confused with Pre-diabetes
    - 3 out of 5
        - Abdominal obesity
        - Low HDL cholesterol
        - Elevated triglyceride level
        - Elevated blood pressure
        - Fasting glucose ≥ 100 mg/dL

Long term complications

- Macrovascular complications

    - Coronary arterial disease (CAD)
    - Cerebrovascular disease
    - Peripheral arterial disease (PAD)
- Microvascular disease
    - Renal insufficiency
    - Retinal neovascularization
        - May occur in pre-diabetes
- Neuropathic disease
    - Peripheral neuropathy
    - Autonomic neuropathy
    - Gastroparesis
- Diabetes mellitus is the leading cause of
    - Blindness
    - ESRD (End-stage renal disease)
    - Lower limb amputations

Symptoms

- Polydipsia
- Polyuria
- Increased appetite
- Weight loss
- Blurred vision
- Yeast infections
- Paresthesias

History

- How long has the patient had diabetes?
- Level of glucose control?
- Are there episodes of hypoglycemia?
- Vascular complications such as renal (elevated creatinine level), cardiac disease, peripheral arterial disease or TIA/CVA?
- Is there home glucose testing and what are the measured levels?
- What was the last HbA1c level?
- Any of the symptoms listed in above section?
- Frequent infections?
- Ulcers or amputations?
- Hyperlipidemia history and treatment?

Evaluation

- Physical examination
    - Assess vital signs
    - Funduscopic exam
    - Foot exam for ulcers, impaired circulation and decreased sensation
- Fasting serum glucose
- Random serum glucose
- HbA1c level
- HbA1c level
    - Screening with Hb1Ac in obese patients with BMI > 25 kg/m² or that have cardiovascular risk factors
- BMP (glucose, electrolytes, creatinine and BUN)
- U/A
    - Evaluate for microalbuminuria which is 30–200 mg/day
    - Ratio of spot urine albumin(mg) to creatinine(gm) ≥ 30 indicates need for a timed collection of urine, either an overnight or 10 hour or 24 hour urine collection
    - Linked to increase in coronary artery disease
    - Microalbuminuria is weaker predictor of future renal disease in type 2 diabetes mellitus than in type 1 diabetes mellitus
- Autoantibodies to islet cells, insulin and glutamic acid decarboxylase are absent in type 2 diabetes

Treatment

- Dietary counseling
- Appropriate weight loss
- Increased activity regimen (> 150 minutes/week recommended if tolerated)
- Hypertension management
- Hyperlipidemia management
    - Statin therapy to reduce cholesterol in males age > 40 years and females age > 45 years by 30–40% with LDL cholesterol target of < 100 mg/dL
    - Younger diabetic patients with risk factors or longstanding disease treat with statins

  - Target of LDL < 70 mg/dL in diabetic patients with known cardiovascular disease
- Manage vascular complications

Lab monitoring

Type 2 treated with insulin

- HbA1c every 3 months
- Fasting lipid profile yearly
- Creatinine level yearly
- Urine microalbumin yearly
- EKG baseline

Type 2 without insulin treatment

- HbA1c every 3–6 months
- Fasting lipid profile yearly
- Creatinine level yearly
- Urine microalbumin measured yearly
- EKG baseline

Pharmacologic Treatment for Type 2 Adult Diabetes

Obese

Monotherapy

- Metformin 500 mg PO bid with or after meals × 1 week, increase weekly by 500 mg to achieve 1000 mg PO bid
  - Decreases HbA1c approximated 1.5%

Second drug if needed

- Glyburide (Micronase) 2.5 mg PO qday after breakfast (elderly 1.25 mg PO) — may need to decrease metformin to prevent hypoglycemia (warn patient about possibility of hypoglycemia)

OR

- Glipizide (Glucotrol) 5 mg PO qday with breakfast (elderly 2.5 mg PO)

OR

- Sitagliptin (Januvia) 50 or 100 mg PO qday

Third drug if needed

- Exenatide (Byetta) 5 mcg SQ bid x 1 month and then may increase as needed to 10 mcg SQ bid
  - Give 1 hr before AM and PM meals

OR

- Insulin glargine 10 units SQ (or 0.2 units/kg) –adjust by 1 unit/day to achieve fasting glucose < 100 mg/dL

Non-obese

Monotherapy

- Metformin 500 mg PO bid with or after meals × 1 week, increase weekly by 500 mg to achieve 1000 mg PO bid

OR

- Glyburide (Micronase) 2.5 mg PO qday after breakfast (elderly 1.25 mg PO)

OR

- Glipizide (Glucotrol) 5mg PO qday (elderly 2.5 mg PO)

Second drug if needed

- Metformin 500 mg PO bid with or after meals × 1 week, increase weekly by 500 mg to achieve 1000 mg PO bid

OR

- Glyburide (Micronase) 2.5 mg PO qday after breakfast (elderly 1.25 mg PO)

OR

- Glipizide 5mg (Glucotrol) PO qday (elderly 2.5 mg PO)

Third drug if needed

- Exenatide (Byetta) 5 mcg SQ bid x 1 month and then may increase as needed to 10 mcg SQ bid
  - Give 1 hr before AM and PM meals

OR

- Insulin glargine 10 units SQ – adjust by 1 unit/day to achieve fasting glucose < 100 mg/dL

Elderly

Monotherapy

- Repaglinide (Prandin) 0.5–4 mg PO up to qid ac (not to exceed 16 mg qday)

Monotherapy failure

- Consider switch to NPH insulin 10 units SQ bedtime

Asians

Monotherapy

- Pioglitazone (Actos) 30 mg PO qday — do not use in bladder cancer, history of bladder cancer, moderate or severe hepatic disease or symptomatic heart failure (NYHA class 3 or 4)

Second drug if needed

- Metformin 500 mg PO bid with or after meals × 1 week, increase weekly by 500 mg to achieve 1,000 mg PO bid

Third drug if needed

- Glyburide (Micronase) 2.5 mg PO qday after breakfast (elderly 1.25 mg PO)

  OR
- Exenatide (Byetta) 5 mcg SQ bid x 1 month and then may increase as needed to 10 mcg SQ bid (not FDA approved with Actos)
  - Give 1 hr before AM and PM meals

  OR
- Insulin glargine 10 units SQ — adjust by 1 unit/day to achieve fasting glucose < 100 mg/dL

Symptomatic patients

- Repaglinide (Prandin) 0.5–4 mg PO up to qid ac (not to exceed 16 mg qday) or insulin to decrease glucose at start of monotherapy initiation

Consult criteria

- HbA1c > 10% after therapy maximization
- Metabolic acidosis
- Progressive renal insufficiency
- Baseline creatinine ≥ 2 mg/dL
- Hypoglycemia complications
- Blood glucose > 450 mg/dL

Notes

CHOLESTEROL MANAGEMENT

When using any management guideline, always follow the Guidelines of Proper Use (page 16).

Considerations

- LDL (low density lipoprotein) cholesterol < 100 mg/dL is optimal
- Lowering LDL cholesterol is the primary target of therapy
- "Low HDL" (high density lipoprotein) is < 40 mg/dL
- Lowering triglycerides from levels ≥ 220 recommended
- Diabetes without CHD (coronary heart disease) is considered raised to CHD risk
- Patients with metabolic syndrome are candidates for lifestyle modification
- Complete lipoprotein profile is recommended as initial screening test

Risk Assessment

Cholesterol

LDL cholesterol

- < 100 mg/dL optimal
- 100–129 mg/dL near optimal
- 130–159 mg/dL borderline high
- 160–189 mg/dL high
- > 190 mg/dL very high

Total cholesterol

- < 200 mg/dL desirable
- 200–239 mg/dL borderline high
- ≥ 240 mg/dL high

HDL cholesterol

- < 40 mg/dL low
- ≥ 60 mg/dL high

Major risk factors (excluding LDL cholesterol)

- Cigarette smoking
- Blood pressure ≥ 140/90 mm Hg or on hypertension medications
- HDL cholesterol < 40 mg/dL
- Diabetes (is a risk equivalent)
- Family history of premature CHD
    - Male 1st degree relative age < 55 years
    - Female 1st degree relative age < 65 years
- Age
    - Men ≥ 45 years
    - Women ≥ 55 years

Categories of risk modifying LDL cholesterol goals

- CHD or CHD risk equivalents — LDL goal < 100
- 2+ risk factors — LDL goal < 130
- 0 to 1 risk factor — LDL goal < 160

CHD risk equivalents

- Peripheral arterial disease
- Aortic aneurysm
- Symptomatic carotid disease
- Diabetes
- Multiple risk factors that confer a 10 year risk of CHD or recurrent CHD > 20%

Secondary causes of increased LDL cholesterol

- Diabetes
- Hypothyroidism
- Obstructive liver disease
- Chronic renal failure
- Drugs
    - Progestins
    - Corticosteroids
    - Anabolic steroids

Metabolic syndrome

Definition

- Lipid and nonlipid risk factors of metabolic origin which enhances the risk for CHD

Risk factors

- Abdominal obesity
  - Men's waist size > 40 inches
  - Women's waist size > 35 inches
- Triglycerides ≥ 150 mg/dL
- HDL cholesterol
  - Men < 40 mg/dL
  - Women < 50 mg/dL
- Blood pressure ≥ 135/ ≥ 85 mm Hg
- Fasting glucose ≥ 110 mg/dL

Treatment

- Weight reduction as appropriate
- Increased physical activity
- A fibrate or nicotinic acid for triglyceride level ≥ 500 mg/dL is recommended

10 year risk estimation for CHD to occur (examples)

Men ≥ 20% risk	Women ≥ 20% risk
Age 55–59	Age 60–64
TC 200–239	TC 200–239
Smoker	Smoker
SBP ≥ 140 mm Hg	SBP ≥ 140 mm Hg

Men's and Women's risk approximately ≤ 10% with above data if not a smoker

Goals of LDL and total cholesterol (minus HDL cholesterol) to modify risk categories

CHD or CHD risk equivalents (or 10 year of CHD risk is > 20%)

- LDL cholesterol < 100 mg/dL
- TC (minus HDL cholesterol) < 130 mg/dL

Multiple CHD risk factors and 10 year CHD risk is < 20%

- LDL cholesterol < 130 mg/dL
- TC (minus HDL cholesterol) < 160 mg/dL

Zero to one CHD risk factor

- LDL < 160 mg/dL
- TC (minus HDL cholesterol) < 190 mg/dL

Treatment to achieve goals

- Treat any secondary causes of increased LDL cholesterol
- Weight loss and increased physical activity
- Low (saturated) fat and low cholesterol diet
- High (soluble) fiber diet 10–25 gms/days
- Recheck in 6 weeks and if target not met
    - Add plant sterols or stanols 2 gms per day (vegetables, fruits, legumes, nuts, and seeds)
    - Increase fiber if possible
- Recheck in 6 weeks and if target not met
    - Start a statin or bile acid sequestrant or nicotinic acid medication
- Recheck in 6 weeks and if target not met
    - Intensify drug therapy
- Recheck in 6 weeks and if target not met
    - Discuss with physician
- Recheck every 4–6 months to monitor response and adherence to therapy
- Monitor side effects and toxicity (myopathy, etc.)

Also treat or modify CHD risk factors

Notes

Reference:

http://www.nhlbi.nih.gov/guidelines/cholesterol/atp3xsum.pdf
Third Report of the National Cholesterol Education Program (NCEP) Expert Panel on Detection, Evaluation, and Treatment of High Blood Cholesterol in Adults (Adult Treatment Panel III)

STROKE PREVENTION MANAGEMENT

When using any management guideline, always follow the Guidelines of Proper Use (page 16).

Considerations

- There are 795,000 strokes in the U.S. each year
- 134,000 stroke deaths per year
- Stroke is the third leading cause of death
- Prevention is most effective approach to manage stroke
- Primary prevention is treatment with no prior history of stroke
- Secondary prevention is treatment of patients with history of stroke

Primary prevention measures include

(In patients with no history of stroke)

- Hypertension treatment
- Platelet inhibitor agents
- Dyslipidemia treatment with statin medications
- Smoking cessation
- Dietary modification
- Weight loss as appropriate
- Exercise

Hypertension

- Most important risk factor to modify
- Target < 140/90 mm Hg
- Diabetic or renal patients the target is < 130/80 mm Hg
- Angiotensin–converting enzyme inhibitor (ACEI) or ARB (angiotensin–receptor blocker) is recommended in hypertension treatment in diabetic patients

Platelet inhibitor agents

- Aspirin 81 mg PO qday may be useful in patients with high risk for cardiovascular events
    - Not useful in low risk patients
- May be used in atrial fibrillation when warfarin cannot be used

Dyslipidemia

- Statins may be useful in diabetic patients
- Target of LDL ≤ 70 mg/dL in diabetic patients is recommended
- Niacin may be considered in patients with low HDL
- See Cholesterol Management section

Smoking cessation

- Counseling
- Oral smoking cessation medications
    - Bupropion (Zyban) 150 mg PO qday for 3 days then increase to 150 mg PO bid
    - Varenicline (Chantix) 0.5 mg PO for 3 days, then 0.5 mg PO bid for 4 days, then 1 mg PO bid for 11 weeks
- Nicotine replacement

Dietary medication

- Low sodium and high potassium diet
- Low fat
- High fruit and vegetable
- Weight reduction in obese patients with BMI > 25 kg/m^2

Imaging evaluation for TIA and new CVA

- Carotid duplex and transcranial doppler, MRI brain and MRA of head and neck, CT brain scan
- Refer to specialist if abnormal
- Refer new CVA or TIA to specialist
- Send to ER immediately if new CVA/TIA < 7 days old or has associated headache or other concerning symptoms

Atrial fibrillation

- Should be screened for at age > 65 years
- Warfarin treatment may be used with target INR of 2.0–3.0
- Aspirin 81 mg PO qday plus clopidogrel (Plavix) 75 mg PO may be used when warfarin adverse effects prohibit its use and is superior to aspirin alone
- Aspirin may be used alone in low to moderate risk patients
- Treatment with warfarin in post–AMI patients with left ventricular thrombus or akinetic segment is reasonable

CHADS2 score

- Used to quantify risk of stroke in atrial fibrillation patients
- Stands for heart failure, hypertension, age, diabetes mellitus and prior stroke/TIA
- 1 point each for heart failure, hypertension, age ≥ 75 years, diabetes mellitus
- 2 points for prior stroke/TIA
- Low risk = 0 points
- Moderate risk = 1–2 points
- High risk = 3–6 points
- Long–term anticoagulation for nonvalvular atrial fibrillation recommended with CHADS score of ≥ 2
    - Warfarin (Coumadin), dabigatran (Pradaxa) or rivaroxaban (Xarelto)
- CHADS score of 0 may use daily aspirin 81–325 mg PO daily
- CHADS score = 1 — may use daily aspirin 81–325 mg PO daily or long–term anticoagulation

Sickle cell disease

- Risk of stroke in children is 1% per year
- Prevalence of stroke by age 20 years is 11%
- Screen with transcranial Doppler ultrasound in children every 2 years

- Children with cerebral blood flow > 200 cm/second by transcranial Doppler ultrasound have stroke rate > 10% per year
    - Red cell long-term transfusion is only therapy in clinical trials shown to prevent stroke

Cardiac conditions associated with an increased risk of stroke

- Atrial arrhythmias
- Cardiac tumors
- Valvular disease
- Prosthetic valves
- Dilated cardiomyopathy
- Coronary artery disease
- Endocarditis
- Congenital cardiac anomalies
- Low left ventricular ejection fraction
    - Also seen in acute coronary syndrome

Secondary prevention

(Patients with history of stroke)

Measures include

- Platelet inhibitor agents
- Hypertension treatment
- Statins
- Lifestyle changes
- Smoking cessation

Warfarin prophylaxis

- High-risk patients
- Age > 75 years
- Target INR 2.0–3.0
- May be used age 65–75 years at discretion of clinician based on underlying disorders such as valvular disease etc.

Dabigatran (Pradaxa)

- 150 mg PO bid for stroke prevention in nonvalvular atrial fibrillation in indicated in patients with CHADS score =2

- Read Physician Desk Reference (PDR) drug information

Rivaroxaban (Xarelto)

- 20 mg PO qday for stroke prevention in nonvalvular atrial fibrillation in indicated in patients with CHADS score =2
- Read Physician Desk Reference (PDR) drug information

Reference:

Guidelines for the Primary Prevention of Stroke

A Guideline for Healthcare Professionals from the American Heart Association/American Stroke Association

ACC/AHA/ESC Practice Guidelines

ACC/AHA/ESC 2006 Guideline for the Management of Patients with Atrial Fibrillation

Notes

Obesity Management

When using any management guideline, always follow the Guidelines of Proper Use (page 16).

Definition

Obesity

- Males with body fat > 25% of body weight
- Females with body fat > 33% of body weight

Overweight classifications

Grade 1 overweight ("overweight")

- BMI (body mass index) 25–29.9 kg/m^2

Grade 2 overweight ("obesity")

- BMI 30–39.9 kg/m^2

Grade 3 overweight ("morbid obesity")

- BMI ≥ 40 kg/m^2

Children

- BMI > 85th percentile for age are "overweight"
- BMI > 95th percentile for age are "obese"

Differential diagnosis

- Hypothyroidism
- Cushing syndrome
- Acromegaly
- Bulimia
- Cardiomyopathy
- Nephrotic syndrome
- Polycystic ovarian syndrome
- Diabetes mellitus
- Medication related obesity — antidepressants, antipsychotics, diabetes treatment with insulin or oral agents, corticosteroids
- Growth hormone deficiency

- Oral contraceptives

Considerations

- A diagnosis of being overweight told to the patient increases the chance of positive behavioral changes with diet and/or activity
- Leptins (an endogenous protein) is involved in weight regulation — leptin resistance with high levels is present in overweight/obese patients
- BMI ≥ 40 kg/m² is associated with decreased life expectancy of 20 years in men and 5 years in women
- 90–95% of weight loss patients regain their weight in 5 years
- 22 kcal/kg per day is needed to sustain patient's present weight
- Clinical judgment should be used in evaluating BMI — for example muscular individuals with high BMI may be healthy
- Weight loss is not necessarily recommended for those with a BMI of 25–29.9 kg/m² or a high waist circumference, unless they have two or more comorbidities

Exclusion from weight loss programs

- Pregnant or breast feeding patients
- Serious and uncontrolled psychiatric illness
- Eating disorder
- Patients with a serious medical condition that may worsen with caloric restriction

High waist circumference and BMI 25–34.9 kg/m²

- Increases cardiovascular disease, diabetes mellitus, hypertension and dyslipidemia risk

Men

- Waist circumference > 94 cm
- Waist to hip ratio > 0.95
    - Severe potential risk with waist circumference > 104 cm

Women

- Waist circumference > 80 cm
- Waist to hip ratio > 0.8

- Severe potential risk with waist circumference > 88 cm

Elderly

- Patients with a BMI 25–29.9 kg/m^2 appear to not be at greater risk of death from all causes

Conditions associated with being overweight

- Coronary artery disease
- Diabetes mellitus
- Stroke
- Hypertension
- Obstructive sleep apnea
- Asthma
- Malignancy (uterine, prostate, breast, gallbladder)
- Increased intracranial pressure
- Meralgia paresthetica
- Urinary (bladder) stress incontinence
- Depression
- Osteoarthritis (DJD — degenerative joint disease)
- Back pain
- Venous stasis disease with edema in legs
- Increased post-surgical complications — pneumonia, wound infections, DVT/PE, and increased surgical risk
- Fatty liver with potential risk for development of cirrhosis

Evaluation

- Lipid panel
- Liver function tests
- Thyroid function tests
- 24 hour urinary free cortisol
- Caliper measured skin thickness and other measurements of waist, hips etc.

Treatment

Preinclusion screening

- Determine patient's expectations
- Determine patient's motivation

- Unrealistic expectations need to be changed prior to starting a weight loss program
- Evaluate for an eating or psychiatric disorder
- Informed consent and written expectations
- Manage co-morbidities

Weight loss program

- Weight loss of 0.9–1.5 kg/week is a reasonable goal
- Weight loss goal must be individualized
- There needs to be a team approach with a motivated patient, with a medical provider, dietician, exercise therapist and psychiatric or behavioral therapy as needed based on the individual needs
- Loss of 10% of body weight in overweight patients with BMI < 40 kg/m^2 is associated with significant benefits and further weight loss may not be needed and may be difficult to sustain

Diet

- Water consumption (500 ml in adults and 10 ml/kg in children) before meals increases weight loss up to 44% more than without water consumption — increases basal metabolic rate
- Diets of ≤ 800 kcal/day are not recommended
- Balanced conventional diets are recommended
    - Reduction of 500–1,000 kcal/day produces 1–2 pounds of weight loss/week
- Reasonable women's diet would be 1,000–1,500 kcal/day depending on activity and BMI (higher BMI and/or activity may have higher caloric intake needs and may change over time) — refer to diet counselor
- Reasonable men's diet would be 1,500–2,400 kcal/day depending on activity and BMI (higher BMI and/or activity may have higher caloric intake needs and may change over time) — refer to diet counselor

Exercise

- Aerobic and resistance exercise is important in building muscle mass and increasing metabolic rate
- Decreases muscle mass loss that occurs with dieting
- Patients should be evaluated for underlying cardiac or respiratory conditions before the exercise program is started to determine its risk

Moderate activity examples

- 45–50 minutes of washing or waxing a car, washing windows, gardening
- Walking 2 miles in 30 minutes
- Swimming laps for 20 minutes
- Fast social dancing for 30 minutes
- Running 1.5 miles in 15 minutes
- Bicycling 5 miles in 30 minutes

Behavioral therapy

- Personal weight monitoring
- Stress management
- Stimulus control
- Cognitive therapy
- Social support

Medications

- For BMI $\geq$ 27 with comorbidities or BMI $\geq$ 30
  - Orlistat 120 mg PO tid with or < 1 hour after a fatty meal
  - Selective serotonin reuptake inhibitors (SSRI's) have been used as an adjunct (fluoxetine, paroxetine)

Weight loss surgery

- Highly motivated individuals
- BMI $\geq$ 40 kg/m^2 may warrant surgical treatment
  - BMI $\geq$ 35 kg/m^2 with severe comorbidities may warrant surgical treatment

Pediatric obesity treatment

- Increase activity

- Adjust diet
- Decrease sedentary activity
- Orlistat 120 mg PO tid with or < 1 hour after a fatty meal only for age 12–16 years

Long term monitoring

- Regular clinic visits
- Group meetings
- Encouragement by email or telephone

Notes

Reference: NHLBI Obesity Education Initiative
Expert Panel on the Identification, Evaluation and Treatment of Overweight and Obesity in Adults.

Asthma Management

When using any management guideline, always follow the Guidelines of Proper Use (page 16).

Definition

- A disorder of variable and recurring symptoms, airflow obstruction, and bronchial hyper-responsiveness with an underlying bronchial inflammation

Differential diagnosis

- Bronchiolitis
- Bronchitis
- COPD
- Airway foreign body
- Vocal cord dysfunction
- Heart failure
- URI
- Pulmonary embolism
- Cystic fibrosis
- Bronchopulmonary dysplasia (premature birth history)

Considerations

- Reversible airway constriction
    - May not be completely reversible over time
- Persistent changes in airways occur
- May be seasonal or perennial
- GERD, OSA (obstructive sleep apnea) and sinusitis may exacerbate asthma

Causes

- Innate immunity changes
- Genetic predisposition
- Environmental factors
    - Allergens and infectious causes (viral URI most common infectious cause)

Signs and symptoms

- Cough (worse at night) — may be only symptom in children
- Wheezing
- Dyspnea
- Chest tightness
- Sputum production

Principles of asthma management

- Assess severity initially
- Assess control of symptoms with treatment to adjust therapy
- Assess severity once control with treatment is achieved
- Identify precipitating factors
- Identify comorbid conditions such as GERD, OSA (obstructive sleep apnea), sinusitis, obesity, emotional stress etc.
- Assess patient's knowledge and ability to self-manage
- Patient instruction for self-monitoring
- Periodic clinic visits to monitor asthma
    - Every 2–6 weeks at start of therapy
    - Every 1–6 months after control is achieved to monitor therapy
- Spirometry — initially, and then after therapy has started, and during periods of exacerbation and every 1–2 years otherwise
- Provide a written asthma plan to patient
- Patient education

Classification of asthma severity

Well controlled

- Symptoms ≤ 2 days/week
- Nighttime awakening ≤ 2 times/month
- No interference with activity
- Short-acting beta–agonist (SABA) use ≤ 2 days/week (excludes exercise-induced asthma)
- FEV1 or peak flow > 80% of predicted or personal best

Not well controlled

- Symptoms > 2 days/week
- Nighttime awakening 1–3 times/week
- Some limitation of normal activity
- SABA use > 2 days/week (excludes exercise-induced asthma)
- FEV1 or peak flow 60–80% of predicted or personal best

Very poorly controlled

- Symptoms throughout the day
- Nighttime awakenings ≥ 4 times/week
- Extremely limited activity
- SABA use several times a day (excludes exercise-induced asthma)
- FEV1 or peak flow < 60% of predicted or personal best

Severe exacerbation

- Dyspnea at rest and interferes with conversation
- Peak expiratory flow (PEF) < 40% of predicted or personal best

Acute treatment

- Inhaled short-acting beta–agonist (albuterol) and ipratropium (if available) — repeat q15minutes × 3 prn or continuous nebulizer awaiting EMS
- Send to emergency department (by ambulance preferentially)

Life threatening exacerbation

- Too dyspneic to speak; diaphoretic
- PEF < 25% of predicted or personal best

Treatment

- Inhaled short-acting beta–agonist (albuterol) and ipratropium (if available) — repeat q15minutes × 3 prn or continuous nebulizer awaiting EMS
- Send by ambulance to emergency department and call emergency department with report

Stepwise approach to asthma management ≥ 12 years of age

- To assist but not replace clinical decision making on individual patients

Step-up as needed

- First check medication adherence, environmental control and comorbid conditions
- Assess control
- Step down when possible and when asthma is controlled for 3 months
- Step up treatment when SABA used > 2 days/week
- Short course oral corticosteroid may be needed for exacerbations

Intermittent asthma

Step 1

Preferred:

- Inhaled short-acting beta–agonist (SABA) prn therapy

Persistent asthma: Daily medication

- Consider SQ immunotherapy for Step 2–4 in patients with allergic asthma

Step 2

- SABA prn

Preferred:

- Low-dose inhaled corticosteroid (ICS)

Alternatives to ICS

- Cromolyn
- Leukotriene receptor antagonist (LTRA)
- Nedocromil
- Theophylline

Step 3

- SABA prn

Preferred:

- Low-dose ICS + long-acting inhaled beta–agonist (LABA)

  OR

- Medium-dose ICS

Alternatives:

- Low-dose ICS + either LTRA, theophylline or zileuton

Step 4 (consult specialist)

- SABA prn

Preferred:

- Medium-dose ICS + LABA

Alternative:

- Medium-dose ICS + either LTRA, theophylline or zileuton

Step 5 (consult specialist)

- SABA prn

Preferred:

- High-dose ICS + LABA

  AND

- Consider omalizumab in allergic asthma patients

Step 6 (consult specialist)

- SABA prn

Preferred:

- High-dose ICS + LABA + oral steroid

  AND

- Consider omalizumab in allergic asthma patients

Stepwise approach to asthma management age 0–4 years of age

- To assist but not replace clinical decision making on individual patients

Step-up as needed

- First check medication adherence, environmental control and comorbid conditions
- Assess control
- Step down when possible and when asthma is controlled for 3 months
- Step up treatment when SABA used > 2 days/week
- Short course oral corticosteroid may be needed for exacerbations

Intermittent asthma

Step 1

Preferred:

- Inhaled short-acting beta–agonist (SABA) prn therapy

Persistent asthma: Daily medication

Step 2 (consider consultation with specialist)

- SABA prn

Preferred:

- Low-dose inhaled corticosteroid (ICS)

Alternatives to ICS

- Cromolyn or montelukast (Singulair)

Step 3 (consult specialist)

- SABA prn

Preferred:

- Medium-dose ICS

Step 4 (consult specialist)

- SABA prn

Preferred:

- Medium-dose ICS + LABA or montelukast (Singulair)

Step 5 (consult specialist)

- SABA prn

Preferred:

- High-dose ICS + LABA or montelukast (Singulair)

Step 6 (consult specialist)

- SABA prn

Preferred:

- High-dose ICS + LABA or montelukast (Singulair) + oral corticosteroid and ICS

Stepwise approach to asthma management age 5–11 years of age

- To assist but not replace clinical decision making on individual patients

Step-up as needed

- First check medication adherence, environmental control and comorbid conditions
- Assess control
- Step down when possible and when asthma is controlled for 3 months
- Step up treatment when SABA used > 2 days/week
- Short course oral corticosteroid may be needed for exacerbations

Intermittent asthma

Step 1

Preferred:

- Inhaled short-acting beta–agonist (SABA) prn therapy

Persistent asthma: Daily medication

- Consider SQ immunotherapy for Step 2–4 in patients with allergic asthma

Step 2

- SABA prn

Preferred:

- Low-dose inhaled corticosteroid (ICS)

Alternatives to ICS

- Cromolyn, LTRA, nedocromil or theophylline

Step 3 (consider consultation with specialist)

SABA prn

Preferred:

- Low-dose ICS + LABA, LTRA or theophylline

  OR

- Medium-dose ICS

Step 4 (consult specialist)

- SABA prn

Preferred:

- Medium-dose ICS + LABA

Alternative:

- Medium-dose ICS + LTRA or theophylline

Step 5 (consult specialist)

- SABA prn

Preferred:

- High-dose ICS + LABA

Alternative:

- High-dose ICS + LTRA or theophylline

Step 6 (consult specialist)

- SABA prn

Preferred:

- High-dose ICS + LABA + oral corticosteroid

Alternative:

- High-dose ICS + LTRA or theophylline + oral corticosteroids

Medications

Short-acting beta–agonist (SABA)

Albuterol HFA inhaler

All ages

- 2 puffs q4–6hr prn
- Spacer recommended

Nebulized albuterol

Age < 5 years

- 0.63–2.5 mg in 3 ml NS q4–8hr prn

Age ≥ 5 years

- 1.25–5 mg in 3 ml NS q4–6hr prn

Inhaled corticosteroid (ICS)

Fluticasone HFA/MDI (Flovent)

Low daily dose

Age < 5 years

- 176 mcg

Age ≥ 5 years

- 88–176 mcg

Medium daily dose

0–11 years

- > 176–352 mcg

Age ≥ 12 years

- > 264–440 mcg

High daily dose

Age ≤ 11 years

- > 352 mcg

Age ≥ 12 years

- > 440 mcg

Short term oral corticosteroids

- Course 3–10 days (no taper needed)

Methylprednisolone, prednisolone and prednisone

Age ≤ 11 years

- 1–2 mg PO qday (NMT 60 mg)

Age ≥ 12 years

- 40–60 mg PO qday

Long-acting beta–agonists (LABA)

Salmeterol DFI 50 mcg/blister

Age ≥ 5 years

- 1 blister q12hr

Formeterol

Age ≥ 5 years

- 1 capsule q12hr

Combination ICS/LABA

Budesonide/formoterol HFA/MDI (Symbicort)

Age ≥ 5 years

- 2 puffs bid (depends on level of control)

Cromolyn

MDI

Age ≥ 5 years

- 2 puffs qid

Nebulizer 20 mg/ampule

Age ≥ 2 years

- 1 ampule qid

Nedocromil MDI

Age ≥ 6 years

- 2 puffs qid

Leukotriene receptor antagonist (LTRA)

Montelukast (Singulair) chewable tablet

Age 1–5 years

- 4 mg qhs

Age 6–14 years

- 5 mg qhs

Age ≥ 15 years

- 10 mg qhs

Zuleuton 600 mg tablet

Age ≥ 12 years

- 600 mg qid

Theophylline

Age < 1 year

- Starting dose 10 mg/kg/day
- Usual maximum dose 0.2 × age in weeks + 5 = mg/kg/day — full term up to 26 weeks divided q8hr and divided q6hr for age 26–52 weeks

Age 1–11 year

- Starting dose 10 mg/kg/day
- Usual maximum 16 mg/kg/day

Age ≥12 years

- Starting dose 10 mg/kg/day up to 300 mg/day
- Usual maximum 800 mg/day

Consult criteria

- As noted in the Stepwise approach above
- Usually Step 3 or higher
- Consider consultation for subspecialty evaluation for:
  - Life-threatening asthma exacerbations or intubation
  - Recurrent hospitalizations or ED visits in patients felt to be adherent to the written action plan — i.e., unresponsive to therapy
  - Atypical features to the patient presentation raising questions as to other problems that mimic asthma such as vocal cord dysfunction syndrome, allergic bronchopulmonary aspergillosis, etc.

Notes

Reference:

Expert Panel Report 3 (EPR-3): Guidelines for the Diagnosis and Management of Asthma - Summary Report 2007

COPD Management

When using any management guideline, always follow the Guidelines of Proper Use (page 16).

Definition

- Disease state with chronic airflow obstruction that is not fully reversible, and is progressive — and includes chronic bronchitis and/or emphysema and/or fixed asthmatic bronchitis and many patients will have substantial overlapping conditions

Differential diagnosis

- Acute bronchitis
- Pulmonary embolism
- Heart failure with bronchospasm
- Bronchiectasis
- Pneumonia
- Chronic asthma

Considerations

- 4th leading cause of death in the U.S.
- Chronic bronchitis defined as 3 months of chronic productive cough each of the past 2 years (other causes of cough excluded)
- Emphysema has permanent enlargement of the airways distal to the terminal bronchioles
- Asthma — see Asthma Management
- Cigarette smoke is leading cause of COPD
- Increase in lung volume occurs

Signs and symptoms

- Productive cough
- Acute chest illness
- Wheezing
- Rhonchi
- Inspiratory crackles
- Dyspnea
- Use of respiratory accessory muscles

- Cor pulmonale (right heart failure and edema)
- Occasional left heart failure
- Barrel chest (emphysema)
- Heart tones distant
- Obesity (more in chronic bronchitis patients)
- Prolonged expiration
- pCO2 retention
- Metabolic alkalosis compensating for chronic respiratory acidosis
- Respiratory failure (end-stage)

Evaluation options

- History and physical examination
- Chest x-ray
- CBC
- Spirometry
    - Forced expiratory volume in 1 second over forced vital capacity (FEV_1/FVC) is less than 70% of predicted commonly
- ABG (pH should be normal; less than 7.30 indicates significant respiratory compromise
    - Any decrease in pH below normal (7.35) from increasing pCO2 is important and needs immediate evaluation and treatment
- Sputum evaluation for acute exacerbations prn
    - Streptococcal pneumonia and hemophilus influenza and moraxella catarrhalis most common bacterial organisms
    - Pseudomonas aeruginosa and enterobacteriaceae may occur in severe obstruction
- CT chest scan prn
- Pulse oximetry

Treatment

- Smoking cessation
- Patient education
- Proton pump inhibitor for GERD
- Long term oxygen for pO2 < 55 mm Hg; or < 59 mm Hg for cor pulmonale or polycythemia

Stage 1 (mild obstruction)

- Influenza vaccine
- Short-acting bronchodilator prn

Stage 2 (moderate obstruction)

- Influenza vaccine
- Short-acting beta–agonist (SABA) prn
- Long-acting bronchodilator
- Cardiopulmonary rehabilitation

Stage 3 (severe obstruction)

- Stage 2 treatment plus inhaled corticosteroids (ICS) for repeated exacerbations
- Consider subspecialty consultation

Stage 4 (very severe obstruction)

- Stage 3 plus oxygen prn
- Surgery options
- Consider subspecialty consultation

Medication options

Short-acting beta–agonist (SABA)

Albuterol HFA inhaler

- 2 puffs q4–6h prn
- Spacer recommended

Long-acting beta–agonists (LABA)

Salmeterol DFI 50 mcg/blister

- 1 blister q12hr

Formeterol

- 1 capsule q12hr

Anticholinergic agents

Ipratropium (Atrovent)

- 2 puffs qid (NMT 12 puffs qday)

Tiotropium (Spiriva)

- 2 inhalations of 1 capsule qday

Inhaled corticosteroid (ICS)

Fluticasone (Flovent)

Low daily dose

- 88–176 mcg

Medium daily dose

- > 264–440 mcg

High daily dose

- > 440 mcg

Short term oral corticosteroids

- Course 3–10 days (no taper needed)

Methylprednisolone, prednisolone and prednisone

- 40–60 mg PO qday

Combination albuterol/ipratropium (Combivent)

MDI

- 2 puffs qid prn (NMT 12 puffs qday)

Combination SABA/ICS

Budesonide/formoterol 160 mcg/4.5 mcg (Symbicort)

- 2 inhalations bid

Fluticasone/salmeterol (Advair diskus) 50 mcg/250 mcg

- 1 inhalation bid

Antibiotic choices for exacerbations

- Azithromycin (Z-pak)
- Doxycycline 100 mg PO bid for 10 days
- Amoxicillin 500 mg PO tid for 10 days
- Septra DS PO bid for 10 days
- Cefuroxime (Zinacef) 250–500 mg PO BID for 10 days

Smoking cessation

- Nicorette
- Zyban
- Chantix

Consult criteria

- Uncontrolled COPD despite maximal medication therapy
- Home oxygen needed
- Respiratory acidosis with a pH < 7.35 (send to emergency department)
- Respiratory fatigue (send to emergency department)
- Progressive weight loss
- Fever ≥ 101.5° F (38.6° C) — remember to evaluate for other causes of fever — UTI, prostatitis, viral syndromes (influenza), etc.

Notes

VENTILATOR MANAGEMENT

When using any management guideline, always follow the Guidelines of Proper Use (page 16).

For clinical settings that permit the practitioner to perform ventilator management and they are trained and experienced to perform those duties

Considerations

- Mechanical ventilation after intubation is a common lifesaving therapy
- Optimization of the ventilation parameters decrease complications and hospital stays
    - Lung protective ventilation — lower tidal volume of 6 mg/kg
- Decreases work of breathing
- Positive pressure is used to inflate lungs
- Positive end–expiratory pressure (PEEP) < 6 cm H2O rarely affects blood pressure and cardiac output
- Oxygen toxicity — not a concern acutely
- Respiratory alkalosis limits minute ventilation adjustments (respiratory rate x tidal volume)
- Check ABG prn and 30 minutes after ventilator adjustment
    - Manipulate one parameter at a time when changes are needed (respiratory rate, tidal volume, PEEP, FiO2 etc.)
- If the practitioner feels that intubation is needed then it most likely is needed
- No absolute contraindications to intubation exist
    - Extreme caution is needed in cervical spine injuries or with cervical spine rheumatoid arthritis or ankylosing spondylitis

Common disease processes requiring intubation when severe

- Asthma
- Heart failure
- COPD exacerbation
- Sepsis

- ARDS
- Pneumonia
- Trauma
- Neuromuscular disorders
- Drug overdose

Complications

Pulmonary

Barotrauma

- High peak pressures > 40 cm H2O
- Pneumothorax
- Pneumomediastinum
- Interstitial emphysema

High oxygen concentration

- Free radical cellular damage
- Absorption atelectasis from nitrogen washout

Cardiovascular effects

- From high PEEP (high intrathoracic pressures)
  - Decreased venous preload and cardiac output
  - Right ventricular dysfunction
- Decreased cardiac output effects
  - Renal blood flow decrease causes decreased urine and sodium excretion
  - Impaired hepatic function
  - Gastrointestinal ischemia

Indications for mechanical ventilation

Clinical indications

- Bradypnea or apnea
- Severe or advanced respiratory fatigue
- Coma
- Obtunded
- Loss of protective airway reflexes (gag reflex)
- Acute lung injury
- ARDS (adult respiratory distress syndrome)
- Shock

Clinical conditions

Hypercapneic respiratory failure

- COPD
- Status asthmaticus
- Neuromuscular disease
- Severe chest wall trauma (flail chest)

Hypoxemic respiratory failure

- Pneumonia
- Pulmonary edema
    - Cardiogenic — heart failure
    - Non-cardiogenic — ARDS
- Diffuse lung disease
    - Interstitial fibrosis or inflammation
    - Pulmonary hemorrhage
- Pulmonary embolism with infarction
- Extreme work of breathing
- Protect airway and control secretions with impaired cough reflex and effort
    - CVA
    - Drug overdose
    - Cervical spine injury

Laboratory indications

- $PaCO_2 > 50$ mm Hg with a $pH < 7.25$
- $PaO_2 < 55$ mm Hg on optimal supplementary oxygen

Pulmonary function test indications

- Vital capacity < 15mL/kg in adults
- Vital capacity < 10 mL/kg in children
- Negative inspiratory force < -20 cm H_2O (normal -65 to -75 cm H_2O
- Forced expiratory volume (FEV_1) < 5 mL/kg

Modes of mechanical ventilation

Volume-cycled

- Delivers a set tidal volume until expiration followed by passive exhalation
- Delivers constant inspiratory flow

- Results in higher pressures delivered than required for lung distension
- Airway pressures vary with changes in pulmonary compliance and resistance
- Ensures a constant minimum minute ventilation
- High airway pressure can occur resulting in barotrauma
    - ARDS or other diffuse lung disease with decreased lung compliance
    - Pneumothorax
    - Right mainstem intubation
    - Increased intra-abdominal pressure
    - Chest wall rigidity
    - "Fighting the ventilator" due to patient agitation

Pressure-cycled

- Set inspiratory pressure is delivered
- When the peak inspiratory pressure is attained passive exhalation occurs
- Useful in ARDS in ICU to limit barotrauma
- Changes in lung function may result in varying tidal volumes which is a disadvantage and requires close monitoring
- Some ventilators allow for volume assured pressure-cycled ventilation with increases in pressure as needed to deliver desired tidal volumes

Tidal volume settings

Volume control mode

- Delivers preset tidal volume regardless of patient effort

Pressure support mode

- Provides inspiratory assistance for patient's spontaneous respirations
- Detects patient's inspiratory effort and applies assist pressure
- Terminates upon detecting patient exhalation
- Requires adequate patient respiratory drive
- Amount of assist pressure is entered in ventilator

Ventilatory support methods

Assist-controlled ventilation

- Ventilator cycles with patient respiratory effort above the set rate
- Independent breathing from ventilator is not allowed
- Can worsen air trapping in COPD with breath stacking

Synchronous intermittent mandatory ventilation (SIMV)

- Preset amount of breaths given per minute
- Independent patient respirations allowed in addition to set ventilator breaths
- Attempts to limit barotrauma

Pressure support ventilation

- For spontaneous breathing patients
- Level of pressure support is set to assist spontaneous respirations
- Decreases barotrauma and respiratory work
- Useful when respiratory failure is not severe
- May improve patient comfort
- Decreases cardiac side effects

Noninvasive ventilation

- Ventilation through a mask
- Useful in mild to moderate respiratory failure
- Patient must be able to follow commands
- CPAP and BiPAP are the modalities
    - BiPAP is a form of CPAP that alternates high and low pressure permitting inspiration and expiration
- Useful in CHF, asthma, COPD and pulmonary edema from volume overload
- Can significantly decrease the need for intubation, and decreases hospital stay and mortality

Commonly used ventilation parameters

- Tidal volume (TV) is amount of air moved in a single breath (5–12 mL/kg)
- Minute ventilation is amount of air moved in a minute (5–10 L/kg)
- Ventilatory rate per minute is 8–12 in adults
    - Too fast rate can cause air trapping (auto–PEEP)
- Peak inspiratory pressure (PIP) < 35 cm H2O
    - Too high may cause barotrauma, poor oxygenation or hemodynamic compromise and too low may cause hypoventilation and atelectasis
- PEEP 2–10 cm H2O
    - May decrease cardiac output from decreased venous return at higher PEEP
    - Maintain at lowest level that achieves desired results for hypoxemia
- Ispiratory:expiratory ratio (I:E ratio) 1:1.5 to 1:4 for time of inspiration to expiration
    - Needed to adequate fill and empty the lungs of air
    - Inadequate expiratory time may lead to air trapping (auto PEEP)
- Plateau pressure is average inspiratory pressure (< 30 cm H2O)
    - Too high may cause barotrauma, poor oxygenation or hemodynamic compromise and too low may cause hypoventilation and atelectasis
- FiO2 (fraction of inspired oxygen) titrated to maintain pO2 over 60 mm Hg or O2 saturation 90% or above (usually set initially at 100% FiO2)
- Inspiratory flow is amount of gas given during inspiration (40–100 L/minute)
- Mean airway pressure is a reflection of mean alveolar pressure

Ventilator settings (initial)

Normal lungs

- Tidal volume 8 mL/kg ideal body weight (may use 5–7 mL/kg)
- Respiratory rate 10–12/minute (max 35/minute)
- I:E ratio 1:2
- PEEP 4 cm H2O

- FiO_2 100% (decrease as permitted to maintain pO_2 60–100 mm Hg or O_2 saturation over 90%)

Asthma/COPD

- Tidal volume 6 mL/kg ideal body weight
- Respiratory rate 10–12/minute
- I:E ratio 1:2 (or possibly higher to avoid auto-PEEP)
- PEEP 4 cm H_2O
- FiO_2 100% (decrease as permitted to maintain pO_2 60–100 mm Hg)

ARDS (adult respiratory distress syndrome)

- Tidal volume 6 mL/kg ideal body weight
- Respiratory rate 10–12/minute
- I:E ratio 1:2
- PEEP 4-15 cm H_2O (start at 4–5 cm H_2O if possible)
- FiO_2 100% (decrease as permitted to maintain pO_2 60–100 mm Hg)
- Plateau pressure < 30 cm H_2O

Hypovolemia (shock)

- Tidal volume 8 mL/kg ideal body weight
- Respiratory rate 10–12/minute
- I:E ratio 1:2
- PEEP 0–4 cm H_2O
- FiO_2 100% (decrease as permitted to maintain pO_2 60–100 mm Hg)

Monitoring ventilator support

- ABG initially and 15–30 minutes after a ventilator change parameter change
  - Maintain pH > 7.3 and < 7.45
    - pH > 7.45 decrease ventilator rate
    - pH 7.15–7.30 increase ventilator rate
  - Maintain pO_2 60–100 mm Hg
  - Maintain pCO_2 35–45 mm Hg unless pH indicates patient is a chronic pCO_2 retainer
    - For example a pH > 7.45 with pCO_2 35–45 mm Hg indicates that the patient may

normally have a higher resting pCO_2 from COPD

- Cardiac monitoring
- Blood pressure monitoring
- Pulse oximetry (maintain O_2 saturation > 90%)
- Peak pressures < 40 cm H_2O
- Plateau pressures < 30 cm H_2O
- Increase PEEP in 2 cm H_2O increments as needed with assessing vital signs for several minutes afterward
- Inspiratory flow 40–100 L/minute

High pO_2 with high FiO_2

- Decrease FiO_2
  - 1% decrease in FiO_2 lowers pO_2 by 7 mm Hg

High pO_2 with lower FiO_2

- Lower PEEP to 3–5 cm H_2O (normal physiologic levels) in 2 cm H_2O increments

High pCO_2

- Increase minute ventilation by increasing respiratory rate or tidal volume

Low pCO_2

- Decrease minute ventilation by decreasing respiratory rate or tidal volume

Ventilator associated pneumonia decreases with

- Elevating head of bed 30°
- Proton-pump inhibitors or histamine-2 blockers

Sedation

- Most patients need sedation by continuous infusion or scheduled dosing
- Daily interruption of sedation when feasible allows for less days of ventilation and better assessment of the patient

Respiratory therapy protocols

- Decrease days on ventilator

- Allow spontaneous breathing trials when patient is a candidate for weaning

Trouble shooting

Sudden respiratory distress

- Disconnect patient from ventilator
- Manual ventilate with ambu bag
- No improvement then check patient

Ventilator problems

- Check tubing for obstruction
- Check for circuit disconnect

Intubation problems

Low resistance check for:

- Endotracheal tube (ET) placement
    - Esophageal location
- Cuff leak if low resistance or low peak inspiratory pressure develops
- Internal tube leak if low resistance or low peak inspiratory pressure develops

High resistance or pressures

- Right mainstem location
- Pneumothorax
- Patient biting ET
- Check tubing for obstruction (suction tube)
- Kinked ET tube

Normal resistance

- CHF (higher pressures)
- Bronchospasms (higher pressures)
- Overly sedated
- AMI
- PE
- Pneumonia (higher pressures)
- Aspiration (higher pressures)

Hypotension treatment options

- IV NS bolus if heart failure or pulmonary edema not present
- Decrease PEEP

- Decrease respiratory rate
- Decrease tidal volume
- If air trapping suspected, increase expiratory time
- Evaluate for pneumothorax or pulmonary embolism as needed

Weaning

- Evaluate patient each day to determine is candidate

Assessment

- Is the respiratory failure process improving?
- Hemodynamic stability
- $PaO_2 > 60$ mm Hg on $FiO_2 < 40\%$ and PEEP < 5 cm H_2O
- Respiratory strength, mental and neuromuscular status adequate?
- Acid-base and electrolyte status optimal
- Afebrile?
- Thyroid and adrenal function sufficient
- Respiratory rate/tidal volume (f/Vt) < 105 usually can be weaned
    - Age > 70 years with f/Vt < 130 may be acceptable

Parameters

- Tidal volume > 5 mL/kg
- Vital capacity > 10 mL/kg
- Respiratory rate < 25/minute
- Minute ventilation < 10 L/minute
- $PaO_2/FiO_2 > 200$
- Shunt < 20%
- Negative inspiratory pressure more negative than -25 cm H_2O

Pressure support weaning

- All breaths are spontaneous
- Gradually decrease pressure support to 5–6 cm H_2O then the patient usually can be extubated

Spontaneous breathing trial (SBT) weaning–preferred

T-piece trial

- Patient disconnected from ventilator with oxygen given through a T-piece
- Respiratory therapy to monitor patient
- Should last 30 to 90 minutes before extubation with assessment of blood pressure, respiratory rate, heart rate and oxygenation
- Should be performed once a day if not successful initially

Consult criteria

- Management under physician's direction
- Requiring mechanical ventilation > 24 hours
- More complicated ventilator or oxygenation problem
- Complex critical illness

Notes

ADULT SEPTIC SHOCK MANAGEMENT

When using any management guideline, always follow the Guidelines of Proper Use (page 16).

For clinical settings that permit the practitioner to perform adult septic shock management and they are trained and experienced to perform those duties

Definitions

Septic Shock

- State of acute circulatory failure characterized by persistent arterial hypotension or by tissue hypoperfusion
  - Documented or strong suspicion for infection
  - SBP (systolic blood pressure) < 90 mm Hg or MAP (mean arterial pressure) < 65 mm Hg
  - Serum lactate elevated (level > 4 mg/dL strongly suggestive of septic shock)
  - SIRS present

Systemic Inflammatory Response Syndrome (SIRS) — 3 or more

- Core temperature > 100.4°F (38° C)
- Heart rate > 90/minute unless on beta-blockers
- Respiratory rate > 20/minute or pCO2 < 32 mm Hg
- WBC > 12,000 or < 4,000 or > 10–15% bands

Sepsis is the presence of infection in addition to SIRS

- Usually has at least one of the following signs of organ hypoperfusion
  - Acute altered mental status
  - Hypoxemia without overt pulmonary disease
  - Elevated plasma lactate levels

- Oliguria (urine output < 30 ml/hour or 0.5 ml/kg over 1 hour

Differential diagnosis

- Heatstroke
- Adrenal crisis and shock
- Cardiogenic shock
- Hypovolemic shock
- Hemorrhagic shock
- DKA
- Neuroleptic malignant syndrome
- Toxic shock syndrome
- Cardiac tamponade
- Massive pulmonary embolism
- Adult respiratory distress syndrome (ARDS)
- Other forms of shock

Considerations

- Culture positive bacteremia occurs in 30–50%
- Not all patients with bacteremia have signs of sepsis
- Serious bacterial infections with or without bacteremia may be associated with changes in all organ systems
    - Change in organ function mediated by host immune system mechanisms against infection
- The continuum of severity is from sepsis to septic shock to multiple organ dysfunction syndrome
- ARDS occurs in 20–40% of septic shock

Early Goal-directed Therapy

(Very important in first 6 hours of treatment)

Treatment goals

- Maintain MAP ≥ 65 mm Hg
- Maintain CVP (central venous pressure) 8–12 mm Hg in nonintubated patients
    - Maintain CVP 12–15 mm Hg in intubated patients
- Keep central venous O2 (ScvO2) saturation ≥ 70%
- Maintain lactate ≤ 2 mmol/L

- Maintain urine output ≥ 0.5 ml/kg/hour in nonrenal failure patients

Monitoring

- Vital signs ≤ every 5 minutes
- Maintain O2 saturation ≥ 90%
- CVP line placement and readings prn
- Place foley

Testing

- ABG
- Lactic acid (lactate) level
- CBC
- BMP
- LFT's
- PT/PTT/INR
- Blood cultures X 2 using different sites if possible
- U/A
- Urine cultures
- Chest x-ray
- EKG
- Troponin and BNP
- Type and screen
- Sputum culture & sensitivity and gram stain if present
- Cortisol level
- Accucheck for glucose

Treatment

IV fluid and pressor treatment

- IV NS boluses 10–20 ml/kg — 500–1,000 ml over 30 minutes
    - Goal is to achieve MAP ≥ 65 and CVP 8–12 mm Hg in nonventilated patients and 12–15 mm Hg in ventilated patients
    - Usually ≥ 4 liters of NS IV is needed
- If CVP target achieved and MAP is < 65 mm Hg then start norepinephrine (Levophed) IV
    - Norepinephrine start at 2–4 mcg/minute IV — usual dosage range 8–12 mcg/minute (may need up to 30 mcg/minute in refractory shock)

- Hematocrit < 30% and ScvO2 < 70% — transfuse packed red blood cells to raise hematocrit > 30%
- Consider using dobutamine IV up to 20 mcg/kg/minute if unable to achieve or maintain ScvO2 > 70% with above measures
- Solucortef 100–200 mg IV if adrenal sufficiency present or suspected
    - 50 mg IV q6hr x 7 days

Empiric antibiotic treatment

- Vancomycin 1 gm IV q12hr (adjust for renal insufficiency

PLUS one beta–lactam

- Piperacillin/tazobactam (Zosyn) 3.375–4.5 gms IV q6hr

OR

- Ampicillin/sulbactam (Unasyn) 3 gm IV q6hr

OR

- Meropenem (Merrem) 1 gm IV q8hr

OR

- Ceftriaxone (Rocephin) 1 gm IV q12hr

OR

- Imipenem (Primaxin) 0.5–1 gm IV q8hr

OR

- Cefepime (Maxipime) 2 gm IV q12hr

OR

- Ceftazidime (Fortaz) 2 gm IV q8–12hr

PLUS one aminoglycoside (adjust for renal insufficiency)

- Gentamycin 5 mg/kg/day IV divided q8hr

OR

- Tobramycin 5 mg/kg/day IV divided q8hr

OR

- Amikacin 15 mg/kg/day IV divided q8–12hr

Pneumonia

- Vancomycin 1 gm IV q12hr (adjust for renal insufficiency

PLUS one beta–lactam

- Piperacillin/tazobactam (Zosyn) 3.375–4.5 gms IV q6hr

  OR
- Ampicillin/sulbactam (Unasyn) 3 gm IV q6hr

  OR
- Meropenem (Merrem) 1 gm IV q8hr

  OR
- Ceftriaxone (Rocephin) 1 gm IV q12hr

  OR
- Imipenem (Primaxin) 0.5–1 gm IV q8hr

  OR
- Cefepime (Maxipime) 2 gm IV q12hr

  OR
- Ceftazidime (Fortaz) 2 gm IV q8–12hr

PLUS fluoroquinolone

- Levofloxacin (Levaquin) 750 mg IV qday — adjust for renal dosing

  OR
- Moxifloxacin (Avelox) 400 mg IV qday

Neutropenia

- Cefepime (Maxipime) 2 gm IV q12hr

  OR
- Ceftazidime (Fortaz) 2 gm IV q8–12hr

  OR
- Imipenem (Primaxin) 0.5–1 gm IV q8hr

May add if desired

(Adjust aminoglycosides for renal insufficiency)

- Gentamycin 5 mg/kg/day IV divided q8hr

  OR
- Tobramycin 5 mg/kg/day IV divided q8hr

  OR
- Amikacin 15 mg/kg/day IV divided q8–12hr

Intra–abdominal sepsis proven or suspected

- Ticarcillin–clavulanate (Timentin) 3.1 gm IV q4-6hr

  OR

- Piperacillin/tazobactam (Zosyn) 3.375–4.5 gms IV q6hr

  OR

- Imipenem (Primaxin) 0.5–1 gm IV q8hr

May add if desired
(Adjust for renal insufficiency)

- Gentamycin 5 mg/kg/day IV divided q8hr

  OR

- Tobramycin 5 mg/kg/day IV divided q8hr

  OR

- Amikacin 15 mg/kg/day IV divided q8–12hr

Fluoroquinolones

- Levofloxacin (Levaquin) 750 mg IV qday — adjust for renal insufficiency

  OR

- Moxifloxacin (Avelox) 400 mg IV qday

Anaerobic coverage if desired

- Metronidazole (Flagyl) 1 gm IV q12hr

  OR

- Clindamycin (Cleocin) 600 mg IV q8hr

Protective lung strategy in ARDS for intubated ventilated patients

- Tidal volumes of 6 ml/kg of ideal body weight
- Plateau pressure < 30 cm H_2O

Consult recommendations

- Close management of patient care with a physician

Notes

Depression Management

When using any management guideline, always follow the Guidelines of Proper Use (page 16).

Definition

- A state of emotional sadness and withdrawal greater and more prolonged than warranted by objective reasons

Differential diagnosis

- Anxiety disorder
- Bipolar affective disorder
- Dementia
- Hypothyroidism
- Hyperthyroidism
- Cushing syndrome
- Addison disease
- Alcoholism
- Drug abuse
- Chronic fatigue syndrome
- Schizophrenia
- Personality disorders
- Sleep apnea
- Adjustment disorder
- Posttraumatic stress disorder
- Premenstrual dysphoric disorder
- Lyme disease
- Syphilis
- Autoimmune diseases
- B-12 deficiency (pernicious anemia)

Considerations

- Lifetime depression incidence is 12% in men and 20% in women
- Most patients with depression do not realize they have a treatable disease
- Antidepressant medication takes 2–6 weeks to achieve therapeutic effect if there is a benefit to be realized

- Antidepressant medication may worsen the depression potentially leading to suicide – close monitoring of treatment needed
- A clearly defined physiologic cause of depression has not been found, though serotonin levels are thought to be an important factor
- Major depressant disorder is multifactorial
- Genetic link for depression exists in some individuals
- Stressors, chronic medical conditions and chronic pain predispose to depression
- Childhood abuse and neglect increases depression incidence in childhood and later in life
- Major depressive disorder has significant morbidity and mortality
- Treatment can help 70–80% of patients, though 50% may not initially respond to treatment
- Males successfully complete suicides 4.5 times as much as females
- 80% of women develop postpartum mood disturbance that is usually self–limited and of short duration lasting 2 weeks
    - Postpartum depression develops over 3 months usually
    - Untreated postpartum depression may cause child development and behavior problems
- Seasonal affective disorder — 2 episodes of a mood disorder in 2 years related to a particular season and outnumbers the nonseasonable episodes
- Severe major depression with psychosis is dangerous and often requires psychiatric admission
- Patient education is very important in depression treatment

Presenting complaints

- Somatic complaints such as fatigue, headache, GI complaints and weight changes
- Elderly may present with confusion
- Irritability
- Social withdrawal
- Dysphoric mood and negative attitude
- Psychosis

Major depressive episode

5 of the following in a 2 week period

- Depressed mood (typically over a 3 month period)
- Anhedonia — diminished interest and pleasure in most activities
- Appetite disturbance or weight change
- Fatigue
- Feelings of worthlessness
- Sleep disturbance
- Decreased concentration ability
- Recurrent thoughts of death or suicide
- Interpersonal rejection or suicide attempts/plans

Caveats

- Must have depressed mood or loss of interest/pleasure
- Symptoms must cause significant distress or impairment of social, occupational or interpersonal relationships
- Symptoms not precipitated by substances or medical conditions
- Symptoms do not meet criteria for bipolar illness
- Symptoms are not accounted for by bereavement
- Should not be coexistent with schizophrenia or other psychotic disorders

Evaluation

- Assess for medical conditions or medications that may cause depression — see Differential diagnosis
- Ask about suicidal or homicidal thoughts/plans

Mental status examination

OMI HAT (OMI = organic disease; HAT = psychiatric or functional)

    - O – Orientation
    - M – Memory
    - I – Intellect
    - H – Hallucinations
    - A – Affect disorder
    - T – Thought disorder
  - Cognitive impairment evaluated by using Mini-Mental Status Examination

Treatment

- Psychotherapy
- Medications
  - Combining medications and psychotherapy most effective and sustained approach

Medications

Selective serotonin reuptake inhibitors (SSRI's)

- Ease of dosing and low toxicity
- Preferred in children, adolescents and late onset depression
  - Studies have indicated an increase in suicidal thoughts on SSRI's, but decreased suicidal attempts
- Common side effects are GI upset, sexual dysfunction and fatigue/restlessness

Citalopram (Celexa)

- Initially 10–20 mg PO qday — may adjust every 2–4 weeks as needed — NMT 40 mg PO qday
- NMT 20 mg PO qday if taking cimetidine, omeprazole, fluconazole or other inhibitors of CYP2C19

Escitalopram (Lexapro)

- Depression
  - 10 mg PO qday — may increase to 20 mg PO qday after 2–4 weeks as needed
- Generalized anxiety disorder and depression in elderly
  - 10 mg PO qday for elderly

Paroxetine (Paxil)

- Depression
  - Initially 10–20 mg PO qday — may increase 10 mg/day q2–4weeks up to 50 mg PO qday as needed
  - Paxil CR: initial 12.5–25 mg PO qday — may increase 12.5 mg PO q2–4 weeks as needed — NMT 62.5 mg PO qday
- Obsessive compulsive disorder
  - Initially 20 mg PO qday — may increase 10 mg/day q2–4weeks up to 60 mg PO qday as needed
- Panic disorder
  - Initially 10–20 mg PO qday — may increase 10 mg/day q2–4weeks up to 60 mg PO qday as needed
  - Paxil CR: initial 12.5–25 mg PO qday — may increase 12.5 mg PO q2–4 weeks — NMT 75 mg PO qday

Vilazodone (Viibryd)

- Initially 10 mg PO qday x 7 days, then 20 mg PO qday x 2–4 weeks, then may increase to 40 mg PO qday as needed
- NMT 20 mg PO qday if taking ketoconazole or other CYP3A4 inhibitors

Other SSRI's

- Fluoxetine (Prozac)
- Sertraline (Zoloft)

Selective serotonin/norepinephrine reuptake inhibitors (SNRI's)

Venlafaxine (Effexor)

- Extended-release: 37.5–75 mg PO qday — may increase 75 mg PO qday every 2–4 weeks — NMT 225 mg PO qday

Desvenlafaxine (Pristiq)

- 50 mg PO qday and may increase as needed to 100 mg PO qday in 2–4 weeks

Duloxetine (Cymbalta)

- 30–60 mg PO qday — NMT 60 mg PO qday
- May be used for diabetic peripheral neuropathy, fibromyalgia and generalized anxiety disorder
- Taper gradually

Atypical antidepressants

Bupropion (Wellbutrin)

- Intermediate-release: 100 mg PO bid — may increase to 100 mg PO tid after 2–4 weeks as needed (NMT 150 mg PO tid)
- Sustained-release (SR): Initially 100 mg PO bid — may increase to 150 mg PO bid after 2–4 weeks — NMT 200 mg PO bid
- Extended-release (XL): 150 mg PO qAM — may increase to 300 mg PO qday after 2–4 weeks (NMT 450 mg PO qday after 4 weeks)

Consult criteria

- Depression with psychosis — schizophrenia or bipolar affective disorder
- Refer patients with suicidal or homicidal ideation for immediate evaluation in emergency department or psychiatric facility
- Severe depression refractory to treatment

Notes

HEADACHE MANAGEMENT

When using any management guideline, always follow the Guidelines of Proper Use (page 16).

Definition

- Cephalic pain disorder

Differential Diagnosis

- Tension headache
- Migraine headache
- Cluster headache
- Sinusitis
- Otitis media
- Trigeminal neuralgia
- Brain tumor
- Subarachnoid hemorrhage
- Subdural hematoma
- Epidural hematoma
- Temporal arteritis
- Chronic daily headache
- Thunderclap headache
- Analgesic rebound headache
- CVA
- Meningitis
- Encephalitis
- Central vein thrombosis
- Normal pressure hydrocephalus
- Pseudotumor cerebri
- Ventricular peritoneal shunt malfunction
- Temporal mandibular joint disorder
- Lyme disease

Considerations

- History is one of the more important tools in headache evaluation
- New headache type in the elderly is suggestive of a higher risk process

- Do not use response to therapy as a judge of the seriousness of the headache

"Functional" or "Primary" headache

- No detectable cause (not uncommon)
- Migraine
- Cluster
- Tension–type headache

"Organic" or "Secondary" headache

From pain sensitive structures; vessels; periosteum

- Postconcussion headaches
- Spinal tap headaches
- Temporal arteritis
- Subarachnoid hemorrhage
- Subdural hematoma
- CVA
- Meningitis
- Encephalitis

Historical red flags

- Sudden onset or onset with exertion
- New, progressive, frequent headaches
- Trauma
- Cancer history
- Immunosuppression/HIV
- Clotting disorders
- First headache
- Worst headache of life
- Fever

Evaluation

- Complete history and physical exam
- Check gait, motor and sensory exam
- Funduscopic exam

Lab *(usually not needed in most headaches)*

- CBC

- ESR/CRP (age > 50 years: temporal arteritis) — usually not needed with no changes in chronic headache pattern
- UCG prn

Tension- type headache

- Pressing or tightening (nonpulsatile quality)
- Frontal-occipital location
- Bilateral: mild/moderate intensity
- Not aggravated by physical activity
- May have trigger points on scalp or cervical muscles

Causes

- Psychological stress
- Sleep deprivation
- Uncomfortable position or bad posture
- Eyestrain
- Irregular meals

Episodic tension–type headache

- Headaches lasting 30 minutes to 7 days
- Less than 15/month
- Pressure or tightening quality — nonpulsatile
- Mild to moderate intensity — may inhibit but not prohibit daily activities
- Bilateral in location
- Not exacerbated by physical activities
- No nausea or vomiting
- Photophobia or phonophonia — absent or one present
- Secondary type headaches not suspected or confirmed

Chronic tension–type headache

- More than 15 per month for more than 6 months
- Same as episodic tension–type headaches above otherwise

Evaluation

- History and physical exam

- Brain MRI if headache is atypical or concerning, or if the patient has a focal neurological exam — CT brain less useful than MRI

Treatment

- Tailored to individual patient
- Regular exercise and meals
- Proper sleep hygiene
- Trigger point injections prn
- Botulinum toxin is not effective

Episodic tension–type headache

- Physical therapy prn
    - Hot and cold applications
    - Stretching
    - Massage
    - Ultrasound therapy
    - TENS
- Psychophysiologic therapy prn
    - Stress management
    - Biofeedback techniques
- NSAID's PO prn
- Tylenol prn
- Fiorinal 1–2 PO q4hr prn not to exceed 6 per 24 hour period
- Midrin 1–2 caps qid PO prn

Chronic tension–type headache or > 2 headaches/week or are > 3 hours or severe enough to disrupt daily activities

Tricyclic antidepressants

- Amitriptyline (Elavil) 10 mg-150 mg PO qday — may give bid-tid
    - Taper gradually when discontinuing
- Nortriptyline (Pamelor) 25–100 mg PO qday — may give bid-tid
    - Taper gradually when discontinuing

Selective serotonin reuptake inhibitors (SSRI)

- Less anticholinergic and cardiovascular side effects than tricyclic antidepressants
- Fluoxetine (Prozac) 20–40 mg PO qday — NMT 60 mg qday
- Sertraline (Zoloft) 50 mg PO qday (may increase 25 mg qweek as needed) — NMT 200 mg qday
- Paroxetine (Paxil) 20 mg PO qday (may increase 10 mg qweek as needed) — NMT 50 mg qday

Migraine headache

Considerations

- 30 million persons in U.S. have at least 1 migraine per year
- Familial prevalence
- Causes are not fully defined
- Chronic migraines may occur with 8 days of opiates per month (more pronounced in males) and barbiturates 5 days per month (more pronounced in females)
- Increased CVA and AMI incidence
- Usually lasts 4-72 hours
- Postdromal symptoms may include tired or refreshed feeling, increased appetite, muscle weakness or myalgias
- May be associated with seizures

Migraine variants

- Hemiplegic migraine — unilateral weakness or paralysis
- Basilar migraine — aphasia, syncope or ataxia
- Ophthalmoplegic migraine — third cranial nerve palsy or visual field cut/monocular blindness
- Chronic migraine — 15 days per month for 3 months

Associated with

- Photophobia
- Phonophobia

- Nausea and vomiting
- May be unilateral or bilateral
- Aura occurs 20%
    - Scotoma (blind spots)
    - Fortification (zigzag patterns)
    - Scintilla (flashing lights)
    - Unilateral paresthesia/weakness
    - Hallucinations
    - Hemianopsia

Precipitants

- Stress
- Sleep disorders
- Vasodilators
- Oral contraceptives
- Menstruation or ovulation
- Smoking
- Strong odors
- Tyramine containing foods — yogurt, soy sauce, sour cream etc.

Evaluation

- Exclude other causes of headaches
- ESR and C-reactive protein in older patients to rule out temporal arteritis
- See CT brain headache criteria later in section

Lumbar puncture considered for

- First or worse headache of life
- Progressive headache
- Rapid onset severe headache
- Unusual chronic intractable headache
- Fever

Acute treatment

- Compazine (prochlorperazine) 5–10 mg IV or IM
- Thorazine (chlorpromazine) 75 mg with Benadryl (diphenhydramine) 25 mg IM
- Ergots DHE 1 mg IV or IM (premedicate with an antiemetic)
- Reglan (metoclopramide) 10 mg IV or IM

- Valproic acid 1 gm IV
- Sumatriptan 6 mg SQ (do not use with history of coronary artery disease) — read drug information
- Maxalt (rizatriptan) 5–10 mg PO q2h prn for headache not to exceed 30 mg/day (do not use with history of coronary artery disease) — read drug information
- Other trpitans
- Midrin 2 caps PO initially then 1 cap PO q1hr prn not to exceed 5 caps/day
- Toradol (ketorolac) 30–60 mg IM (do not use if creatinine is elevated)
- Compazine suppository (prochlorperazine) 25 mg PR bid prn (may cause extrapyramidal reaction)
- Acetaminophen
- Aspirin
- Narcotic prn (not preferred)
- Uninterrupted sleep may resolve episode

Prophylactic treatment

- Remove migraine triggers
- Biofeedback and/or cognitive behavior therapy prn
- Naproxen 250 mg PO tid or 500 mg PO bid
- Topiramate (Topamax) 50 mg bid — start at 25mg/day and titrate up over 2 weeks — doses greater than 100 mg daily are rarely effective
- Valproic acid (Depakote) start at 500 mg PO qday for 1 week, then increase to 500–1,000 mg PO divided into a daily or BID dosing — NMT 1,000 mg daily
    - Valproic acid adverse reactions
        - Hepatic failure (monitor liver function tests especially in first 6 months of therapy)
        - Pancreatitis
        - Pregnancy fetal risks — especially in first trimester
- Amitriptyline (Elavil) 10 mg-150 mg PO qday — may give bid-tid
    - Taper gradually when discontinuing

- Propranolol 20 mg PO qid may progress up to 80 mg PO tid
- Fluoxetine (Prozac) 20–40 mg PO qday — NMT 60 mg qday
- Sertraline (Zoloft) 50 mg PO qday (may increase 25 mg qweek as needed) — NMT 200 mg qday
- Paroxetine (Paxil) 20 mg PO qday (may increase 10 mg qweek as needed) — NMT 50 mg qday

Cluster headaches

- More common in males
- Lancinating and severe
- Sudden onset — peaks in 10–15 minutes
- Unilateral facial location
- Duration: 10 minutes to 3 hours per episode
- Character: boring and lancinating to eye
- Distribution: first and second divisions of the trigeminal nerve (approximately 18–20% of patients complain of pain in extratrigeminal regions)
- Autonomic symptoms such as ptosis, conjunctival injection, rhinorrhea, nasal congestion and lacrimation that are ipsilateral to the pain
- Frequency: may occur several times a day for 1–4 months (often nocturnal)
- Patients are very restless (unlike migraine)
- Periodicity: circadian regularity in 47% of patients
- Remission: long symptom-free intervals occur in some patients for 2 months to 20 years

Treatment options

- O2 8 LPM face mask or 100% nonrebreather mask
- Sumatriptan 6 mg SQ (do not use with history of coronary artery disease) — read drug information
- Lidocaine 1 cc of a 10% solution placed on a swab in each nostril for 5 minutes is potentially helpful
- Capsaicin applied intranasally (has a burning sensation side effect)
- Verapamil 240 mg-480 mg daily for preventative therapy

Trigeminal neuralgia

- Commonly idiopathic
- Shock like severe pains in the distribution of trigeminal nerve
- Onset usually around age 60–70 years of age
- If it occurs at a younger age, work-up including MRI of the brain is warranted
- Pains last seconds to less than 2 minutes
- Can be triggered by specific activities such as eating, talking, brushing teeth, etc.
- No associated neurologic deficits
    - A sensory deficit excludes the diagnosis

Glossopharyngeal neuralgia

- Pain is over the distribution of glossopharyngeal nerve triggered by coughing, yawning, swallowing cold liquids

Occipital neuralgia

- Pain is in the posterior scalp region

Treatment options of cranial neuralgias

- Carbamazepine 200 mg PO bid to start (DOC)
    - Titrate increasing dose every 3 days by 200 mg
    - Effective dose is usually 600–1200 mg qday
    - Instruct patient they will need monitoring for aplastic anemia and severe leucopenia
- Dilantin (phenytoin) for carbamazepine failures (lower rate of success in treating neuralgia)
    - Dose of 300–600 mg PO qday (levels need monitoring)
    - Cerebyx (fosphenytoin) 250 mg IV for severe attack
- Lamictal (lamotrigine) 100–400 mg PO qday (NMT 250 mg PO qday in children) — read drug information
- Treatment includes occipital nerve blocks

Discharge instructions

- Trigeminal neuralgia aftercare instructions

Consult criteria

- Complicated cranial neuralgias

Temporal arteritis

- True emergency of the elderly
    - Age of onset 50–70 years of age
    - Six times more common in females than in males
- Headache localized over eye or to scalp
- Fever, malaise and weight loss are associated symptoms
- Jaw claudication is an important associated symptom
- Frequently associated with polymyalgia rheumatica (joint and muscles aches)
- ESR 50–100
- C-reactive protein elevated usually
- Vision loss can occur early in course of disease

Treatment

- Prednisone 40–80 mg PO qday or divided bid for several months to one year

Discharge criteria

- Minimal symptoms
- Severe symptoms or question of eye involvement should be admitted with IV high dose steroid treatment and ophthalmology consultation obtained

Discharge instructions

- Temporal arteritis aftercare instructions
- Follow up within 1 day
- Return for visual changes

Consult criteria

- Discuss all temporal arteritis cases with a physician

Subarachnoid hemorrhage (SAH)

- "Thunderclap" headache
- Sudden onset and reaching maximal intensity in seconds to minutes

- 1/3 not exertional
- May awake with SAH
- Sentinel leak in SAH headache may improve over time
- May cause EKG abnormalities

Evaluation

- CT brain scan (3rd generation scanner)
    - Nearly 100% accurate in the first 6 hours
    - Sensitivity (true positives) 93% at 24 hours after onset, 83% at 3 days and 50% at 1 week
    - False negative may occur with severe anemia or small hemorrhage
- Lumbar puncture
    - If CT brain scan negative and SAH suspected as possible cause of headache
    - May be falsely negative within 2 hours of SAH onset
    - Xanthochromia will appears 2–4 hours after bleed and remain for 2 weeks at least, up to 4 weeks in 40% of patients
    - May be negative in 10–15% of patients
- Cerebral angiography
    - If CT brain and lumbar puncture nondiagnostic and diagnostic uncertainly persists
- CT angiography — sensitivity and specificity comparable to cerebral angiography
- MRI brain may be used, but not as accurate as above imaging
- Monitor for acute hydrocephalus in SAH involving the CSF spaces

Headaches Prompting CT Brain Scan Consideration

- Worst headache of life — consider lumbar puncture if CT negative
- Change in headache from previous headache symptoms/patterns
- Focal deficits
- Acute neurologic complaints

- New onset seizure with headache
- Complaints of altered mental status
- Migraine aura that is sensory or motor
- Change in migraine aura
- Headache > 24 hours
- Thunderclap headache
- Headache in elderly
- Historical "Red Flag" headaches
- Minor head trauma on anticoagulation
- Anticoagulation patient with new headache symptoms

Consider "Don't Miss Diagnoses"

(Perform testing for possible diagnoses when suspected)

- Subarachnoid hemorrhage
- Meningitis and encephalitis
- Temporal arteritis
- Acute narrow angle closure glaucoma
- Hypertensive emergencies
- Carbon monoxide poisoning
- Cerebral venous sinus thrombosis (seen, for example, with OCP use or with patients with coagulopathy)
- Pseudotumor cerebri
- Acute strokes
- Mass lesions

Consult Criteria

- Headaches refractory to treatment
- Headache with fever unless consistent with a benign process
- Acute neurologic complaints or findings
- Above diagnosis suspected in the "Don't miss diagnosis" section
- Questionable diagnosis
- Status migrainosus (> 24 hours; dehydration)
- "Historical Red Flag" headache

Notes

SEIZURE MANAGEMENT

When using any management guideline, always follow the Guidelines of Proper Use (page 16).

Definition

- Focal or generalized electrical depolarization's of the brain resulting in focal or generalized neurologic and motor findings with or without loss of consciousness
- Epilepsy is defined as 2 of more seizures not provoked by other illness or causations, or a first time seizure that has a predisposition to recur

Differential Diagnosis

- Pseudoseizures
- Migraines
- Encephalitis
- Meningitis
- Transient global amnesia (TGA)
- Psychogenic unresponsiveness
- TIA (rare TIA's can present with focal motor activity or unresponsiveness)
- Cardiogenic syncope
- Hypoglycemia
- Conversion reaction

Considerations

Generalized seizures (most common)

Classic tonic-clonic ("grand mal")

- Sustained generalized muscle contractions followed by loss of consciousness

Absence seizures ("petit mal")

- Brief episodes of sudden immobility and blank stares

Partial seizures

Simple

- Brief sensory or motor symptoms without loss of consciousness
    - Focal motor seizures is an example

Complex

- Mental or psychiatric symptoms
- Affect changes
- Confusion
- Automatisms
- Hallucinations
- Impaired consciousness

Status epilepticus (SE)

- Newly defined as seizure > 5 minutes or 2 or more seizures in which patient does not recover consciousness
- Older definition > 30 minutes or 2 or more seizures in which patient does not recover consciousness (controversy exists about definition)
- Mortality of 10–12%
- Failure to recognize nonconvulsive SE increases poor outcomes
- Prolonged SE leads to electromechanical dissociation
    - Exhibits minor movements: twitching of eyes, face, hands, feet;
    - Coma

Prolactin level

- Helpful if drawn within 10–20 minutes of seizure and elevated 2 times normal
    - Syncope can also elevate prolactin levels
- Normal prolactin level favors pseudoseizure but cannot differentiate seizure from syncope
- Normal prolactin does not rule out seizure

Pseudoseizures

- Closed eyes during seizure: 96% sensitive; 98% specific in indicating pseudoseizure

- Open eyes during seizure: 98% sensitive; 96% specific in indicating true seizure
- Can also occur 10–20% of the time in patients with epilepsy

First–time seizure recurrence risk depends on

- Brain MRI abnormality
- Abnormal EEG
- Partial–onset seizure/focal neurological exam

30–50% recurrence if 1 present

80% recurrence if all 3 present

15% recurrence if none present – may withhold anticonvulsant therapy

- Anticonvulsant treatment decreases the recurrence of first–time grand mal seizure

Causes

- Idiopathic
- Genetic/congenital malformations
- Hypoglycemia or hyperglycemia
- Hypernatremia and hyponatremia
- CVA
- Cerebral mass
- Intracranial hemorrhage — especially subarachnoid or intraparenchymal
- Traumatic brain injury
- Cocaine
- Meningitis
- Encephalitis
- Eclampsia
- Fever
- Prescribed drugs (lowered seizure threshold especially with some antibiotics and analgesics)
- Withdrawal syndromes (drugs and alcohol)

Evaluation

Seizure history

- Any warning before the seizure ("spell") occurred?
- What did patient do during seizure?

- How long did the seizure last?
- Was patient relating to environment during seizure?
- Does the patient recall the seizure?
- How long did it take till the patient was "back to normal" after the seizure (spell) occurred and how did the patient feel after the seizure or spell?
- How frequent do the "spells" or seizures occur?
- Any precipitating events or actions associated with the seizure?
- Any treatment response of seizure disorder?

- Obtain history of associated symptoms
- Drug abuse history

Patients baseline lab

- BMP
- Seizure drug levels if measurable

Seizure patients with comorbid considerations and new onset seizures

- CMP, Mg^{++} in select patients
- Pregnancy test in childbearing age women
- Consider lumbar puncture (LP) in immunocompromised patient or with meningitis signs
- Consider LP in patients with seizure and fever
- CBC; U/A; chest x-ray as indicated by associated symptoms or findings
- Blood alcohol and drug screen as indicated
- Serum anticonvulsant levels if measurable

Monitoring anticonvulsant levels

- Determine anticonvulsant level that achieves seizure control
- Determine maximal amount of anticonvulsant the patient can tolerate without toxic side effects
- Determine if patient's anticonvulsant levels are therapeutic before accepting medication failure
- Around 30% of patients miss at least 1 dose of anticonvulsant medication per month

- Pharmacokinetic changes may occur with hepatic metabolism over several weeks resulting in decreased anticonvulsant levels
- Some patients are controlled at subtherapeutic anticonvulsant levels

Neuroimaging

- Brain magnetic resonance imaging) with and without contrast (MRI) is the preferred imaging modality
- CT brain scanning may be ordered if MRI not performed
- CT brain scan on elderly or patients taking Coumadin (warfarin)
- CT brain scan for head trauma

Electroencephalography (EEG)

- Strengthens diagnosis
- Assists with determining prognosis

Treatment

- Goal is to achieve seizure free state without adverse medication effects
    - Achieved in 60% of patients
- Monotherapy is preferred to decrease adverse side-effects and cost, and increase compliance
- Vocational and social rehabilitation may be needed

Precautions

Driving motor vehicles

- Check state laws
- More restricted for commercial vehicle drivers — 5 year seizure-free period usually required
- Usually need to have a State specified seizure-free interval

Water activities

- Do not swim alone
- Wear life preserver
- Be monitored taking baths

Heights and power tools

- Should be avoided

Anticonvulsant medications

(Read adverse reactions and contraindications)

Generalized seizures

Valproic acid (Depakote, Depacon)

- 125 mg PO tid — increase every 3–7 days by 125 mg a day (usual daily dose 750–4,000 mg total) — NMT 60mg/kg/day
- Therapeutic range 50–100 mcg/mL
- Adverse reactions
  - Hepatic failure (monitor liver function tests especially in first 6 months of therapy)
  - Pancreatitis
  - Pregnancy fetal risks — especially in first trimester

Phenytoin (Dilantin)

- 100 mg PO bid–qid (may dose qday)
- Therapeutic range 10–20 mcg/mL
- Second–line drug

Carbamazepine (Tegretol)

- 200 mg PO bid — may increase qweek by 200 mg total daily dose split tid–qid
- NMT 1600 mg PO qday total dose usually needed
- Therapeutic range 5–12 mcg/mL
- Second–line drug

Levetiracetam (Keppra)

- 500 mg PO bid — may increase 1,000 mg daily q2weeks to achieve control
- NMT 1,500 mg PO bid

Lamotrigine (Lamictal)

- Dose varies depending on co–existent anticonvulsant treatment — read drug insert or reference information

- Watch for a new skin rash

Absence seizures

Ethosuximide (Zarontin)

- 500 mg PO qday — increase 250 mg q4-7 days to achieve therapeutic range
- NMT 1,500 mg qday
- Therapeutic range 40–100mcg/mL

Valproic acid (Depakote, Depacon)

- 15mg/kg/day — increase 5–10 mg/kg/day to achieve control (usually < 60 mg/kg/day needed)
- Therapeutic range 50–100 mcg/mL
- Second line drug — for atypical absence seizures

Focal seizures

Carbamazepine (Tegretol)

- 200 mg PO bid — may increase qweek by 200 mg total daily dose split tid–qid
- NMT 1600 mg PO qday total dose usually needed
- Therapeutic range 4-12 mcg/mL
- First–line drug

Phenytoin (Dilantin)

- 100 mg PO bid–qid (may dose qday)
- Therapeutic range 10–20 mcg/mL
- Second–line drug

Oxcarbazepine (Trileptal)

- Adjunct or monotherapy
- Dose varies depending on co-existent anticonvulsant treatment — read drug insert or reference information

Levetiracetam (Keppra)

- 500 mg PO bid — may increase 1,000 mg daily q2weeks
- NMT 1,500 mg PO bid

- Adjunctive therapy when first-line treatment failure

Zonisamide (Zonegran)

- 100 mg/day — increase to 200mg/day after 2 weeks
  - Can increase to 400mg/day with at least 2 weeks between each 100mg increase
- Adjunct therapy

Switching anticonvulsant medications

- Requires a period of overlap
- Give patient a written schedule of the taper to discontinue the medication day-by-day or week-by-week

Consult criteria

- Intractable seizures
- When surgery contemplated for seizure management
- Discontinuing anticonvulsant therapy
- Patient on multiple anticonvulsants

Notes

ARTHRITIS MANAGEMENT

When using any management guideline, always follow the Guidelines of Proper Use (page 16).

Osteoarthritis (OA)

Definition

- Focal degeneration of the articular cartilage often with bony hypertrophy characterized by:
    - Morning stiffness
    - Joint stiffness after prolonged rest
    - Joint pain with activity relieved by rest
    - Joint range of motion often reduced
    - Gradual onset progressing over years
    - Often leads to disuse muscle atrophy and a feeling of joint instability
    - Joint effusions may occur, but are non-inflammatory with less than 2,000 WBC's/ml

Differential diagnosis

- Rheumatoid arthritis
- Psoriatic arthritis
- Avascular necrosis
- Ankylosing spondylitis
- Bursitis/tendonitis/muscle pain
- Gout or pseudogout
- Referred pain — especially with knee and hip pain
- Septic arthritis
- Hemochromatosis

Considerations

- Prevalence of 15% in the US population — most common in ages > 65 years
- Affects over 20 million in the U.S.
- Most common arthritic problem > 50 years of age
- Progression is slow, occurring over years to decades
- Predominantly a non-inflammatory condition arising from degenerative changes and

progressive loss of cartilage with subsequent hypertrophic bone changes

- Mostly primary and idiopathic — secondary causes include trauma, obesity, inflammatory arthropathy and severe neuropathy
- There is an inverse relationship between OA and bone mass
- From age related "wear and tear" or injury with loss or damage to cartilage and synovial membrane allowing bones to come into contact
- Therapy, both medical and physical, is directed at symptom relief and slowing down the disease progression
- Incidence increases with age
- More common in females over males by 2–3 to 1

Risk factors (* = most common)

- Age*
- Female gender
- Joint instability/muscle weakness
- Heredity*
- Obesity*
- Overuse
- Peripheral neuropathy
- Trauma
- Joint infection
- Hypermobility

Evaluation

History

Keys to diagnosis — 2 primary patterns are seen:

- Patients with Heberden and Bouchard nodes with involvement of first CMC joint
- Patients with a noninflammatory asymmetric oligo or monoarthritis affecting the hip, knee, MTP joints or spine

- Most commonly involved joints are knee (medial > lateral), hips, hands, spine, and 1st MTP joint of foot

- Involved hand joints are distal interphalangeal(DIP)/proximal interphalangeal(PIP)/carpometacarpal (CMC)

Physical examination

- Look for bony overgrowth around the joint, crepitus, and reduced ROM

Plain x–rays (preferred imaging modality)

- Look for non–uniform joint space narrowing, bone sclerosis and osteophytes
- Look for calcium deposits (chrondrocalcinosis), erosions (rheumatoid arthritis and psoriatic arthritis), and fractures (trauma)
- Check for patellofemoral joint space narrowing
- X–ray changes of OA correlate poorly with the degree of disability or pain

Other imaging as needed

- MRI for in–depth evaluation of cartilage or ligament damage
- Bone scans to differentiate osteoarthritis from other diseases as indicated

Labs

- Used to rule out other diseases or infections
- CBC
- ESR/C–reactive protein
- Uric acid
- Creatinine
- If needed to further clarify the arthritic process — rheumatoid factor/ACPA (positive anticitrullinated peptide antibody), ANA, T4, and joint aspiration

- Arthrocentesis if needed to differentiate from septic, inflammatory and crystal arthritis — synovial fluid is usually amber, clear, with normal viscosity and less than 2000 WBCs/ml

Treatment — directed at symptomatic relief and slowing down disease progression

- Patient education in joint protection

- Muscle strengthening and stretching exercises
- Physical and occupational therapy prn
- Weight reduction to ideal body weight
- Adaptive aids — canes, braces, splints
- Acetaminophen or NSAID's to maximum dose (caution in renal disease with NSAID's)
    - Try 3 or 4 different NSAID's before giving up on this type of medication — a patient may respond to one NSAID but not another
    - Glucosamine chondroitin PO — benefits unclear
    - Intra-articular corticosteroid injections when effusion present — NMT 3 per year (relief lasts up to 4-6 weeks)
    - Sodium hyaluronate (Synvisc) knee injections
    - Topical agents (Aspercreme or capsaicin)
    - Tramadol for mild to moderate OA pain
    - Arthroplasty (joint replacement) for disabling disease

Consult criteria

- Failure to respond to medical therapy
- If OA pain severe enough to require narcotics, refer to a physician or rheumatologist for a consult or approval
- Septic arthritis found or suspected — consult immediately
- Joint effusion in a prosthetic joint
- Symptoms/pain out of proportion to findings

Psoriatic arthritis

Definition

- Chronic inflammatory arthritis that usually occurs with established cutaneous psoriasis, with or without nail changes

Differential diagnosis

- Erosive osteoarthritis
- Gout
- Rheumatoid arthritis
- Ankylosing spondylitis

- Reactive arthritis
- Septic arthritis
- Secondary syphilis
- Systemic lupus erythematosus
- Pauciarticular juvenile arthritis

Considerations

- Psoriasis occurs in 1–2% of the population with psoriatic arthritis found in 5–20% of them
- Psoriasis occurs before arthritis in 75% of patients
- Psoriasis occurs after arthritis in 13–15% of patients
- Psoriasis occurs simultaneously in 8–10% of patients
- Genetic association with HLA B27 leukocyte antigen with spondylitis-type
- Accounts for 2–20% of childhood arthritis and is monoarticular with onset
- DIP joints are affected as opposed to MCP/PIP joints in rheumatoid arthritis
- Distal interphalangeal joints are asymmetrically affected as opposed to symmetrical involvement with rheumatoid arthritis
- Increased risk of arthritis with psoriatic nail involvement or widespread skin rash

Presentations — five variants of psoriatic arthritis have been described:

- Asymmetric oligoarthritis of large or small joints is seen in 30–40 % of patients
- DIP arthritis is seen in 10–15% of patients usually in association with nail pitting
- RA-like symmetrical polyarthritis in 25–50% patients
- Psoriatic spondylitis in 20% of patients — 50% of whom are HLA-B27 positive
- Arthritis mutilans in less than 5% of patients

Associated extra-articular manifestations

- Conjunctivitis 20%
- Iritis/uveitis 7%

    - Approximately 40% of iritis patients will have sacroiliitis
  - Dactylitis of finger or toe is common

Evaluation

- History and physical examination
- X-rays may reveal asymmetric erosive changes in small joints of feet and hands
- Lab tests are not very helpful
  - ESR may be best guide to disease activity
  - Hyperuricemia may be found in patients with extensive skin disease

X–ray changes

- Asymmetric soft tissue swelling
- Periostitis
- Bony fusion of DIP/PIP joints
- Bony erosions
- Severe joint space narrowing

Treatment

- Treatment should be aimed at reducing symptoms of inflammation, preserving joint function by halting disease progression
- Therapeutic principles should include patient education, joint protection, physical therapy and vocational counseling
- Cold and heat treatments

Mild disease

- NSAID's to maximum dose (caution in renal disease with NSAID's)
- Judicious use intra-articular corticosteroid injections for inflamed joint avoiding psoriatic plaques

Moderate or severe disease

Disease–modifying antirheumatic drugs (DMARD's) — initiated if NSAID's and joint intra–articular corticosteroids failure to control arthritis

Caveats

- **Specialists work in tandem with referring clinics**
- **Read drug information in literature and be familiar with effects and side effects of medications as listed in the literature and/or Physician Desk Reference (PDR)**
- Joint surgery referral only for advanced disabling disease in an attempt to regain some function

Considerations

- Check CBC, creatinine, LFT's and investigate abnormalities before DMARD or Biologics medications are used
- Document negative pregnancy test and discussion of contraception in fertile females before treatment
- Consider pneumovax vaccination
- Document PPD results before Biologics therapy

DMARD's

Considerations

- Use lowest effective dose
- Monitor for myelosuppression, immunodeficiency, infections, hepatic disease — read drug information in literature
- Contraindicated in pregnancy
- Check blood tests q4-6weeks — and more frequent testing when initiated

Medications

- Methotrexate
- Sulfasalazine (Azulfidine)

    - Avoid in sulfa allergic patients
    - Agranulocytosis in 1% of patients
    - Check for G6PD deficiency before treatment
    - Monitor LFT's and CBC
- Leflunamide
    - GI side effects most common
    - If AST or ALT > 2 times normal of upper limit of normal (ULN) then reduce drug
    - If AST or ALT > 3 times normal of upper limit of normal (ULN) then stop drug
    - Monitor for hypertension
    - Monitor for renal dysfunction
- Cyclosporine and/or etretinate may also be used in conjunction with a physician for treatment of psoriasis/psoriatic arthritis
- Plaquenil use contraindicated because it may precipitate skin disease flares

Biologics (tumor necrosis factor inhibitors) for failure to respond to DMARD's (methotrexate at a minimum)

- Anti-TNFs are noted for dramatic improvement in skin and articular manifestations of the disease

Caveats

- **Specialists work in tandem with referring clinics**
- **Read drug information in literature and be familiar with effects and side effects of medications as listed in the literature and/or Physician Desk Reference (PDR)**

Cautions

- Severe infection risk exists
- Stop all DMARDs and Biologics if infection identified or suspected until treated and resolved
- Malignancy risks may be increased

- Do not use in optic neuritis or multiple sclerosis patients or in a first degree relative of these patients
- Do not use in patients with significant heart failure
- Avoid live vaccines
- Biologics may be used with or without DMARDs

Biologic medications

- Etanercept (Enbrel)
- Inflximab (Remicade)
- Adalimumab (Humira)
- Golimumab (Simponi)

Rheumatology referral criteria

- Evaluation and initiation of DMARDs or Biologic therapy
- Failure to respond to treatment
- Pregnancy despite previous warnings
- Surgery referral contemplated
- Psoriatic arthritis refractory to treatment
- Significant side effects of therapy or other unexpected complications

Rheumatoid arthritis (RA)

Definition

- Chronic systemic inflammatory process of unknown etiology primarily involving the peripheral joints characterized by:
  - Symmetrical joint swelling/pain
  - Morning stiffness > 60 minutes
  - Symptoms present > 6 weeks
  - Polyarthritis (> 4 joints) more so than an oligoarthritis (1–4 joints)
  - Positive anticitrullinated peptide antibody (ACPA)

Differential diagnosis

Acutely:

- Reactive arthritis

- Infections (Parvovirus B19, EBV, Lyme disease)
- Systemic lupus erythematosus
- Early scleroderma

Chronic:

- Systemic lupus erythematosus
- Psoriatic arthritis
- Lyme disease
- Reactive arthritis
- Erosive OA
- Polyarticular gout
- Polymyalgia rheumatica
- Sarcoidosis

Considerations

- Common initial site of onset — hands (MCP/PIP/wrist), foot (MTP), knee but may involve any joint with a synovial membrane
- Cervical vertebrae 1 and 2 most common spine involvement — may cause neurologic deficits/symptoms (caution with endotracheal intubation)
- Persistent synovitis weakens the periarticular support structures leading to subluxations and joint deformities, i.e., Boutonniere and Swan neck deformities of the hands
- Genetics account for 50% of occurrence
- Peak onset typically 20–40 years of age, with a female to male prevalence of 3:1, and a second peak at 60 years of age, with prevalence of female: male of 1:1
- Juvenile rheumatoid arthritis is the most common cause of arthritis in children
- Mortality increased 2–3 times over background due to immunosuppression, infection, disability, heart and lung disease, steroids and malignancy
    - Cardiovascular causes are followed in order by infection, respiratory disease and malignancy

Findings and symptoms

Constitutional

- Generalized morning stiffness, malaise

Joint findings

- Soft tissue swelling/pain in the typical joints
- Joint deformities, i.e., subluxations of joints and reduced ROM
- Tendon rupture may occur
- Joint effusion, especially in the knee — look for Baker's cyst

Extra–articular findings

- Pleuritis and pleural effusions
- Interstitial pulmonary fibrosis
- Vasculitis
- Pericarditis/pericardial effusion
- Rheumatoid (subcutaneous) nodules usually found on extensor surfaces and fingers/toes
- Anemia of chronic disease — hemoglobin typically ~ 10 gm/dL (if less then check for iron deficiency anemia and/or blood loss)
- Felty's syndrome (granulocytopenia and splenomegaly) in patients with long standing rheumatoid arthritis
- Eye symptoms — episcleritis, scleritis and keratoconjunctivitis sicca
- Fever (juvenile rheumatoid arthritis)

Rheumatoid arthritis 2010 classification criteria

A score of ≥ 6 out of 10

- 1 large joint — no points
- 2–10 large joints — 1 point
- 1–3 small joints — 2 points
- 4-10 small joints — 3 points
- Greater than 10 small (with 1 small joint) — 5 points
- Negative rheumatoid factor (RF) and anti-citrullinated peptide antibody (ACPA) — 0 points
- Low positive RF or ACPA — 2 points
- High positive RF or ACPA — 3 points

- Normal C-reactive protein (CRP) and erythrocyte sedimentation rate (ESR) — no points
- Elevated CRP or ESR — 1 point
- Symptoms < 6 weeks — no points
- Symptoms ≥ 6 weeks — 1 point

History and physical examination

- Evaluate the whole patient and the effect of joint symptoms on life, work and activity

Labs

- CBC
- Creatinine level
- LFTs
- CRP or ESR
- ACPA and rheumatoid factor (RF)

Lab considerations

- ANA may be positive in ~ 10–30% of RA patients usually in low titer with negative double-stranded DNA (dsDNA)
- RF positive in ~75–80% of patients with RA
- ACPA positive in 100% of RA patients (false positive rate 5–6%)
- CRP/ESR correlate with inflammation and can be used as a crude guide for response to treatment, but RA patients may have inflammation due to other causes that is partially suppressed by RA treatment with DMARD's or Biologics

X–rays

- Look for soft tissue swelling and osteopenia around the joints, bone erosions and joint space narrowing
- Earliest bone erosions often seen on 2nd or 3rd MCP heads, 3rd finger PIP joint or 5th MTP joint
- MRI if C1–2 needs evaluation

Treatment

- Treatment should be aimed at reducing symptoms of inflammation and preserving joint function by halting disease progression

- Therapeutic principles should include patient education, joint protection, physical therapy and vocational counseling
- Occupational therapy for orthotics and splints
- Cold and heat treatments
- Patient education

Early disease

- NSAID's — these may improve symptoms but they do not suppress disease progression (caution with renal disease)
- Judicious use of intra-articular (IA) steroids — infrequently used
- Systemic steroids should be reserved for severe uncontrolled arthritis or corticosteroid bridging therapy till DMARD's take effect
- Analgesics prn besides NSAID's
- Do not use both oral and IA steroids

See DMARDs under Psoriatic Arthritis section for considerations and monitoring

- Treatment with DMARDs and Biologics require periodic toxicity checks
- Specialists work in tandem with referring clinics — earliest possible referral to a rheumatologist is preferable
- Methotrexate — preferred first line agent
- Sulfasalazine (Azulfidine)
- Cyclosporine
    - May be used by a rheumatologist
- Leflunamide
- Minocycline 100 mg PO bid
- Plaquenil

See Biologics (tumor necrosis factor inhibitors) for failure to respond to DMARD's under Psoriatic Arthritis section

- Etanercept (Enbrel)
- Infliximab (Remicade
    - May use with methotrexate
- Adalimumab (Humira)
- Golimumab (Simponi)

Rheumatology referral criteria

- Evaluation and initiation of DMARDs or Biologic therapy
- Failure to respond to treatment
- Pregnancy despite previous warnings
- Surgery referral contemplated
- Rheumatoid arthritis refractory to treatment
- Significant side effects of therapy or other unexpected complications

Notes

Reference: Arthritis and Rheumatism
Vol. 62, No. 9, September 2010, pp 2569 - 2581
DOI 10.1002/art.27584
c 2010, American College of Rheumatology

Glossary

ABG — arterial blood gas

ABI — ankle brachial index

AC — acromioclavicular

ACEI — angiotensin converting enzyme inhibitor

ADT — adult diphtheria tetanus

Anaphylaxis — IgE antibody release of various mediators such as histamine causing varying degrees of symptoms such as rash, pruritus, bronchospasm, GI symptoms, hypoxia, upper airway compromise, hypotension and potentially death

Angina — cardiac chest discomfort, or other discomfort or symptoms, from deficit of blood flow and oxygen delivery to the heart

Anion gap — sodium minus chloride and CO2 (serum bicarbonate)

Anti-HBS — antibody to hepatitis B surface antigen

Aortic dissection — tearing of the wall of the aorta

ARB — Angiotensin receptor blocker

ASA — aspirin

Asthma — reversible constriction of pulmonary small airways

Asymptomatic hypertension — elevated blood pressure with no acute end-organ compromise of function

Bandemia — increased white blood cell bands from stress, infection, or inflammation

BB — beta-blocker

B-HCG — beta human chorionic gonadotropin

BID (bid) — twice a day

BMP — basic metabolic profile including sodium, potassium, chloride, carbon dioxide (CO2), glucose, creatinine and BUN (blood urea nitrogen)

BNP – B-type natriuretic peptide, determined by stretch of cardiac muscle from CHF. Elevated in many other conditions that cause strain on the heart in addition to CHF

Bronchitis – reversible constriction of pulmonary small airways from an infection in the lungs

BSA – body surface area

Burst fracture – fracture through entire vertebral body (unstable)

CBC – complete blood count

CCB – calcium channel blocker

CHD – coronary heart disease

CHF – (Congestive heart failure) Cardiac dysfunction secondary to decreased ability of the left ventricle (LV) to eject or fill with blood

COPD – chronic obstructive pulmonary disease, usually chronic bronchitis or emphysema, or mixture of both

CPK – creatine phosphokinase (a muscle enzyme)

C-RP – C reactive protein (nonspecific marker of inflammation)

CSF – cerebral spinal fluid

C-spine – cervical spine

CXR – chest x-ray

CVA – brain neuronal death from a deficit of cerebral perfusion resulting in lack of oxygen to parts of the brain

DBP – diastolic blood pressure

D-dimer – a measurable byproduct of fibrinogen pathway indicating some level of blood clot formation

DIC – disseminated intravascular coagulation

DIP – distal interphalangeal

DJD – degenerative joint disease (osteoarthritis)

DKA – diabetic ketoacidosis (a metabolic acidotic diabetic condition resulting from insulin resistance or severe deficit of insulin, and fatty acids metabolism for energy needs, that is associated with potential mortality)

DOC – drug of choice

DUB — dysfunctional uterine bleeding

DVT — deep vein thrombosis

Dyspnea — shortness of breath

EBV — Epstein-Barr virus

Emergency hypertension — acute end-organ injury secondary to elevated blood pressure

Epley maneuver — treatment of BPV (moves otoliths out of semicircular canals). Avoid with recent neck fracture, instability or surgery, carotid disease or recent retinal detachment

ESR — erythrocyte sedimentation rate (nonspecific marker of inflammation)

ESRD — end stage renal disease

FFP — fresh frozen plasma

GC — gonococcal or gonococcus

GERD — Gastroesophageal reflux

GI — gastrointestinal

gm(s) — gram or grams

gtt — drop

HAART — highly active antiretroviral therapy with 2 NRTIs and either a protease inhibitor or NNRTI

Hallpike maneuver — patient going from sitting position to supine position rapidly with head below horizontal plane of body and head rotated quickly and carefully to the left or right. Any nystagmus and symptoms induced represent a positive test.

HBIG — hepatitis B immune globulin

HHS — hyperglycemic hyperosmolar syndrome

HIV — human immunodeficiency

HR — heart rate

HSV — herpes simplex virus

IBS — irritable bowel syndrome

IG — immune globulin

IM — intramuscular

INR — international normalized ratio (measures Coumadin – warfarin therapy)

IOP — intraocular pressure

IUP — intrauterine pregnancy

IV — intravenous

Jugular venous distension — distension of the external jugular vein in the neck due to increased pressure in the right side of the heart or in the lungs (pulmonary hypertension, COPD, CHF)

KUB — kidney, ureter and bladder plain x-ray

LES — lower esophageal sphincter

LFT's — liver function tests

LP — lumbar puncture

LOC — loss of consciousness

MDI — metered dose inhaler

Metabolic acidosis — decreased serum bicarbonate

mmol/L = mEq/L on serum test levels

MP — metacarpophalangeal

MRSA — methacillin resistance staphylococcus aureus

NaHCO3 — sodium bicarbonate

NMT — no more than

Nonspecific chest pain — chest pain without evident specific cause

NNRTI — non-nucleoside reverse transcriptase inhibitor

NRTI — nucleoside reverse transcriptase inhibitor

NS — normal saline

NSAID's — nonsteroidal anti-inflammatory drugs

Nystagmus — rhythmic involuntary eye movements named for the quick component

O2 saturation — percent of hemoglobin carrying oxygen

ORT — oral rehydration therapy

Osmolol gap — the difference between calculated and measured osmolality in the blood, usually less than 10

PAD — peripheral arterial disease

Panic disorder — state of hyperventilation causing decreased pCO2 measurement on blood gas (respiratory alkalosis), elevated pH, resulting in feeling short of breath, acute calcium shifts into cells (can cause carpospasm), hypokalemia, paresthesias, and a sense of impending doom when more severe

PCP — primary care provider

PCR — polymerase chain reaction

PE — physical examination or pulmonary embolism (use context)

PEP — postexposure prophylaxis

PERC — pulmonary embolism rule out criteria

PID — pelvic inflammatory disease

PIP — proximal interphalangeal

PMN — polymorphonuclear neutrophil

PN — peripheral neuropathy

PO — per oral

POC — products of conception

PPI — proton pump inhibitor

PR — per rectum

PRBC — packed red blood cells

Presyncope — state of feeling that a fainting or syncopal episode will occur

prn — as needed

Pseudoaddiction — a condition caused by under-treatment of pain where the patient engages in an active and often repetitive search for pain medications

Pseudoseizures — seizure-like activity caused by psychiatric or functional considerations that is not a true seizure

PSVT — paroxysmal supraventricular tachycardia

Pulmonary embolism — blood clot(s) located in the lung's blood vessels that originated elsewhere, usually from veins in pelvis or proximal legs

Q or **q** — every

QID (qid) — four times a day

RCT — rotator cuff tear

Respiratory acidosis — increased pCO2 on blood gas measurement

Respiratory alkalosis — decreased pCO2 and elevated pH on blood gas from increased minute ventilation or hyperventilation

Respiratory failure — increasing blood gas pCO2 and respiratory fatigue with decreasing pH, resulting in increasing somnolence, altered mental status and hypoxemia

RSV — respiratory syncytial virus

SBO — small bowel obstruction

SBP — systolic blood pressure

Sepsis — usually a bacterial infection frequently used to mean invasion of the blood stream

SLR — straight leg raise

SQ — subcutaneous

SS disease — sickle cell homozygous disease

SSRI — selective serotonin reuptake inhibitor

STD — sexual transmitted disease

SVT — supraventricular tachycardia

Syncope — loss of consciousness from decreased cerebral perfusion

TBSA — total body surface area

TC — total cholesterol

Tdap — tetanus, diphtheria and acellular pertussis vaccine

TGA — transient global amnesia

Thrombocytopenia — low platelet count

TIA — transient ischemic attack

TID (tid) — three times a day

TM — tympanic membrane

Troponin — breakdown cardiac muscle component indicating injury or death to cardiac muscle depending on level

TSH — thyroid stimulating hormone most commonly elevated in primary hypothyroidism

U/A — urine analysis

UCG — urine pregnancy test (urinary chorionic gonadotropin)

UDS — urine drug screen

UGI — upper gastrointestinal

UTI — urinary tract infection

Valsalva — straining of abdomen causing increase in intracranial and intraocular pressure

WBC — white blood count

Well's criteria — criteria developed to assess level of probability of VTE (venous thromboembolic) disease either in extremities or lungs (pulmonary embolism)

Whole bowel irrigation — giving polyethylene glycol (Miralax or Go-lytely) to flush out the intestines

Index

A

A CAT MUDPILES, 299
Abdominal Pain Protocol, 180
Abscess - soft tissue, 607
Accelerated idioventricular rhythm, 48
Accident Protocol – Motor Vehicle, 368
Acromioclavicular (AC) injuries, 434
Acute Bronchitis Protocol – Adult, 79
Acute chest syndrome in sickle cell anemia, 683
Acute mountain sickness, 742
Acute urethral syndrome, 262
Acyclovir, 152
Adenosine, 43
Adolescent Psychiatric Protocol, 698
Adult and Adolescent Psychiatric Protocol, 698
Adult Asthma/Acute Bronchitis Protocol, 79
Adult Gastroenteritis Protocol, 195
Adult Minor Head Trauma Protocol, 304
Adult Psychiatric Protocol, 698
Adult Seizure Protocol, 154
Adult Septic Shock Management, 848
Albuterol aerosol, 89
Alcohol Intoxicated Patient Protocol, 703
Aldosterone antagonists, 786
Allergy Protocol, 84
Alpha-1 blockers, 767
Altitude Illness Protocol, 741
Amiodarone, 49
Anal fissure, 241
Anaphylactoid reactions, 84
Anaphylaxis, 86
Angina medication treatment, 772
Angina/AMI, 24

Angioedema, 86
Angioedema of oropharyngeal area, 350
Angiotensin converting enzyme inhibitor (ACEI), 762
Angiotensin converting enzyme inhibitors (ACEI), 766
Angiotensin receptor blockers, 766
Animal and Human Bite Protocol, 586
Anion gap calculation, 299
Anion gap mnemonic, 120
Ankle Sprain Protocol, 462
Anorectal Disorder Protocol, 239
Antibiotic-associated Colitis Protocol, 209
Anticoagulation, 787
Anticonvulsant medications, 878
Antidotes, 122
Antihypertensive Medications, 765
Antivenom complications, 601
Aortic dissection, 25
Aplastic crisis in sickle cell anemia, 683
Apley's test of knee, 452
Appendicitis in children, 186, 206
Appendicitis in elderly, 185, 205
Appendicitis Protocol, 205
Arthritis Management, 881
Aspirin, 40
Asthma, 70
Asthma Management, 820
Asthma management principles, 821
Asthma medications, 828
Asthma Protocol – Adult, 79
Asthma Protocol – Pediatric, 497
Asthma treatement, 821
Asthma treatment, 80
Athlete's Foot (Tinea Pedis) Protocol, 639
Atopic Dermatitis/Eczema Protocol, 622
Atopic Eczema/Dermatitis Protocol, 622
Atrial fibrillation, 37
AV block, 45
Avulsion of the central extensor slip, 473
Avulsion of the volar carpal plate, 473

B

Babesiosis, 658
Back Pain Protocol, 172
Back section, 171
Baker's cyst, 457
Bees, wasps, and fire ants bites or stings, 596
Bell's Palsy Protocol, 150
Benadryl, 89
Benign Febrile Seizure Protocol, 480
Beta-blocker, 772
Beta-blockers, 31, 766, 775
Bicipital tendonitis, 428
Biologics, 626, 887, 888, 893
Black widow spider bites, 594
Bleeding Protocol, 385
Blepharitis, 331
Blood/fluid replacement for hemorrhage, 370
Bowel Disease Protocol, 212
Boxer's fracture, 467
Bronchiolitis Protocol, 502
Bronchitis, 70
Bronchitis treatment, 80
Brown recluse spider bite, 593
B-type natriuretic peptide (BNP), 781
Burn Protocol, 388
Burst fracture, 404
Button battery, 237

C

Calcium channel blockers, 766, 777
Cancer Emergency Protocol, 687
Cardiac Dysrhythmia Protocol, 35
Cardiovascular section, 23
Cardizem, 39, 766
Cat bites, 589
Cellulitis Protocol, 603
Cellutitis causes, 603
Centor criteria, 320

Central alpha-2 agonists, 767
Central retinal artery occlusion, 342
Central retinal vein occlusion, 342
Cervical spine trauma, 315
Cervical spine trauma in motor vehicle accidents, 373
CHADS2 score, 811
Chalazion, 331
Chemical burns, 393
Chemical eye injuries, 338
Chest Pain Protocol, 24
Chicken Pox (Varicella) Protocol, 665
Chilblains, 739
Child Abuse Protocol, 719
Cholesterol Management, 805
Cholesterol risk assessment, 805
Chondromalacia patella, 458
Chronic renal disease, 764
Chronic Renal Failure Protocol, 266
Classification of heart failure, 55
Clavicle fractures, 435
Clavicle fractures and dislocations, 434
Cluster headache, 129, 867
Colic – pediatric, 486
Colitis Protocol (antibiotic-associated), 209
Collateral ligament tear of finger, 473
Colles fracture, 469
Compartment syndrome, 391, 410, 466
Compartment syndrome in electrical burns, 391, 410, 466
Complex febrile seizure treatment, 481
Compression fracture, 404
Concussion, 304, 312
Congestive Heart Failure Protocol, 54
Conjunctivitis, 327
Constipation Protocol, 250
Contact Dermatitis Protocol, 628
COPD exacerbation, 68
COPD Management, 832
COPD medications, 834
Coral snake (eastern) antivenom, 601
Coral snake envenomation, 599

Corneal abrasion, 334
Corneal foreign body, 335
Corneal ulcer, 333
Coronary Artery Disease Management, 768
Coumadin, 40, 122, 143, 177
Croup Protocol, 505
Croup severity assessment, 506
Crying Infant Protocol, 485
CSF rhinorrhea, 356
CT Abdominal Scan Issues, 192
CT brain scan in headaches, 132, 870
CVA, 38, 139
CVA/TIA Protocol, 139

D

Dabigatran (Pradaxa), 812
D-dimer in chest pain, 26, 677
D-dimer in syncope, 60
Deep venous thrombosis, 398
Dehydration Protocol – Pediatric, 509
Delirium causes, 166
Delirium in the elderly, 525
Delirium Protocol, 166
Delirium tremens, 708
Dental Injury Protocols, 361
Dental Pain Protocol, 365
Depression, 701
Depression Management, 854
Dermatitis Protocol (Contact), 628
Dermatology section, 585
Diabete type 2 treatments, 102
Diabetes complications, 791, 798
Diabetes evaluation, 791, 800
Diabetes history, 799
Diabetes insipitus, 288
Diabetes Protocol, 94
Diabetes symptoms, 799
Dialysis disequilibrium syndrome, 267
Diarrhea, 198

Diarrhea Protocol – Pediatric, 515
Diltiazem, 39, 43, 766
Disease Management section, 759
Diuretics, 765
Dizziness Protocol, 135
DKA, 94
DMARD, 887, 888, 893
Dog bites, 587
Domestic Violence Protocol, 717
Drug Interactions, 755
Drug seeking behavior, 752
DVT prophylaxis, 680
Dysfunctional uterine bleeding, 533
Dyshidrotic Eczema Protocol, 620
Dyspnea Protocol, 66

E

Early Goal-directed Therapy, 849
Early withdrawal symptoms, 708
Eclampsia, 544
Ectopic pregnancy, 542
Eczema Protocol, 622
Ehrlichiosis, 658
Elbow Protocol, 442
Elder Abuse Protocol, 722
Elderly abdominal pain, 185
Electrical burns, 391
Electrolyte and Acid/Base Disturbances section, 281
Endocarditis Protocol, 576
Endocrine section, 93
Endometriosis, 541
ENT Emergency Protocol, 348
Environmental section, 725
Epididymoorchitis, 271, 559
Epiglottis, 321
Epinephrine, 71, 81, 86, 87, 90, 277, 351, 376, 498, 507, 601, 642
Erythema multiforme, 614
Erythema Multiforme Protocol, 614

Erythema Nodosum Protocol, 618
Estimated blood and fluid losses (adults), 369
Ethanol related seizures, 708
Exposure Skin and Frostbite Injury Protocol, 737
Extremity Disorders section, 397
Extremity Medical Disorder Protocol, 398
Eye Protocols, 327
Eyelid lacerations, 337

F

Facial Fractures Protocol, 356
Falls in elderly, 528
Febrile seizere - simple, 481
Febrile seizure - complex, 481
Febrile Seizure Protocol - Benign, 480
Felon, 668
Fever Protocol - Pediatric, 476
FFP, 232, 370, 550
Finger Injury Protocol, 472
First degree burn, 388
Flank Pain Protocol, 176
Flexion-extension plain films, 316
Flexor tenosynovitis, 672
Flomax, 257
Foot fractures and dislocations, 421
Forearm fractures, 416
Forearm Injury Protocol, 465
Foreign Body (Intestinal) Protocol, 236
Fourth degree burn, 389
Fracture Protocol, 410
Frostbite and Exposure Skin Injury Protocol, 737
Frostnip, 740

G

Gallbladder Disease Protocol, 223
Gamekeeper thumb, 473
Gastritis Protocol, 219
Gastroenteritis Protocol - Adult, 195
Gastroenteritis Protocol - Pediatric, 509

Gastroesophageal Reflux Disease (GERD) Protocol, 216
Gastrointestinal Bleeding Protocol, 231
Gastrointestinal Foreign Body Protocol, 236
Gastrointestinal section, 179
General Patient Criteria Protocol, 20
Generalized seizures, 154, 160, 873
Genital Herpes Protocol, 650
Geodon, 701
GERD (Gastroesophageal Reflux Disease) Protocol, 216
Geriatrics Protocol, 522
Geriatrics section, 521
Glaucoma, 339
Glucagon, 90
Glucose home monitoring, 795
Gonococcal disease, 554
Gout, 402
Gout in knee, 459
Guidelines of Proper Use, 16
Gynecology section, 531

H

H. pylori, 219
Haldon, 701
Hand Infection Protocol, 667
Hand Injury Protocol, 465
Hand, Wrist, and Distal Forearm Injury Protocol, 465
Head in hand sign, 315
Head trauma, 371
Head Trauma and Neck Pain section, 303
Head Trauma Protocol – Adult, 304
Head Trauma Protocol – Pediatric, 309
Headache Management, 860
Headache Protocol, 126
Heart block, 45
Heart Failure Management, 780
Heartburn, 217
Heat cramps, 728
Heat exhaustion, 728
Heat Illness Protocol, 726

Heat stroke, 729
HEENT section, 317
Hematology and Oncology section, 673
Hematuria in kidney stones, 256
Hemodialysis for ingestions, 121
Hemorrhoids, 239
Henoch-Schonlein Purpura Protocol, 611
Hepatitis B and HIV Postexposure Prophylaxis Recommendations, 570
Hepatitis B postexposure prophylaxis, 574
Hepatitis Protocol, 227
Hernia, 184
Herpes Simplex Gingivostomatitis Protocol, 646
Herpes Zoster (Shingles) Protocol, 652
Herpetic Whitlow Protocol, 648
High pressure injection injuries, 468
High-altitude cerebral edema, 743
High-altitude pulmonary edema, 744, 746
Hip dislocation, 450
Hip Fracture, 449
Hip Protocol, 446
Historical red flag headaches, 132, 871
HIV and Hepatitis B Postexposure Prophylaxis Recommendations, 570
HIV postexposure prophylaxis for mucosal membrane and nonintact skin exposures, 572
HIV postexposure prophylaxis percutaneous injuries, 570
HIV Protocol, 565
Home glucose monitoring, 795
Hordeolum, 331
Human and Animal Bite Protocol, 586
Human bite, 467
Human bites, 586
Human Immunodeficiency Virus (HIV) Protocol, 565
Humerus fractures, 437
Humerus fractures and dislocations, 434
Hydrocele, 279
Hyperglycemic hyperosmolar syndrome, 97
Hyperkalemia Protocol, 282
Hyperkalemia treatment, 283

Hypernatremia Protocol, 288
Hypertension Management, 760
Hypertension medication, 762
Hypertension Protocol, 51
Hypertension treatment, 52, 53
Hypertensive emergency, 51
Hypertensive urgency, 51
Hyperthyroidism Protocol, 110
Hyperviscosity syndrome, 692
Hyphema, 343
Hypoglycemia, 99
Hypoglycemia management, 794
Hypoglycemia Protocol, 94
Hypokalemia Protocol, 285
Hypokalemia treatment, 286
Hyponatremia Protocol, 294
Hyponatremia treatment, 297
Hypothermia Protocol, 732
Hypothyroidism Protocol, 106

I

Immune reconstitution inflammatory syndrome, 567
Impetigo Protocol, 630
Incomplete abortion, 544
Indigestion, 25
Inevitable abortion, 544
Infectious Disease section, 553
Inflammatory Bowel Disease Protocol, 212
Insect Sting and Spider Bite Protocol, 593
Insulin therapy, 790, 793
Insulin therapy in DKA, 97
Intestinal angina, 183
Iritis, 333
Irritable Bowel Syndrome Protocol, 201

J

Junctional rhythm, 43

K

Keratitis, 330
Kidney Stone Protocol, 256
Kidney stone treatment, 258
Knee Disorders Protocol, 454
Knee Soft Tissue Injury Protocol, 451

L

Labetalol, 143
Laceration and Cutaneous Wound Protocol, 376
Lachman's test of knee, 452
Lateral epicondylitis, 442
Legg-Calve-Perthes' disease, 447, 448
Leukostasis, 693
Lidocaine, 49, 130, 158, 376, 429, 867
Ludwig's Angina, 348
Lumbar radiculopathy (sciatica), 403
Lyme Disease Protocol, 661

M

Male Genitourinary Protocol, 271
Male Genitourinary section, 255
Malignant Otitis Externa, 324
Mallet finger, 472
Mandible fracture, 358
Marcaine, 376
McMurray's test of knee, 452
Medial epicondylitis, 442
Medications section, 751
Mental status examination, 167, 856
Metabolic Acidosis, 299
Metabolic Acidosis Protocol, 299
Metabolic syndrome, 798
Metacarpal fractures, 418
Metacarpal joint dislocation, 468
Metoprolol, 40, 766
MgSO4, 71, 81, 286, 499, 547, 705
Migraine headache, 864

Migraine prophylactic treatment, 866
Missed abortion, 544
Mobitz type 1 second degree heart block, 45
Mobitz type 2 second degree heart block, 45
Mood disorders, 701
Motor Vehicle Accident Protocol, 368
MRSA in abscess, 607
Myopericarditis, 25
Myxedema coma, 108

N

Nasal and Facial Fractures Protocol, 356
Near Drowning Protocol, 747
Neck Pain Protocol, 313
Neck trauma, 315
Needlestick, 570
Neoplastic cardiac tamponade, 691
Nephropathy – contrast induced, 193
Neurology section, 125
Neutropenic fever, 687
New Orleans CT brain criteria, 306
New York Heart Association classification for heart failure, 782
Nicardipine, 143
Nitrates, 774
Nonanion gap acidosis, 299
Non-freezing environmental injuries, 739
Nosebleed Protocol, 344
Notice, 15
NSAID's in peptic ulcer disease, 219
Nursemaid elbow, 444

O

Obesity Management, 814
Olecranon bursitis, 443
Opioid withdrawal, 711
Oral Rehydration Therapy exclusion criteria, 517
Oral Rehydration Therapy in adults, 197
Oral Rehydration Therapy in children, 291

Orbital blowout fractures, 357
Orbital cellulitis, 332
Orlowski score in near drowning, 748
Osgood-Schlatter's disease, 455
Osmolol gap, 120, 300, 705
Osteoarthritis (DJD), 458
Osteoarthritis (OA), 881
Otitis Externa Protocol, 324
Otitis Media Protocol, 493
Ottawa knee rule, 451
Ottawa Rule for ordering ankle x-rays, 462
Ovarian cysts, 539

P

Paraphimosis, 277
Paronychia, 667
Partial seizures, 154, 160, 874
Patella fracture and dislocation, 419
Patellar bursitis, 456
Patellar grind test, 458
Peak flow, 70, 80
Pediatric abdominal pain, 186
Pediatric Asthma Protocol, 497
Pediatric dehydration assessment, 290, 510
Pediatric Dehydration Protocol, 509
Pediatric Diarrhea Protocol, 515
Pediatric Fever Protocol, 476
Pediatric Gastroenteritis Protocol, 509
Pediatric Minor Head Trauma Protocol, 309
Pediatric Seizure Protocol, 160
Pediatrics section, 475
Pelvic inflammatory disease, 537
Pelvic Pain Protocol, 536
Pepcid, 89
Peptic Ulcer Disease and Gastritis Protocol, 219
Peptic Ulcer Disease Protocol, 219
Perianal abscess, 243
Pericarditis, 25
Periorbital (preseptal) cellulitis, 331

Peripheral arterial disease, 400
Perirectal abscess, 244
Peritonsillar abscess, 321
Pernio, 739
Pharmacology in the elderly, 522
Phimosis, 278
Phlegmasia alba dolens, 676
phlegmasia cerulea dolens, 676
Pilonidal cyst/abscess, 248
PIP Joint dislocation, 473
Pit viper antivenom, 600
Pit viper envenomation grading, 598
Pityriasis Rosea Protocol, 644
Placenta abruption, 547
Placenta previa, 548
Pleurisy, 25
Pneumonia causes, 75
Pneumonia Protocol, 75
Pneumonia treatment, 76
POC (products of conception), 544
Position of function, 472
Postconcussion syndrome, 305
Pre-diabetes, 798
Preeclampsia, 544
Pregnancy Complications Protocol, 544
Premature ventricular contractions, 46
Priapism, 276, 683
Primary survey in trauma, 368
Prolactin level, 155, 161, 874
Prostatitis, 274, 560
Protocol Supervisory Agreement, 18
Pruritus ani, 247
Pseudoaddiction, 752
Pseudoseizures, 155, 161, 874
Psoriasis Protocol, 624
Psoriatic arthritis, 884
Psychiatric and Social section, 697
Psychiatric Protocol – Adult and Adolescent, 698
Psychosis, 700
Pulmonary embolism, 24

Pulmonary Embolism Rule-out Criteria (PERC Rule), 28, 678

Q

QT interval prolongation, 755

R

Rectal prolapse, 245
Respiratory section, 65
Retinal detachment, 341
Retropharyngeal abscess, 321
Return-to-sports recommendations, 312
Rheumatoid arthritis (RA), 889
Rib fractures, 415
Rivaroxaban (Xarelto), 813
Rocky Mountain Spotted Fever, 657
Rotator cuff tear, 431

S

Salter fracture pneumonic, 423
Salter Harris Fracture Protocol, 423
Scabies Protocol, 632
Scapular fractures, 436
Scapular fractures and dislocations, 434
Schizophrenia, 701
Second degree deep partial thickness burn, 388
Second degree superficial partial thickness burn, 388
Secondary survey in trauma, 369
Seizure Management, 873
Seizure Protocol – Adult, 154
Seizure Protocol – Pediatric, 160
Selective serotonin reuptake inhibitors (SSRI's), 857
Sentinel leak, 127, 870
Septic abortion, 544
Septic arthritis, 401
Septic arthritis in knee, 460
Septic hip, 446
Septic Shock, 848
Septic shock antibiotic therapy, 850

Septic Shock Management, 848
Serotonin syndrome, 756
Serum osmolality in DKA, 96
Serum sickness, 601
Severe severity, 508
Severe uncontrolled hypertension, 51
Sexual Assault Protocol, 714
Sexually Transmitted Disease Protocol, 554
Shaken baby syndrome, 720
Shingles (Herpes Zoster) Protocol, 652
Shoulder (glenohumeral) dislocation, 438
Shoulder and Arm Trauma Protocol, 434
Shoulder Protocol, 428
Sickle Cell Anemia Protocol, 682
Sinus bradycardia, 44
Sinus tachycardia, 36
Sinusitis Protocol, 489
Sinusitis signs, 490
SIRS, 848
Slipped capital femoral epiphysis, 448
Smith fracture, 469
Snake Bite Protocol, 597
Sniff position, 507
Soft Tissue Abscess Protocol, 607
Sore Throat Protocol, 318
Spider Bite and Insect Sting Protocol, 593
Spinal cord compression, 172, 689
Statins, 772
Status epilepticus, 155, 161, 874
Status epilepticus in pediatrics, 482
Status epilepticus treatment, 158
Status epilepticus treatment in children, 163
Steroids, 89
Stevens Johnson Syndrome, 614
Strep throat, 320
Stroke prevention (primary), 809
Stroke prevention (secondary), 812
Stroke Prevention Management, 809
Stye, 331
Subacromial bursitis, 428

Subarachnoid hemorrhage (SAH), 869
Subconjunctival hemorrhage, 341
Superior vena cava syndrome, 690
Superventricular tachycardia, 41
Supraspinatus tendonitis, 428
Suture and staple removal times, 381
Suture types, 377
Syncope evaluation, 59
Syncope/Presyncope Protocol, 58
Syndrome of Inappropriate Antidiuretic Hormone Secretion (SIADH), 694
Synovial Fluid Analysis, 426
Syphilis, 562

T

Temporal arteritis, 869
Tension headache, 128
Tension-type headache, 862
Testicular torsion, 272
Tetanus prophylaxis, 582
Tetanus Protocol, 580
TGA, 141
Thermal burns, 389
Third degree burn, 389
Third degree heart block, 45
Thoracic outlet syndrome, 429
Thought disorders, 700
Threatened abortion, 544
TIA, 139
TIA mimics, 140
TIA treatment, 143
Tick Bite Protocol, 655
Tinea Capitis Protocol, 635
Tinea Corporis Protocol, 637
Tinea Pedis (Athlete's Foot) Protocol, 639
Tissue adhesives, 378
Tooth fractures, 361
Torticollis, 313
Toxic Epidermal Necrolysis, 615

Toxic Ingestions section, 115
Toxicology Protocol, 116
Toxidromes, 117
Transient synovitis of hip, 446
Trauma section, 367
Trench foot, 739
Trigeminal neuralgia, 868
Troponin in kidney failure, 282
Type 1 Diabetes Mellitus Management, 789
Type 2 Diabetes Mellitus Management, 797
Type 2 diabetes mellitus medication treatment, 800

U

Ultraviolet keratitis, 334
Urethritis, 271, 559
URI and Sinusitis Protocol, 489
URI Protocol, 489
Urinary and Male Genitourinary section, 255
Urinary Tract Infection Protocol, 261
Urine culture, 263
Urticaria, 85
Urticaria Protocol, 641
UTI complicated, 262
UTI in pregnancy, 549

V

Vaginal Bleeding Protocol, 532
Valtrex, 150, 152, 647, 648, 650, 654, 670
Varicella (Chicken Pox) Protocol, 665
Venereal warts, 562
Venous Thromboembolic Disease Protocol, 674
Ventilator indications, 838
Ventilator Management, 837
Ventricular dysrhythmias, 46
Ventricular tachycardia, 49
Vertigo, 136
Vitamin K, 386

W

Warfarin, 812
Weight loss program, 817
Well's DVT criteria in chest pain, 27, 677
Well's DVT criteria in syncope, 61
Well's Pulmonary Embolism Criteria, 67
Wernicke's encephalopathy, 709
Wild animal bites, 591
Withdrawal Protocol, 707
Worst headache of life, 132, 870
Wrist Injury Protocol, 465

CPSIA information can be obtained at www.ICGtesting.com
Printed in the USA
BVOW000446080713

324915BV00003B/7/P

9 780984 917396